AF868526

Practical Handbook of Thoracic Anesthesia

Practical Handbook of Thoracic Anesthesia

Philip M. Hartigan
Editor

Steven J. Mentzer
Consulting Surgical Editor

Springer

Editor
Philip M. Hartigan, MD
Assistant Professor of Anaesthesia
Harvard Medical School
Director, Division of Thoracic Anesthesia
Department of Anesthesiology, Perioperative and Pain Medicinea
Brigham and Women's Hospital
Boston, MA USA

ISBN 978-0-387-88492-9 e-ISBN 978-0-387-88493-6
DOI 10.1007/978-0-387-88493-6
Springer New York Dordrecht Heidelberg London

Library of Congress Control Number: 2011943746

Printed on acid-free paper

Springer is part of Springer Science+Business Media (www.springer.com)

Preface

Why This Book?

The vast majority of the roughly 200,000 thoracic surgical procedures this year will take place in centers where there is no dedicated, subspecialized thoracic anesthesia service. A considerable hunger for guidance and pearls is present among skilled generalists who occasionally find themselves thrust into thoracic cases with unfamiliar problems to solve. Similarly, fellows, residents, and medical students have expressed a need for efficiently accessible, essential principles, and specific management guidance for thoracic cases. All have experienced the frustration of wading through large, thickly referenced tomes that are reluctant to take a stand on controversial issues.

- When should one use PEEP vs. CPAP during one-lung ventilation?
- What else can one do if the patient desaturates? What really works?
- How do you know when it is safe to induce a patient with an anterior mediastinal mass?
- How do I decide whether an epidural is indicated?
- There is a tracheal resection/reconstruction in my room tomorrow. What do I need to know? What are my ventilation options while the airway is divided?
- How should the ventilator be set for patients with severe COPD during one-lung ventilation?
- What is the bottom line on fluids and post-pneumonectomy pulmonary edema?

We, as authors and editors, sought to distinguish this text in several respects. **First**, issues such as those above which are germane to concrete management decisions have been addressed directly, along with an assessment of the degree of certainty behind the positions which we take several respects. **Second**, we have deliberately included insights from the thoracic surgical perspective. Just as we perceive surgeons to be enlightened when they demonstrate some understanding of our issues, we believe that anesthesiologists elevate their own performance and perception when they understand key surgical considerations. **Third**, we have sought to make the information as practical and accessible as possible; heavy on bottom lines, and somewhat lighter on the evidence basis. This is not to suggest that the evidence basis was not diligently vetted. We have simply chosen to spare the reader most of the digestion process. **Fourth**, knowledge and technical skills at the fringes of thoracic anesthesia are given relatively more attention. The skilled thoracic anesthesiologist needs to understand respiratory therapy equipment (including delivery devices for inhaled nitric oxide), basic thoracic radiology, common ICU management issues following thoracic surgery, positioning issues, chronic post-thoracotomy pain syndrome, and other related aspects of total patient care. **Fifth**, the reader will find abundant illustrations; in particular, nearly 40 bronchoscopic images which will help advance his or her ability to recognize anomolies, guide surgery, and correct airway device malpositions.

How to Use This Book

Nobody reads medical textbooks cover-to-cover. We understand that. Most will open this book because they have a specific thoracic surgical case assigned which they are unfamiliar or uncomfortable with.

In that case, **Part IV** will quickly take you to a summary of the essential anesthetic management issues for some 30 specific procedures. Authors were asked to "get to the point" efficiently, and to make the essentials easy to extract. The surgical editor was asked to coedit this section with the following question in mind: "For each procedure, what surgical issues do you wish that anesthesiologists understood?" You will also find the chapters in Part IV richly cross-referenced in order to connect the reader to deeper explanations of key points.

A challenge in putting this book together was the fact that so many issues were relevant to multiple specific surgical procedures. How to make each chapter of Part IV reasonably complete, without making the section horrendously redundant? **Start by reading Chapter 16**.

Chapter 16 (**Part III**) takes the reader step-by-step through a typical pulmonary resection case. The sequence of events, common decision points, common problems and their solutions, and essential principles are summarized. Many of these serve as foundations for the other specific surgical procedures which follow in Part IV. It is included in Part III because it is an overview chapter, but it also specifically addresses lobectomy and lesser resections, such as segmentectomy and wedge resection. Other chapters in Part III provide overviews of preoperative, postoperative, and surgical considerations for thoracic surgical patients.

Part I provides essential foundation concepts, principally respiratory physiology, targeted specifically to those which are relevant to thoracic anesthesia management. Radiology for thoracic anesthesia is inserted here as is a chapter specifically addressing the controversy of acute lung injury following pulmonary resection. While the latter is a hotly controversial topic, it is addressed here because of its very practical implications with regard to fluid management and management of one-lung ventilation; central, practical issues for so many thoracic cases.

Part II addresses very technical issues, and will be useful as a "how-to" manual for many procedures and pieces of equipment fairly specific to thoracic anesthesia.

Part V provides a practical summary of thoracic pain management issues, both acute and chronic.

Boston, MA, USA Philip M. Hartigan

Acknowledgments

First and foremost, the contributing authors deserve my deepest heartfelt gratitude for their contributions. The idea for this project bubbled up from them during a team meeting and took off by dint of their commitment and hard work. Their tolerance of my editing has been nothing short of heroic. A special note of deep personal gratitude is due Dr. Steven J. Mentzer, Professor of Surgery, Harvard Medical School, for his surgical insights in Chapter 15 and throughout Part IV. That "surgical dimension" to this project was a critical distinguishing feature. The "MVP Award" for this talented team must go to Dr. Ju-Mei Ng, author of 7 chapters, and source of invaluable editorial support.

Several ingredients made the soil particularly fertile at Brigham and Women's Hospital for the growth of this project. The sheer volume and acuity of thoracic surgical cases here (>3,000/year) are a testimony to the leadership and talents of Dr. David J. Sugarbaker, who built the Department of Thoracic Surgery here from the ground up and created a collaborative, challenging environment in which the Thoracic Anesthesia Division could grow and thrive. The creation of a dedicated Thoracic Anesthesia subdivision was the vision of Dr. Simon Gelman, Professor and Chairman of Anesthesia during the 1990s when the division was created, possibly the first such division in the world. Dr. Gelman remains a beacon of insight and vision for this department, and for me personally. Dr. Charles Vacanti, the current Department Chairman, has generously provided support, without which this book would not have been possible. The constant parade of extraordinary thoracic anesthesia fellows-in-training has continually injected energy and kept us honest. Perhaps most importantly, the giants whose shoulders we stand on are Drs. Simon Body and Stanley LeeSon, founding leaders of the Division of Thoracic Anesthesia here at Brigham and Women's Hospital, who lit the torch that we carry.

I would like to especially thank Meghan Leary for excellent organizational and graphics help. We were very lucky to have the help of superb illustrators in Marcia Williams and Sara Krause. Thanks are also due to many at Springer, including Shelley Reinhardt, Wendy Vetter, and particularly Kevin Wright, Development Editor, as well as Brian Belval, who initially sealed the deal and put so much trust in us.

Finally, and most importantly, on behalf of all the authors, I wish to thank the families and loved ones for their patience, sacrifices, and support.

Table of Contents

Contributors

Teresa M. Bean, MD

Instructor in Anaesthesia, Harvard Medical School, Cardiothoracic Anaesthesiologist, Department of Anaesthesiology, Perioperative and Pain Medicine, Brigham and Women's Hospital, Boston, MA USA

Thomas Edrich, MD, PhD

Assistant Professor of Anaesthesia, Harvard Medical School, Cardiothoracic Anaesthesiologist and Intensivist, Department of Anaesthesiology, Perioperative and Pain Medicine, Brigham and Women's Hospital, Boston, MA USA

Vladimir Formanek, MD

Assistant Professor of Anaesthesia, Harvard Medical School, Cardiothoracic Anaesthesiologist, Department of Anaesthesiology, Perioperative and Pain Medicine, Brigham and Women's Hospital, Boston, MA USA

Gyorgy Frendl, MD, PhD

Assistant Professor of Anaesthesia, Harvard Medical School, Director, Surgical Critical Care Translational Research Center, Thoracic Anaesthesiologist and Intensivist, Department of Anaesthesiology, Perioperative and Pain Medicine, Brigham and Women's Hospital, Boston, MA USA

Andrew D. Friedrich, MD

Associate Professor of Anesthesiology, University of Cincinnati School of Medicine, Director of Perioperative Medicine, Department of Anesthesiology, University of Cincinnati Hospital, Cincinnati, OH USA

Peter Gerner, MD

Professor and Chairman, Department of Anesthesiology, Critical Care and Pain Medicine, Paracelsus Medical University, Salzburg General Hospital, Salzburg, Austria, Associate Professor of Anaesthesia, Harvard Medical School, Boston, MA USA

Philip M. Hartigan, MD

Assistant Professor of Anaesthesia, Harvard Medical School, Director, Division of Thoracic Anaesthesia, Department of Anaesthesiology, Perioperative and Pain Medicine, Brigham and Women's Hospital, Boston, MA USA

Juan C. Ibla, MD

Assistant Professor of Anaesthesia, Harvard Medical School, Director of Anaesthesia for Lung Transplantation, Cardiac Anaesthesiologist, Department of Anaesthesiology and Perioperative Medicine, Boston Children's Hospital, Boston, MA USA

Shannon S. McKenna, MD

Assistant Professor of Anaesthesia, Harvard Medical School, Medical Director of Surgical Intensive Care Units, Thoracic Anaesthesiologist and Intensivist, Department of Anaesthesiology, Perioperative and Pain Medicine, Brigham and Women's Hospital, Boston, MA USA

Steven J. Mentzer, MD

Professor of Surgery, Harvard Medical School, Senior Thoracic Surgeon, Division of Thoracic Surgery, Brigham and Women's Hospital, Boston, MA USA

Ju-Mei Ng, F.A.N.Z.A.

Assistant Professor of Anaesthesia, Harvard Medical School, Thoracic Anaesthesiologist, Department of Anaesthesiology, Perioperative, and Pain Medicine, Brigham and Women's Hospital, Boston, MA USA

Michael Nurok, MB, ChB, PhD

Clinical Associate Professor, Weill Cornell Medical College, Associate Attending Anesthesiologist, Department of Anesthesiology, Hospital for Special Surgery, New York, NY USA

Nicholas Sadovnikoff, MD

Assistant Professor of Anaesthesia, Harvard Medical School, Director of Anaesthesia Critical Care Fellowship Program, Co-Director of Surgical Intensive Care Units, Department of Anaesthesiology, Perioperative, and Pain Medicine, Brigham and Women's Hospital, Boston, MA USA

David A. Silver, MD

Instructor in Anaesthesia, Harvard Medical School, Director of Education, Associate Director of Cardiothoracic Fellowship Program, Cardiothoracic Anaesthesiologist and Intensivist, Department of Anaesthesiology, Perioperative, and Pain Medicine, Brigham and Women's Hospital, Boston, MA USA

Eric D. Skolnick, MD

Assistant Professor of Clinical Anesthesia, Georgetown University, Director of Thoracic Anesthesia, Department of Anesthesiology, Washington Hospital Center, Washington D.C., USA

Nelson L. Thaemert, MD

Instructor in Anaesthesiology, Harvard Medical School, Cardiothoracic Anaesthesiologist, Department of Anaesthesiology, Perioperative, and Pain Medicine, Brigham and Women's Hospital, Boston, MA USA

George P. Topulos, MD

Associate Professor of Anaesthesia, Harvard Medical School, Department of Anaesthesiology, Perioperative, and Pain Medicine, Brigham and Women's Hospital, Boston, MA USA

Beatrice Trotman-Dickenson, MB.BS., MRCP, FRCR

Instructor in Radiology, Harvard Medical School, Fellowship Program Director, Division of Thoracic Imaging, Department of Radiology, Brigham and Women's Hospital, Boston, MA USA

Sarah H. Wiser

Instructor in Anaesthesia, Harvard Medical School, Thoracic Anaesthesiologist, Department of Anaesthesiology, Perioperative, and Pain Medicine, Brigham and Women's Hospital, Boston, MA USA

I

Essential Foundations

Chapter 1
Thoracic Radiology

Thomas Edrich and Beatrice Trotman-Dickenson

Keywords Thoracic radiology • Intraoperative oxygen desaturation • Air trapping • Respiratory acidosis • Mediastinal lipomatosis • Atelectasis • Pleural effusions • Pulmonary edema • Interstitial pulmonary disease • Hypercapnia (permissive hypercapnia) • Airway management • V/Q-scans • Ventilation–perfusion scintigraphy

Introduction

Patients undergoing thoracic surgery typically have chest X-ray (CXR) films and computed tomography (CT) for detailed preoperative surgical planning. Increasingly, electronic picture archiving and communications system (PACS) enables viewing of these studies at any computer terminal in hospital. The thoracic anesthesiologist viewing these images for preoperative evaluation is particularly interested in identifying patients at risk for intraoperative oxygen desaturation or air trapping with risk of respiratory acidosis. Evidence to predict the ease of intubation and lung isolation should also be sought. Significant mass effects within the chest may also affect anesthetic management, but are discussed elsewhere in this text (Chapter 20).

P.M. Hartigan (ed.), *Practical Handbook of Thoracic Anesthesia*,
DOI 10.1007/978-0-387-88493-6_1,

Normal Findings

The "normal CXR" has standard landmarks. Basic aspects should be identified, such as the mediastinal and cardiac borders, airways, and lung volumes, as shown in Fig 1-1. Identification of all support devices is important. Of note, when the chin is flexed down, the tip of the endotracheal tube (ETT) migrates deeper (about 2 cm) into the trachea. In Fig 1-1, the chin is not visible on the CXR and thus the neck is not flexed forward. Since the ETT tip is 3 cm above the carina, the risk of right-mainstem intubation is minimal even if the neck were to be flexed forward.

A common variant is the azygous lobe as seen in the CXR and a coronal CT slice in Fig 1-2. This may complicate surgery of the right upper lobe. A tracheal bronchus (incidence 0.1–2%) is another common variant. A right apical tracheal bronchus is shown in Fig 1-3. Here, the apical segmental bronchus departs directly from the distal trachea rather than from the right upper lobe. If the tracheal bronchus exits high up in the trachea, it may become obstructed by the tracheal cuff of a double-lumen ETT.

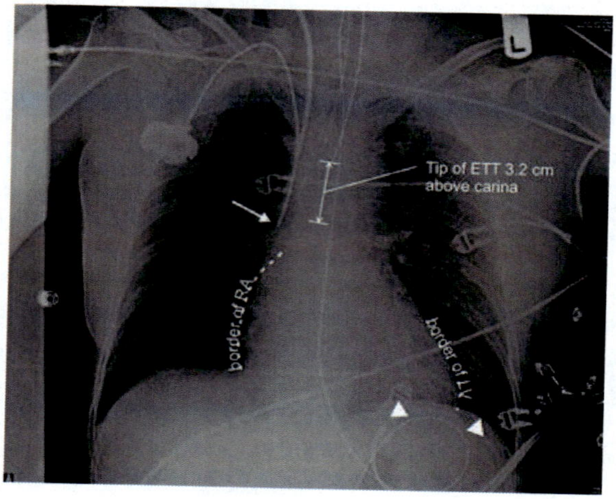

Figure 1-1 – Portable CXR with sketched right atrial (RA) and left ventricular (LV) borders. Note the presence of a well-positioned central venous line (CVL) and portacath with the tips lying near the junction of the superior vena cava and the right atrium (*arrow*). The tip of the endotracheal tube (ETT) is positioned approximately 3 cm above the carina. The nasogastric tube (NGT) is positioned appropriately crossing the diaphragm into the stomach. The NGT remains in midline until crossing the diaphragm (*arrowheads*) indicating that it is not in the airways.

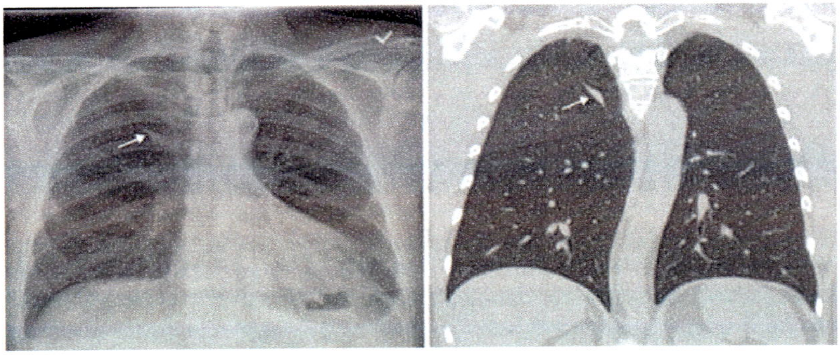

Figure 1-2 – CXR and CT image of a patient with an azygous lobe. The azygous vein (*arrow*) lies in a fold of the fissure in the *right upper lobe*.

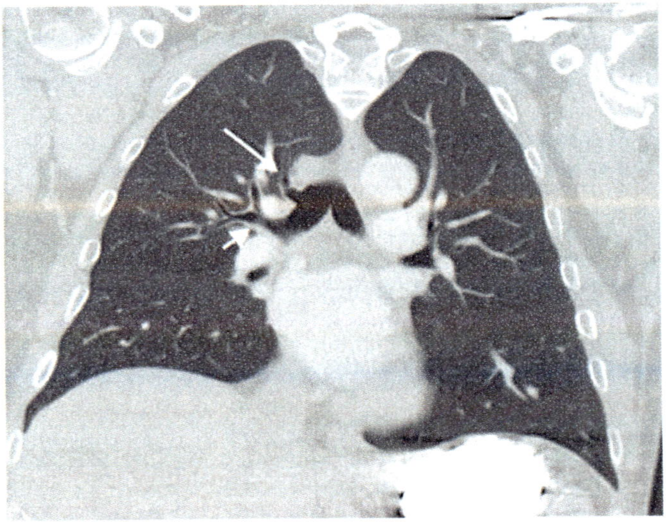

Figure 1-3 – Coronal CT image displaying an apical bronchus. The segmental bronchus for the apical segment of the *right upper lobe* (*long arrow*) does not depart from the *right upper lobe* bronchus (*short arrow*), but rather from the trachea itself (see Chapter 10 for corresponding bronchoscopic images).

Bronchial variants and their implications for lung isolation are further discussed in Chapters 8 and 9.

Figure 1-4 shows mediastinal lipomatosis ("fat pad") at the junction of the cardiac base and the diaphragm. Since this obscures the silhouette of the right heart border, it may be mistaken for a right middle lobe consolidation, mass, or atelectasis.

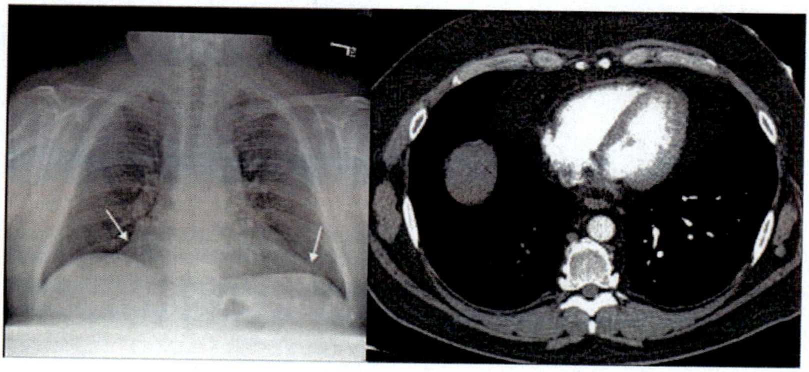

Figure 1-4 – CXR and CT depicting mediastinal lipomatosis ("fat pad") around the base of heart (*arrows* in CXR). This normal variant must be differentiated from atelectasis or consolidation of the *right middle* lobe since it obscures the right heart border. In the CT, the Hounsfield units of the fat pad are similar to the subcutaneous fat.

Causes for Intraoperative Oxygen Desaturation

Atelectasis represents loss of ventilation through collapsed lung regions. Although hypoxic pulmonary vasoconstriction occurs to reduce blood flow, considerable shunting can persist leading to oxygen desaturation. Atelectasis can be identified by an opacity associated with volume loss and localized by the loss of a normal cardiac or diaphragmatic silhouette, since the atelectatic lung abutting these structures is of similar opacity. Figure 1-5 shows a loss of the normal right heart border due to atelectasis of the right middle lobe (RML). A triangular opacification behind the heart indicates atelectasis of the left lower lobe (LLL) as well. In the lateral CXR, the collapsed RML is delimited by the minor and major fissures. The corresponding CT reveals both atelectatic lobes.

In Fig 1-6, the combinations of RML and right lower lobe (RLL) atelectasis mimic an elevated diaphragm or a pleural effusion – here, the inferior border of aerated lung in the right thorax consists of the minor fissure, not the hemidiaphragm.

Complete collapse (atelectasis) of the lung can be difficult to differentiate from pleural effusion or consolidation. Volume loss and

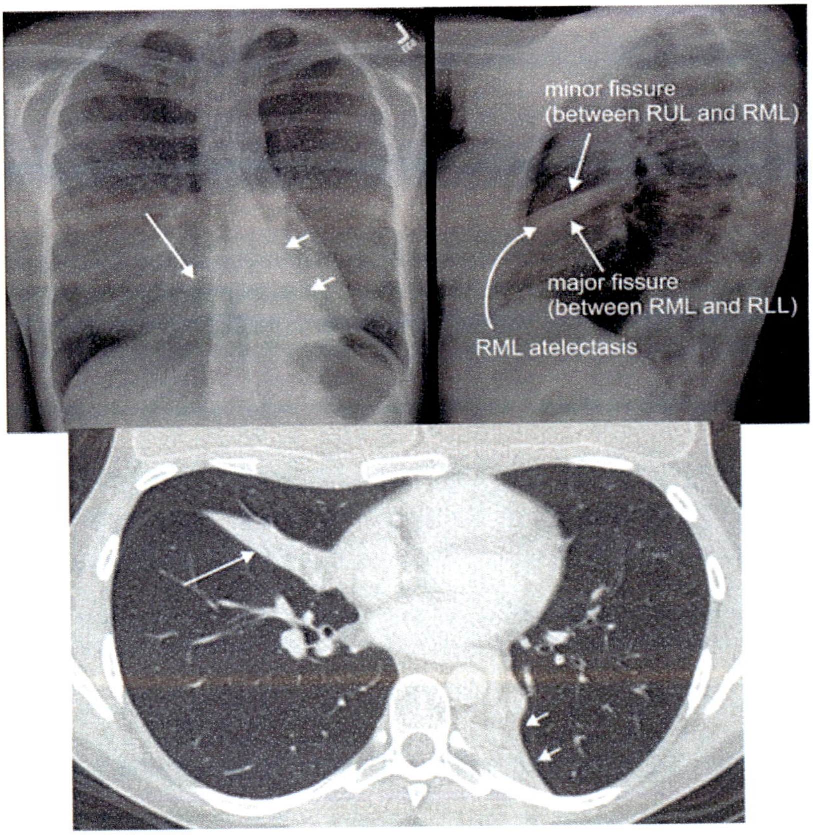

Figure 1-5 – *Right middle lobe* (RML) atelectasis obscuring the right heart border in the posterior–anterior CXR (*large arrow*). There is also atelectasis of the *left lower lobe* causing a triangular opacification medially along the left mediastinum (*small arrows*). The CT shows the corresponding regions. In the lateral CXR, the volume loss due to RML atelectasis can be recognized by the unusual proximity of the minor and major fissure.

mediastinal displacement in the ipsilateral direction are key findings. Mediastinal displacement is apparent in Fig 1-7A as the central venous line (CVL) and the trachea are displaced toward the opacified lung. Bronchoscopy was performed on this patient to remove mucous plugging resulting in reinflation of the lung Fig 1-7B. The mediastinum with CVL and trachea returned to midline. However, moderate bilateral effusions can be seen. Since this CXR was taken with the patient in a semirecumbent position, the pleural effusion

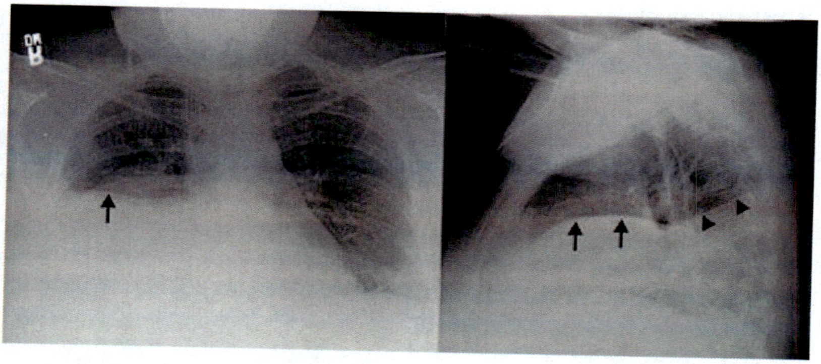

Figure 1-6 – Atelectasis of RML and RLL. In the left image, the curvilinear border of the minor fissure (*arrow*) can mimic an elevated hemidiaphragm or an effusion. In the lateral CXR, the *posterior upward* sloping opacity (*arrowheads*) represents the major fissure with the collapsed RLL beneath it. The *large arrows* mark the minor fissure with the collapsed RML below it.

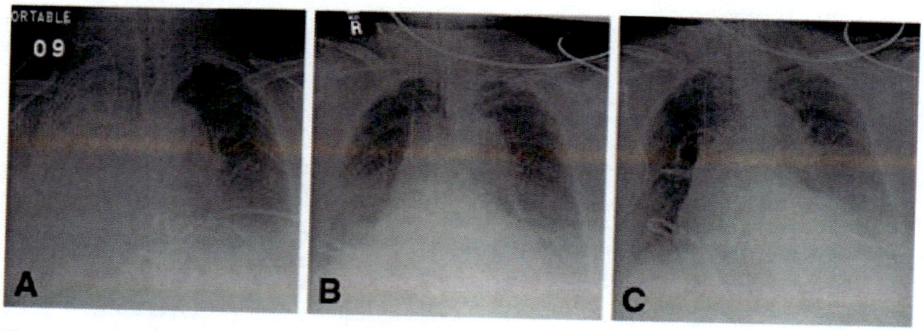

Figure 1-7 – Atelectasis of the entire lung with ipsilateral deviation of the trachea and the central venous line indicating that significant volume loss has occurred (**A**). After bronchoscopy and removal of mucous plugs, the lung is reinflated and the position of the CVL returns to normal. However, bilateral effusions remain extending into the minor fissure (**B**). Placement of a pigtail catheter successfully drains the right effusion (**C**).

does not obscure the costophrenic angle. However, the pleural effusion has a layering appearance and extends into the minor fissure (i.e., between the RUL and the RML). Subsequent drainage with a pigtail catheter was successful (Fig 1-7C).

Pleural effusions often accompany atelectasis of the adjacent lung as can be seen in Fig 1-7b. In extreme cases, pressure from pleural effusions can cause mediastinal shift to the opposite side, as illustrated in Fig 1-8. Any mediastinal shift is significant to the anesthesiologist because the resulting traction on the inferior vena cava (IVC) and pressure on the heart may cause hemodynamic compromise.

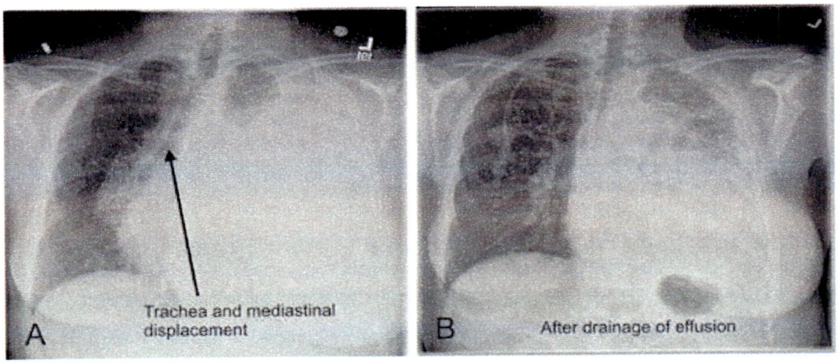

Figure 1-8 – A large malignant pleural effusion causing shift of the mediastinum to the contralateral side (**A**). After drainage, the trachea and mediastinum return to midline (**B**).

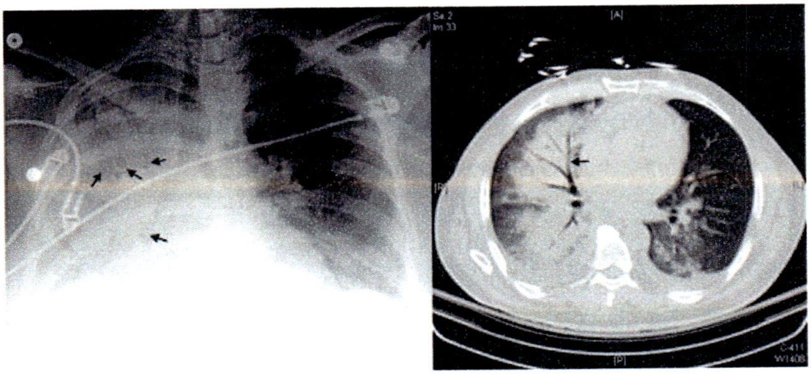

Figure 1-9 – Consolidation in the setting of pneumonia. Fluid-filled alveoli provide contrast against the air-filled bronchi ("air bronchograms") in both CXR and CT. See *arrows*.

This is accentuated when the patient is placed in the lateral decubitus position with the affected side up.

In contrast to atelectasis, consolidation of the lung occurs when fluid and infiltrate fills alveolar spaces, but no significant volume loss occurs. This may occur in the setting of pneumonia. Larger airways may not fill and are visible on CXR and CT imaging because they are contrasted by the consolidated surrounding lung ("air bronchograms"). Clinically, this leads to shunting of blood and desaturation. Figure 1-9 shows such a patient with pneumonia and "air bronchograms."

Pulmonary edema also increases shunting of blood perfusion past fluid-filled alveoli. This can be caused by pulmonary venous congestion in the setting of heart failure (cardiogenic pulmonary edema) or other volume overload situations, such as acute renal failure. Iatrogenic volume overload is not uncommon after certain thoracic procedures, such as esophagectomy. Upper lobe vessel redistribution and signs of interstitial edema, such as Kerley B lines (lymphatic distension of interlobular septa), may develop as shown in the CXR of Fig 1-10.

Noncardiogenic pulmonary edema, such as acute lung injury/acute respiratory distress syndrome (ALI/ARDS), can develop in the setting of systemic inflammation causing increased pulmonary vascular permeability and edema. Typical radiographic findings include patchy bilateral infiltrates as seen in Fig 1-11. CT imaging reveals inhomogeneous, dependent infiltrates that can shift with changes in body position. Difficulties with both oxygenation and ventilation occur as the lungs lose compliance with edema and then form hyaline membranes.

Patients with interstitial pulmonary disease may present with stiff, small, noncompliant lungs and a preoperative oxygen requirement. CXR radiographic findings are reticular opacities associated with low lung volumes as shown in Fig 1-12.

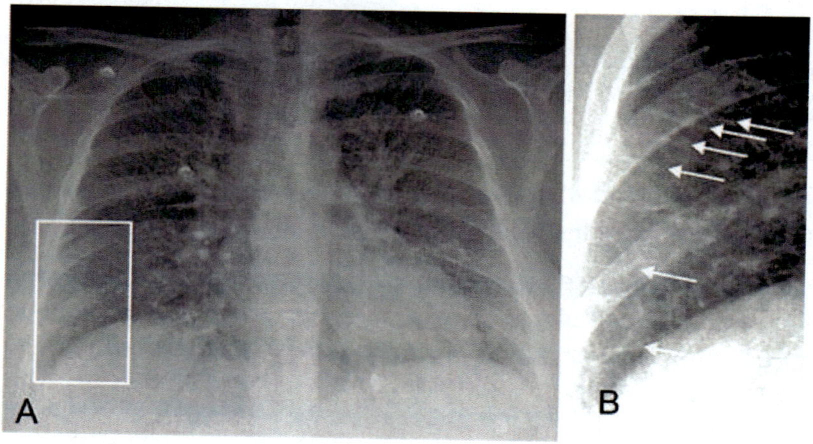

Figure 1-10 – Pulmonary edema with upper-lobe vessel redistribution and Kerley B lines which indicate interstitial septal thickening due to edema (**A**). Magnification of the right lateral lung field shows Kerley B lines in more detail (*white arrows*) (**B**).

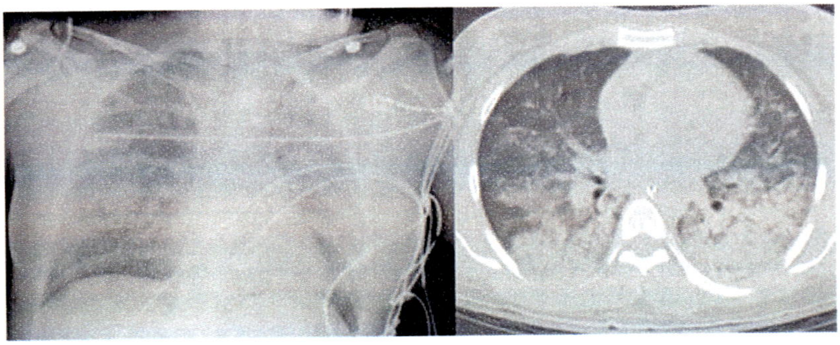

Figure 1-11 – CXR and CT with patchy, bilateral inhomogeneous infiltrates consistent with acute respiratory distress syndrome (ARDS). The dependent infiltrates in the CT can shift with changes in body position. Clinically, lung compliance decreases and high ventilation pressures may be necessary to prevent derecruitment of alveoli and to maintain adequate oxygenation.

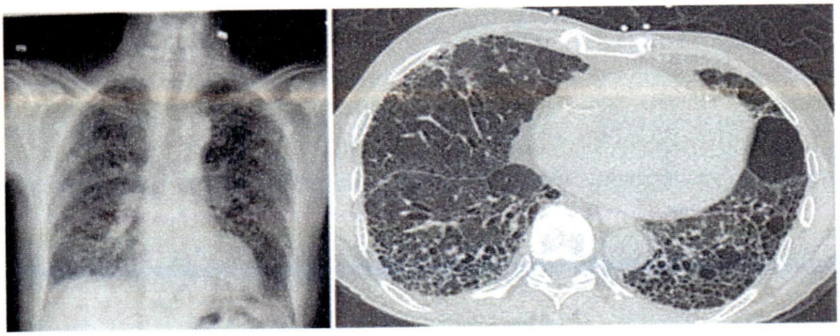

Figure 1-12 – Interstitial disease due to idiopathic pulmonary fibrosis (IPF). CXR reveals low lung volumes associated with reticular opacities. The CT shows widespread destruction of normal alveolar architecture resulting in a "honey-comb" appearance. Clinically, the lungs are noncompliant and oxygenation can be challenging.

Causes for CO_2 Retention and Air Trapping

In patients with chronic obstructive pulmonary disease (COPD) and emphysema, bronchiolar walls are weakened and collapse during expiratory flow (flow limitation). This causes air trapping and hyperinflation of the chest. For the anesthesiologist, primary

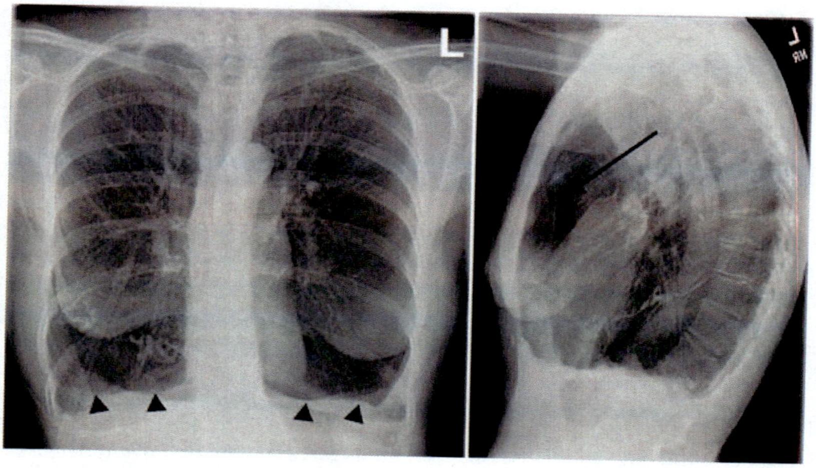

Figure 1-13 – Typical findings in a patient with COPD, including hyperinflated lungs, flattened diaphragms (*arrowheads*), and increased retrosternal space (*arrow*). Respiratory acidosis and hemodynamic effects of air trapping are the principal clinical challenges for the anesthesiologist.

concerns are the inability to ventilate sufficiently to eliminate carbon dioxide and the phenomenon of air trapping potentially decreasing the preload to the heart. Often, a controlled degree of hypercapnia (permissive hypercapnia) and associated respiratory acidosis must be tolerated to avoid excessive airway pressures and hemodynamic compromise due to decreased cardiac preload. Radiographic signs of COPD are hyperinflation of the lungs, flat diaphragms, a bell-shaped thorax, and increased retrosternal space as shown in Fig 1-13.

Conditions that Pose Other Specific Risks for Anesthesia

Conditions that pose specific risks while undergoing anesthesia include pneumothorax, anterior mediastinal mass, tracheal strictures, endotracheal and bronchial tumors, and tracheoesophageal fistulas. A simple pneumothorax (Fig 1-14) may develop tension when positive-pressure ventilation is initiated. One should consider tube thoracostomy before inducing anesthesia and applying positive-pressure ventilation.

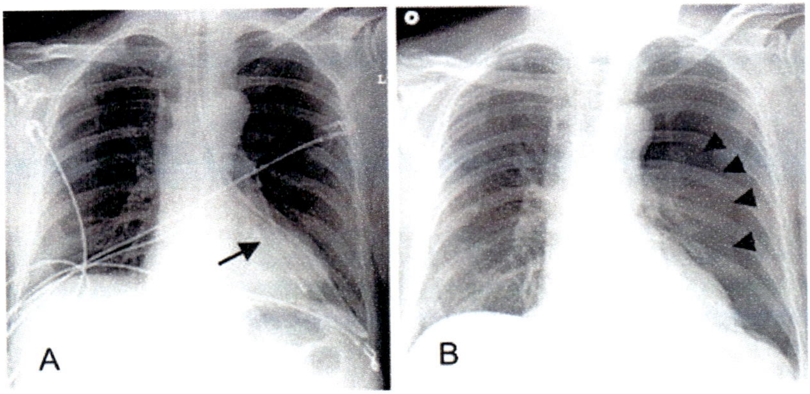

Figure 1-14 – Pneumothorax (PTX) caused by a misplaced Dobhoff feeding tube (DHT). *Panel A* shows the misplaced DHT (*arrow*) entering the left lung and perforating into the left pleural space. The PTX is still small, apical, and subtle. After removal of the DHT (*panel B*), the pneumothorax enlarges and becomes apparent (*arrowheads*).

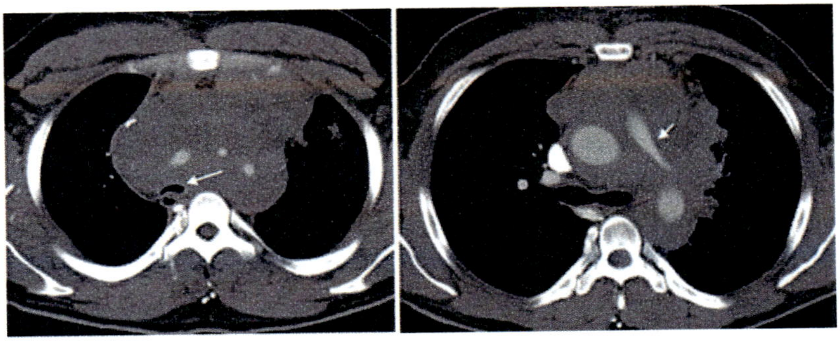

Figure 1-15 – CT images of a mediastinal mass positioned anteriorly and compressing both the pulmonary artery (*short arrow*) and the trachea (*long arrow*). After induction of anesthesia and muscle relaxation, the thoracic diameter decreases with the attendant risk that the mass may completely compress the great vessels or the airway and cause cardiovascular and respiratory collapse.

An anterior mediastinal mass (Fig 1-15) may cause compression of the heart, the great vessels, or the airways when anesthesia is induced and the thoracic volume decreases (Chapter 20). Also, the anesthesiologist must be aware that the mediastinal mass could be a thymoma with associated myasthenia gravis and implications for muscle paralysis. Furthermore, intraoperative manual compression

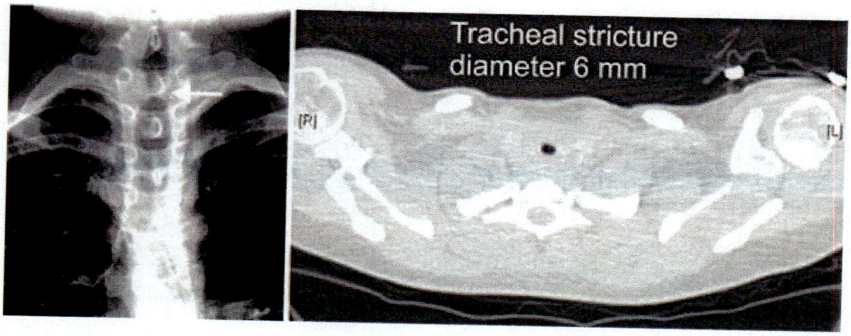

Figure 1-16 – Tracheal stricture visible on CXR (*arrow*) with a corresponding CT slice. Since the stricture occurs only 2.5 cm below the cords, it may be difficult to advance the endotracheal tube into proper position.

by the surgeon during the resection may obstruct blood flow through the superior vena cava. Therefore, intravenous access in the lower extremities may be necessary in order to administer medications. In general, any mass effect on the chest threatening airway patency, venous return, or cardiac output should be assessed by the anesthesiologist prior to induction. The CT scan is a helpful tool for this, but precise cutoff criteria delineating excessive vs. acceptable risk for induction are not available.

Tracheal strictures, deviation, or tortuosity may pose difficulties when advancing an endotracheal tube or attempting lung isolation. A stricture is visible in the CT but also may be visible on plain CXR as shown in Fig 1-16. Note that the degree of tracheal stenosis tends to be somewhat exaggerated by CT scans.

When planning airway management for patients with endotracheal or bronchial tumors or tracheoesophageal fistulas, CT images are useful. Three-dimensional reconstructions and virtual bronchoscopy of complicated airway pathology can be valuable for anesthetic as well as surgical planning (Fig 1-17). For example, the distance between the carina and a tracheoesophageal fistula can be calculated to determine whether the cuff of an endotracheal tube lies at or below the fistula and to isolate it from the lower airways.

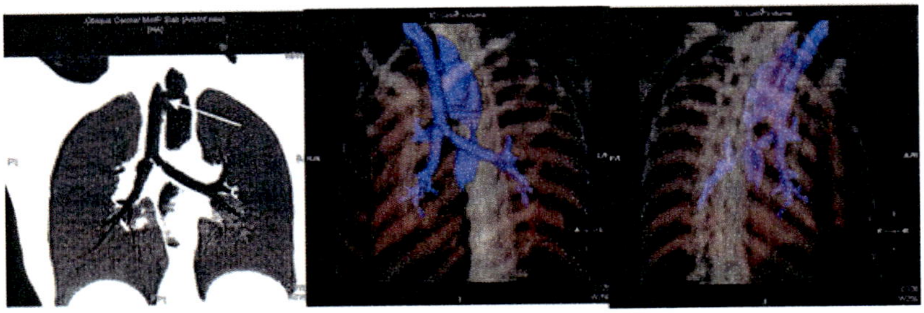

Figure 1-17 – Imaging of a tracheoesophageal fistula. The coronal reconstruction of the CT at *left* shows the actual fistula (*arrow*). The three-dimensional reconstruction allows rotation (*middle* and *right* images) to investigate the relationship of the esophagus to the tracheal tree more precisely.

Accessory Exams

Ventilation–perfusion scintigraphy (V/Q-scanning) is frequently performed before pneumonectomies (or lesser resections in patients with marginal lung function) to more accurately predict postoperative lung function. V/Q-scans require both an intravenous injection of radioactive technetium-labeled macroaggregated albumin (Tc 99m-MAA) and inhalation of a radioactive gas Xenon-133 or aerosolized compounds with technetium DTPA. The uptake of radioactive ions is measured by a gamma camera and the percentage of radioactivity contributed by each lung correlates with the contribution to the function of that lung. The scan displays the pattern of both perfusion and ventilation as shown in Fig 1-18.

V/Q scans allow calculation of predicted postoperative FEV_1, an important predictor of postoperative pulmonary function and cardiopulmonary reserve. Pneumonectomy in a patient with minimal perfusion to the affected lung has little impact. Normal or excessive perfusion to the operative lung, on the other hand, predicts a proportional reduction in FEV_1 and increased right heart stress following pneumonectomy. Normal or increased perfusion of the operative lung also predicts difficulty with gas exchange during one-lung ventilation (Chapter 5).

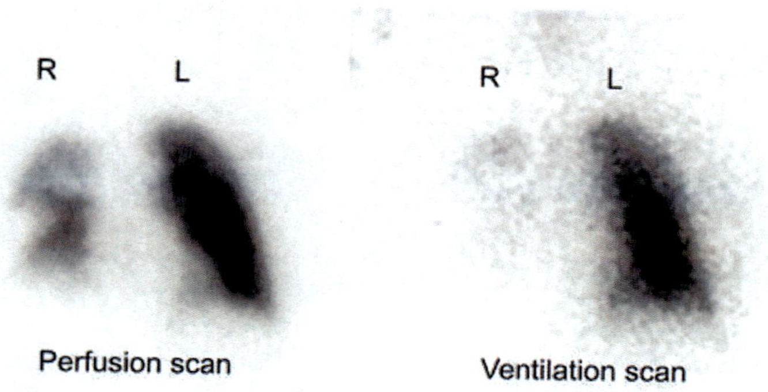

Figure 1-18 – Ventilation–perfusion (V/Q) scan in a patient with right mesothelioma. Perfusion to the affected lung is reduced considerably. Ventilation is minimal. Clinically, this patient had poor oxygenation due to V/Q mismatch and shunting of blood through the nonventilated lung. Right pneumonectomy was tolerated well because there was no significant increase in RV afterload – the right lung had only been receiving 18% of total cardiac output.

Suggested Reading

Trotman-Dickenson B. Radiology in the intensive care unit (part I). J Intensive Care Med. 2003a;18(4):198–210.

Trotman-Dickenson B. Radiology in the intensive care unit (part 2). J Intensive Care Med. 2003b;18(5):239–52.

Jacobson FL. Chest imaging: role of CT, PET/CT, and MRI. In: Sugarbaker DJ, editor. Adult chest surgery. New York: McGraw-Hill; 2009. p. 19–34. Chapter 3.

Chapter 2
Respiratory Physiology

Michael Nurok and George P. Topulos

Keywords Respiratory system • Ventilation • Inspiration • Expiration • Pleural and transmural pressure • Lung volumes • FEV_1 • FRC • Functional residual capacity • Hysteresis • Diffusing • Diffusing capacity • Miget diagrams • Hypoxic pulmonary vasoconstriction

Introduction

The primary function of the respiratory system is to exchange carbon dioxide and oxygen in order to support metabolism. The respiratory system accomplishes this by bringing blood and air in close proximity across a large, diffusive surface area. Two bulk flow pumps, the heart and lungs move blood and gas, respectively. Two diffusion systems allow exchange of blood and gas between the lungs and pulmonary capillaries, and then tissue capillaries and cells (Fig 2-1).

Ventilation

Components of the Lung

The respiratory system is made of two components, the lung and chest wall. Functionally, the lung is divided into two regions: a conducting zone comprised of airways larger than respiratory

P.M. Hartigan (ed.), *Practical Handbook of Thoracic Anesthesia*,
DOI 10.1007/978-0-387-88493-6_2, © Springer Science+Business Media, LLC 2012

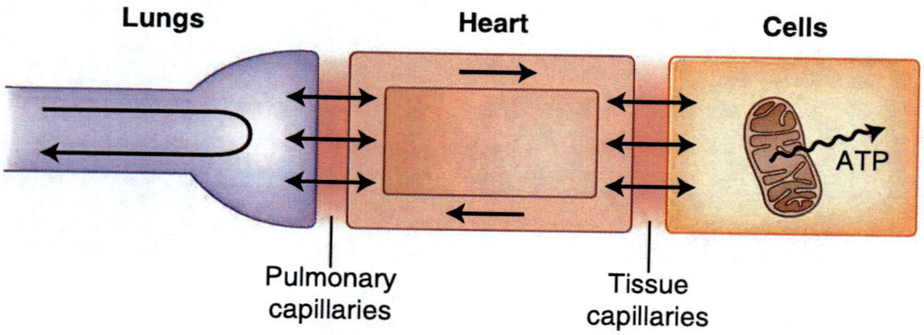

Figure 2-1 – Weibel diagram.

bronchioles, and a respiratory zone containing smaller airways with gas exchanging units called alveoli. The chest wall includes the rib cage, abdomen, and diaphragm. A continuous envelope of parietal and visceral pleura separates the chest wall from the lung with a potential pleural space between.

Inspiration and Expiration

The diaphragm is the primary muscle of inspiration. It is a dome-shaped structure that forces abdominal contents downward and forward with contraction resulting in an increase in volume of the thorax. Contraction of external intercostal muscles between adjacent ribs also aids in increasing the thoracic volume.

Expiration is passive during quiet breathing and *always passive* during mechanical ventilation in relaxed or anesthetized patients. During expiration the respiratory system returns toward its resting volume as determined by the intrinsic elastic properties of the lung and chest wall. When ventilation is increased, expiration becomes active and the muscles of the abdominal wall and internal intercostals contract with a resultant decrease in the diameter and volume of the thorax.

A number of accessory muscles contribute to ventilation when the respiratory system is taxed. These include the sternocleidomastoids, pectoralis, trapezius, and muscles of the vertebral column.

Pleural and Transmural Pressure

The pressure inbetween the visceral and parietal pleura of the lung (pleural pressure) is transmitted to regions continuous with the pleural space including the pericardium and great vessels. As a result pleural pressure significantly influences cardiac physiology.

The transmural pressure across the lung parenchyma is alveolar pressure, the pressure inside the lung, minus pleural pressure. As seen in Fig 2-2, the change in pleural pressure required for a given volume change during spontaneous ventilation is dominated by the mechanical properties of the lung and is negative during inspiration. During mechanical ventilation the change in pleural pressure required for a given volume change is dominated by chest wall mechanical properties and is positive during lung inflation. However, unlike pleural pressure, the change in transmural pressure across the lung parenchyma required for a given volume change is the same during both spontaneous and mechanical ventilation (see graph in Fig 2-2).

Control of Breathing

Details regarding the control of respiration remain topics of controversy. It is thought that an intrinsic respiratory rhythm is generated in the central nervous system (CNS), analogous to cardiac pacemakers. Rate and depth of breathing are altered by $PaCO_2$, PaO_2, and pH.

$PaCO_2$ is normally the dominant factor governing moment-to-moment respiration. Changes in $PaCO_2$ from a set point result in increased or decreased respiratory drive. CO_2 diffuses freely across the blood brain barrier resulting in similar changes in cerebro-spinal fluid (CSF) $PaCO_2$, HCO_3, and H^+. *Central* chemo-receptors in the pons and medulla respond to changes in CSF $PaCO_2$ and hydrogen ion concentration.

PaO_2 modulates respiration through *peripheral* chemoreceptors (principally carotid and aortic bodies). Some patients exhibit complete loss of hypoxic respiratory drive following bilateral carotid

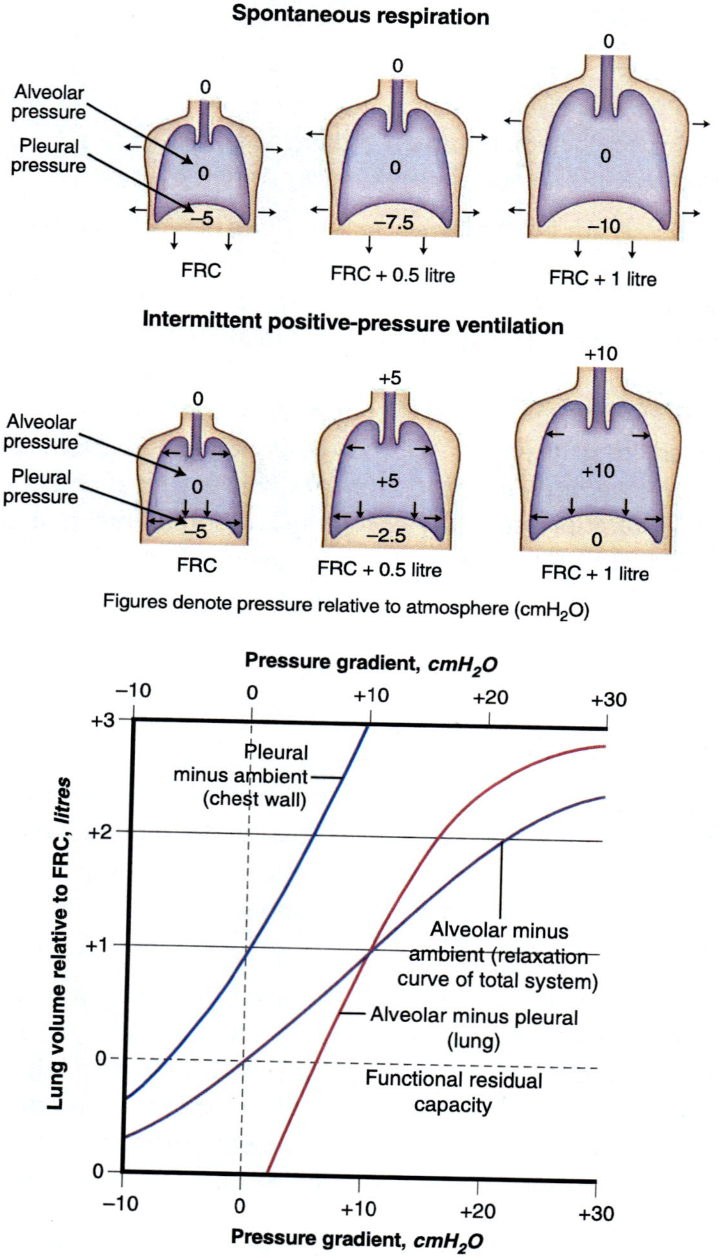

Figure 2-2 – Diagram showing different pleural pressures with mechanical and spontaneous ventilation and diagram of lung volume vs. transmural pressure.

body resection. Peripheral chemoreceptors also respond to $PaCO_2$, but this is less important than the central response to $PaCO_2$. Carotid, but not aortic bodies respond to changes in pH.

Ventilation may additionally be influenced by other peripheral chemoreceptors, pulmonary stretch receptors, juxta-capillary receptors, pain, temperature, blood pressure, conscious volition, and other inputs. The integration of these factors is complex and poorly understood. At normal $PaCO_2$, hypoxia must be severe (50 mmHg) to drive respiration, whereas minor fluxes in $PaCO_2$ prompt compensatory ventilatory changes, defending $PaCO_2$ within a tight range. However, the CO_2 ventilatory response curve is left-shifted and steeper at decreased PaO_2.

In some disease states, notably COPD, the sensitivity to increased $PaCO_2$ is diminished. Such patients are frequently labeled as dependent on hypoxic drive, and supplemental oxygen is withheld for fear of depressing ventilation. Evidence exists that such patients exhibit near baseline minute ventilation despite increased FiO_2, and that the observed increase in $PaCO_2$ is due to disruption of $\dot{V}/\dot{Q}$ matching (increased dead space due to inhibition of hypoxic pulmonary vasoconstriction (HPV)), rather than hypoventilation (1, 2). The clinical pearl is that if a COPD patient is hypoventilating following surgery, withdrawal of supplemental oxygen is *not* the solution. Other causes should be sought (narcotics, pain, residual volatile agent, residual paralytic, obstruction, etc.).

Lung Volumes

The following static lung volumes are conventionally defined. A capacity is the sum of two volumes.

- *Residual volume* (RV) is the volume of gas remaining in the lungs after a maximal expiration. It is approximately 1.2 l in a 70-kg human.
- *Tidal volume* (Vt) is the volume of gas exhaled from inspiration to expiration. Vt can also be measured during inhalation. It is approximately 0.5 l in a 70-kg human.

- *Total lung capacity* (TLC) is the volume of gas in the lungs following a maximal inspiration (Vital capacity + RV). It is approximately 6.0 l in a 70-kg human.
- *Vital capacity* (VC) is the volume of gas exhaled from a maximal inspiration to maximal expiration (TLC–RV). It is approximately 4.6 l in a 70 kg human. TLC and RV are set by the mechanical properties of the respiratory system.

FEV_1 and FVC

Two particularly useful pulmonary function tests are the forced volume of gas exhaled in one second (FEV_1) and the forced vital capacity (FVC). In health, FEV_1 is approximately 80% of FVC. In restrictive lung diseases both FEV_1 and FVC are reduced but the ratio of FEV_1/FVC is normal. In obstructive diseases FEV_1 is disproportionately reduced compared to FVC. In addition, the flow volume loop is typically concave toward the volume axis in obstructive, but not restrictive disease. All lung volumes and flows should always be examined as a percentage of predicted values based on height, age, sex, and ethnicity.

Compliance, Elastance

Compliance is volume change as a function of transmural pressure change, or the slope of a volume pressure curve. *Elastance* is the reciprocal of compliance. Elastic recoil is the transmural pressure at a specific volume.

Each of these quantities may be measured for the lung or chest wall alone, or for the sum of the respiratory system. They are static properties and are measured with the respiratory muscles relaxed, with no gas flow and an open airway.

Relaxation Volume and Functional Residual Capacity

The volume of a structure when its transmural pressure is zero is its *relaxation volume*. When the transmural pressure across an isolated relaxed chest wall is zero it contains approximately 75% of its TLC volume, whereas the isolated lung contains a volume slightly below RV when its transmural pressure is zero. The volume at which the elastic recoil of the lung and chest wall are equal, and opposite is the relaxation volume of the respiratory system.

Functional Residual Capacity (FRC) is the volume of gas in the lung at end expiration. It should be distinguished from the relaxation volume defined above. In healthy adults at rest FRC is essentially equal to the relaxation volume of the respiratory system, and FRC is usually treated as synonymous with relaxation volume. This is a source of confusion as the two volumes can be different. FRC is variously used to refer to:

1. Relaxation volume of the respiratory system
2. The volume of gas in the lung at the end of a "normal" expiration
3. The volume of gas in the lung at the end of any expiration

The reader is often required to decide which meaning was intended by context. In many situations these volumes are different. For example, the neonatal chest wall is much more compliant than in adults; while this may facilitate passage through the birth canal, it lowers the relaxation volume of the respiratory system. To prevent closing of airways that would occur if FRC were to drop to relaxation volume, neonates end expiration by closing the glottis. Another example where FRC and relaxation volume may differ is in obstructive lung disease where FRC is dynamically determined and may be considerably above relaxation volume.

Although the elastic properties and relaxation volumes of the lung and chest wall are different, the compliances or slopes of the curve of the two structures are very similar throughout the midlung volumes. The compliance of the chest wall falls at low lung volumes, and the compliance of the lung falls at high lung volumes. See Fig 2-2.

FRC and relaxation volume are affected by body size, sex, age, diaphragmatic muscle tone, posture, anesthesia, and various pathologic states that affect the lung, chest wall, or muscle tone.

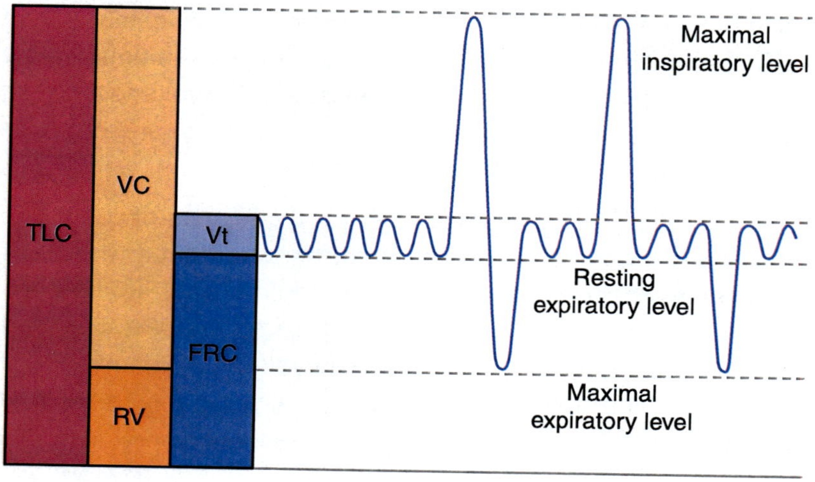

Figure 2-3 – Lung volumes.

FRC is measured using either a nitrogen washout technique, the wash-in of a tracer gas, or whole body plethysmography.

The clinical significance of FRC is twofold. First, it represents a reservoir of gas which may provide oxygen to the circulation during periods of apnea (e.g., during intubation). Second, maintaining an adequate lung volume at end expiration is critical to keeping airways open. If airways close during expiration and do not open on a subsequent inspiration, alveoli distal to the closure will undergo absorption atelectasis resulting in shunt. Small airways lacking cartilage depend on radial traction of the lung to stay open, and this radial traction falls as lung volume falls.

Closing Capacity

Closing capacity (CC) is the lung volume during expiration at which airways begin to close. FRC falls below CC resulting in airways closure in patients who are elderly, obese, or supine and anesthetized. FRC declines with supine position; CC does not. Approaching age 55, FRC falls below CC in the supine position resulting in a decrease in oxygenation.

Hysteresis

The inflation and deflation characteristics of the lung are not identical. At a given volume the transmural pressure is higher during inflation and lower during deflation. The faster the volume is changed the greater the difference in pressure. This behavior is called hysteresis (Fig 2-4) and is caused predominantly by the surface tension at the gas liquid interface.

Alveolar Ventilation

Several forms of ventilation are conventionally described. The total ventilation, V_E, is the volume of gas leaving the lung during expiration. Alveolar ventilation (V_A) = total ventilation − dead space ventilation.

Dead Space

A proportion of ventilation, *physiologic dead space*, does not participate in gas exchange. Physiologic dead space is the sum of anatomic and alveolar dead space. Anatomic dead space is the

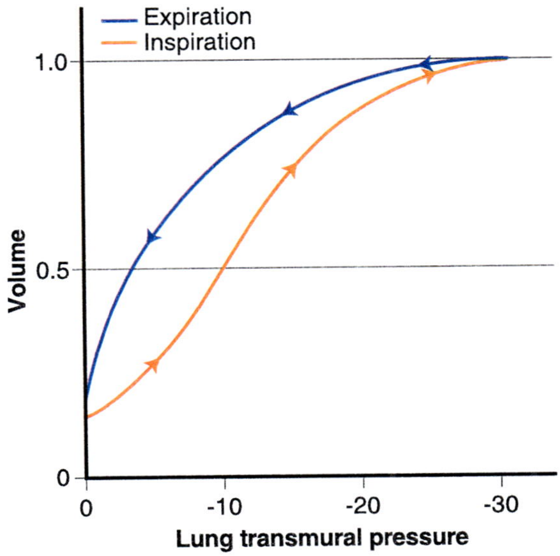

Figure 2-4 – Hysteresis.

volume of gas in the conducting airways. Alveolar dead space is the change in volume of gas in alveoli that are not functionally perfused. In health the alveolar dead space approximates zero and therefore physiologic and anatomic dead spaces are almost identical. When dead space is increased in disease, it is essentially always due to an increase in alveolar dead space.

Resistance and Gas Flow

Airway resistance is predominantly affected by airway cross-sectional area, which in turn is influenced by lung volume, elastic recoil, and airway smooth muscle tone. In any individual the primary modifiable determinant of airways resistance is lung volume. The intrinsic elastic properties of the lung cannot be changed. Therefore, maximum flows are greater at high lung volumes, and may be diminished by airway constriction or compression, secretions, foreign bodies, and increased lung water. In healthy subjects, intermediate-sized bronchi contribute most of the resistance to flow, and small airways contribute the least.

In a given airway, gas flow may be laminar or turbulent (3). Characteristics that promote turbulence include high flow rates, tubes that are not long and straight (i.e., curved, branching, changing in diameter), and fluids with high density or low viscosity. At a given flow turbulence is more likely in a smaller tube. In laminar flow states, the pressure drop required for a given flow is proportional to the flow, inversely proportional to the fourth power of the radius, the flow profile is parabolic with highest velocity in the center of the airway, and viscosity is the dominant fluid characteristic. Turbulent flow is less efficient, the pressure drop required for a given flow is proportional to the flow squared, inversely proportional to the fifth power of the radius, the flow profile is flat, and density is the dominant fluid characteristic.

Expiratory Flow Limitation

During expiration as lung volume falls so does elastic recoil and airway transmural pressure. Consequently, airway diameter decreases and resistance increases. Maximum expiratory airflow

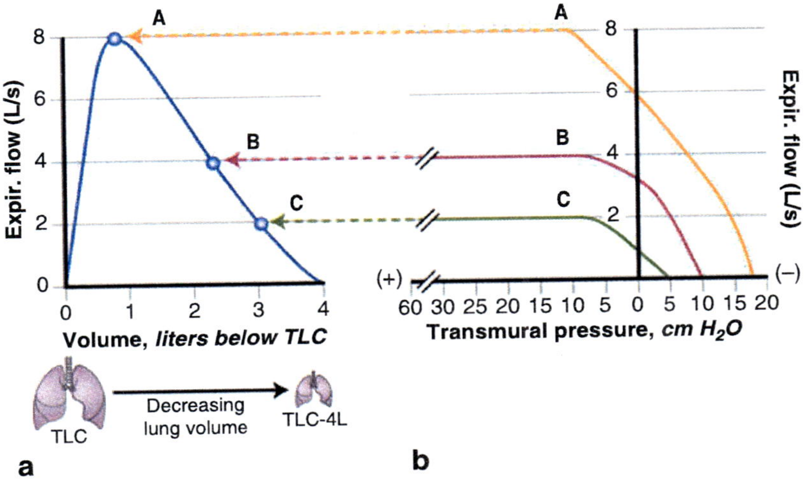

Figure 2-5 – (**a**) Expiratory phase of a flow-volume loop. (**b**) Expiratory flow becomes relatively fixed (independent of positive transmural pressure or effort) at different rates depending on lung volume (Compare A vs. B vs C). modified from West JB; Respiratory Physiology - the essentials (7th Edition) Lippencott, Williams & Wilkins, 2005.

falls and becomes "effort independent"; that is independent of increased effort beyond a modest threshold. These factors give rise to the characteristic outer envelope of the expiratory portion of the flow-volume loop. See Fig 2-5.

The mechanisms that limit maximum flow through compressible tubes, both airways and blood vessels, are complex. The *equal pressure point model* (Fig 2-6) describes the phenomenon in airways as follows. The pressure outside intrathoracic airways is Ppl, the pressure within the airway begins at alveolar pressure (Ppl + Lung elastic recoil pressure, which depends upon lung volume) and ends at zero (atmospheric) at the mouth. As gas flows from alveolus to mouth, the pressure within the airway falls due to resistance. Therefore, during a forced expiration the pressure within the airway will at some point equal Ppl (the equal pressure point). Downstream (mouthward) of the EPP the airway transmural pressure will be negative, and the airway is compressed. Increased expiratory effort increases Ppl but not lung elastic recoil pressure, further compressing the airway so flow does not increase. The loss of elastic recoil and therefore lung elastic recoil pressure in obstructive lung disease causes expiratory airflow limitation to become more severe and more

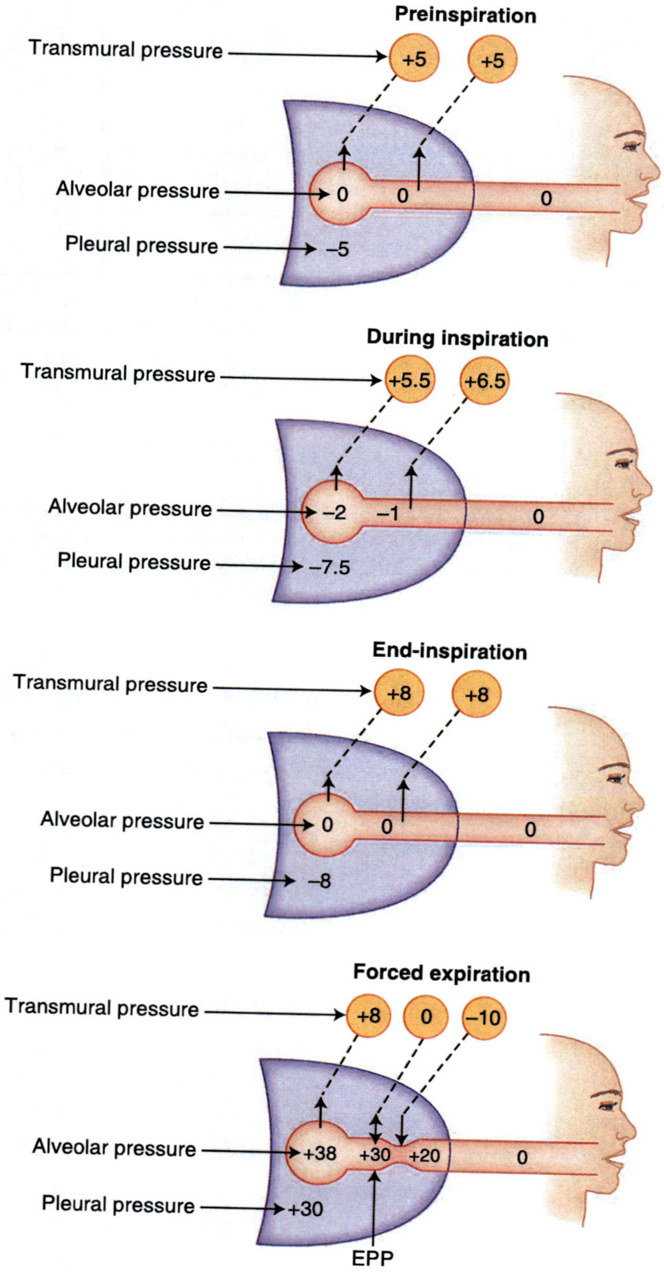

Figure 2-6 – Flow limitation in a single alveolus (equal pressure point model).

heterogenous. This phenomenon is clinically relevant to obstructive pulmonary disease, and to air trapping, and its consequences.

Work of Breathing

A variety of forces must be overcome to move gas, the lung, and chest wall. The work of breathing is the measure of work involved in overcoming these forces. The amount of work required is dependent on airways resistance (see above) and the physical properties of the tissues and liquids comprising and contained in the respiratory system, the gas that is being breathed, and the interfaces of gases, liquids, and tissues contained in the thorax.

Diffusion

Gas transport across the alveolar wall is via passive diffusion. Diffusion rates are influenced by the partial pressure difference between alveolar gas and blood, the surface area of alveoli available for diffusion, the distance over which the gas must diffuse, the solubility of the gas in the alveolar wall, and their molecular weights.

In healthy lungs there is an estimated 50–100 m^2 of alveolar-capillary surface area, and the thickness of the tissue barrier through which gases must diffuse is less than half of a micrometer. Transit time of blood in the lung is determined by the ratio of pulmonary capillary volume to cardiac output. At rest blood spends approximately three-fourth of a second in the pulmonary capillaries.

Doubling cardiac output (e.g., exercise) does not halve transit time because the increased pulmonary artery pressure causes pulmonary capillary blood volume to increase by a combination of recruitment and distension. This design provides an enormous capacity for gas exchange, and in healthy individuals pulmonary end capillary blood and alveolar gas are in equilibrium for all gases even at high flows. *Gas exchange is rarely diffusion-limited*. Under rare circumstances, such as very high cardiac output states, transit time may be reduced enough that diffusion limitation becomes important.

CO_2 is much more soluble in water and tissue than O_2, and as a result, CO_2 diffuses approximately 20 times faster. Consequently, diffusion limitation of carbon dioxide is even more uncommon than for oxygen.

Diffusing capacity (DL) of the lung is measured using uptake of carbon monoxide (CO) because of its very high affinity for hemoglobin. DLCO is measured as CO uptake (V_{CO})/alveolar partial pressure of CO (P_ACO).

Ventilation Perfusion Relationships

The respiratory system accomplishes exchange of gas by having blood and air in close proximity across a large diffusive surface area. Efficient exchange of oxygen and carbon dioxide depends on the regional matching of ventilation and perfusion in all areas of the lung. A spectrum of possible $\dot{V}/\dot{Q}$ ratios exists within each of the roughly 480 million alveoli of the lung. At the extremes are shunt – a state of perfusion without ventilation ($\dot{V}/\dot{Q}=0$), and dead space – ventilation without perfusion ($\dot{V}/\dot{Q}=$infinity).

Shunt

The reader should note that shunt is variously used to refer to:

1. Pure or true shunt as defined above ($\dot{V}/\dot{Q}=0$)
2. The solution to the shunt equation for venous admixture or virtual shunt (see below)
3. Areas of very low $\dot{V}/\dot{Q}$ ratios

The mixed venous blood that flows through true shunt mixes with pulmonary capillary blood and reduces the oxygen content of arterial blood. Increasing the FiO_2 has no impact on the hypoxic effect of true shunt. Sources of shunt may be physiologic or pathologic (Table 2-1).

Table 2-1 – Sources of true shunt

Physiologic shunt (1–3% of CO)
- Bronchial circulation
- Pleural circulation
- Thebesian veins

Pathologic sources of shunt
- Intrapulmonary
  - Atelectasis
  - Intrapulmonary arteriovenous malformations
- Extrapulmonary
  - Cardiac right to left shunts (requires abnormal communication between right and left heart and elevated right heart pressure)

Arterial oxygen content is reduced by true shunt as well as perfusion of regions of low $\dot{V}/\dot{Q}$ ratio. Examination of PaO_2 or A-a gradient fails to distinguish these causes. The shunt equation quantifies the amount of shunt that would exist if true shunt alone explained the degree of arterial oxygen deficiency. Ventilation with 100% O_2 will restore oxygenation in areas with very low $\dot{V}/\dot{Q}$ ratios, and the shunt equation will yield a better estimate of true shunt. The shunt and dead space equation (see below) are derived from simplified two-compartment models where blood flow is either ideal or shunt, and ventilation is either ideal or dead space.

$$Qs/Qt = [(Cc'O_2 - CaO_2)/(Cc'O_2 - CvO_2)]$$

Qs = shunt blood flow;

Qt = total blood flow;

$Cc'O_2$ = end pulmonary capillary oxygen content;

CaO_2 = arterial oxygen content;

CvO_2 = mixed venous oxygen content.

Dead Space

Like the term shunt, dead space is variously used to refer to:

1. Pure dead space as defined above ($\dot{V}/\dot{Q}$ = infinity)
2. The solution to the dead space equation (see below) or virtual dead space
3. Areas of very high $\dot{V}/\dot{Q}$ ratios

Dead space was defined earlier as the volume of gas that is not available for exchange with blood. Physiologic dead space is measured using the modified Bohr equation and is defined as $V_D/V_T = PaCO_2\text{-}P_ECO_2/\ PaCO_2$.

V_D = dead space ventilation;

V_T = total ventilation;

$PaCO_2$ = partial pressure of carbon dioxide in arterial blood;

P_ECO_2 = partial pressure of carbon dioxide in end tidal gas;

$PaCO_2$ = partial pressure of carbon dioxide in arterial gas.

Physiologic dead space is composed of anatomic dead space and alveolar dead space which is usually negligible in health. Anatomic dead space is measured by the Fowler's method where a subject inspires a single breath of pure oxygen and the washout of dead space gas is plotted by the accumulation of nitrogen to a plateau consistent with that of pure alveolar gas and is approximately 2 ml/pound lean body weight.

In normal upright subjects at rest, approximately 80% of ventilation and perfusion go to lung regions with a $\dot{V}/\dot{Q}$ ratio of 0.3–1.0. Shunt predominantly affects oxygenation, demonstrated by a low PaO_2 due to a widening of the alveolar to arterial (A–a) gradient. An increase in alveolar dead space predominantly affects CO_2 and is demonstrated by an increase in total ventilation needed to achieve a given $PaCO_2$, due to a widening of the arterial to end-tidal gradient.

$\dot{V}/\dot{Q}$ heterogeneity always results in an increased (A–a) gradient because the oxyhemoglobin dissociation curve plateaus, and blood flow through regions with high $\dot{V}/\dot{Q}$ ratios cannot compensate for the low O_2 content of blood coming from lung regions with low $\dot{V}/\dot{Q}$ ratios (Fig 2-7). However, the same is not true for CO_2 because the CO_2 content vs. partial pressure relationship is nearly linear.

Distribution of ventilation and perfusion is modeled using the multiple inert gas elimination technique (MIGET) in which six inert gases of different solubility are injected intravenously, and measured in arterial and mixed venous blood and expired gas. The lung is modeled as a set of 50 respiratory units, each with a different V/Q ratio. The amount of ventilation to regions of pure dead space, of perfusion to regions of pure shunt, and of ventilation and perfusion to lung regions with the intermediate values of $\dot{V}/\dot{Q}$ matching can be graphically illustrated. MIGET diagrams thus subdivide the lung based on function ($\dot{V}/\dot{Q}$ matching) rather than structure, and illustrate the functional distribution of ventilation and perfusion.

In Fig 2-8, $\dot{V}/\dot{Q}$ relationships derived from MIGET are depicted in a young healthy patient in the upright position and breathing spontaneously. Note that ventilation and perfusion are tightly matched to one another, and exhibit little spread (dispersion) to regions of inefficient $\dot{V}/\dot{Q}$ relationships.

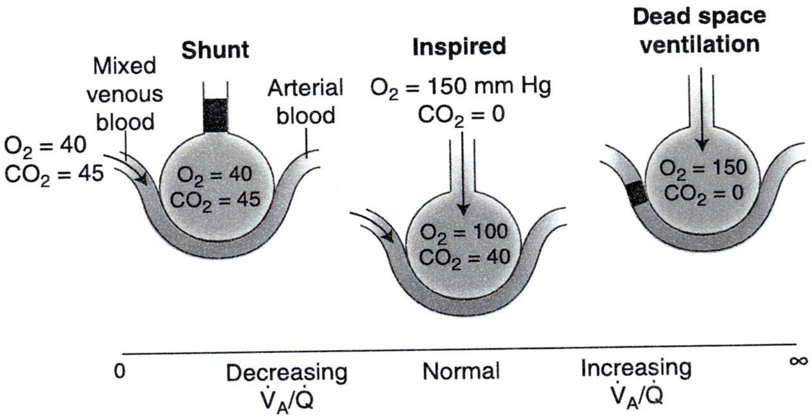

Figure 2-7 – Effects of different $\dot{V}/\dot{Q}$ ratios.

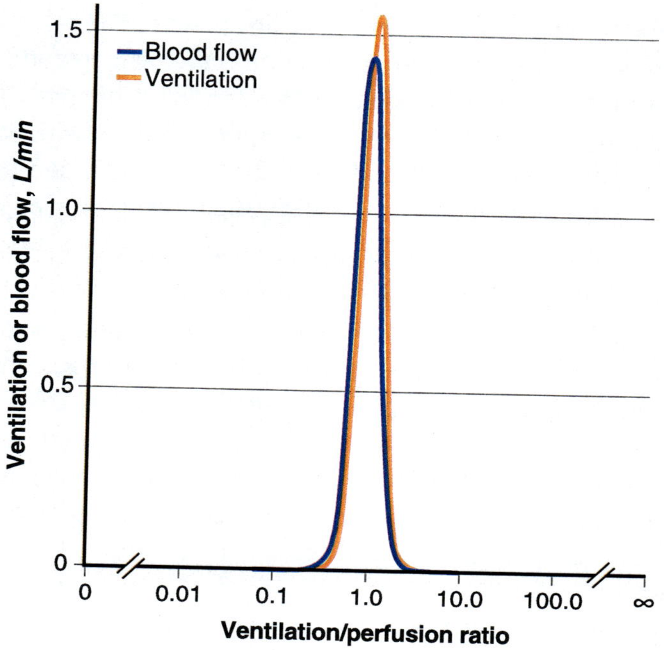

Figure 2-8 – Distribution of ventilation and perfusion in a patient aged 22 years.

The remarkable degree of $\dot{V}/\dot{Q}$ matching normally achieved in the topographically complex lung is incompletely understood. Prominent mechanisms include gravity, HPV, and the congruence of the geometry between the pulmonary arterial and tracheobroncheal arborizations.

Gravitational Effects

Both perfusion and ventilation are greater in dependent portions of the lung due to gravity. Because blood has greater density than lung tissue, the effect on perfusion exceeds that on ventilation. While both $\dot{Q}$ and $\dot{V}$ increase from non-dependent regions to dependent regions, $\dot{Q}$ increases faster, and the $\dot{V}/\dot{Q}$ ratio falls. This results in lower $\dot{V}/\dot{Q}$ ratios in dependent regions and higher ratios in nondependent regions.

The effects of gravity on regional distribution of local pulmonary artery and pulmonary vein pressure in relation to each other and to alveolar pressure (the pressure outside pulmonary capillaries) result in a vertical gradient of flow. The effects are often described as West zones of the lung. There is no blood flow in zone 1 where Palv > Ppa > Ppv. Moving down the lung, in zone 2 where Ppa > Palv > Ppv, flow increases quickly as the driving pressure (Ppa–Palv, *not* Ppa–Ppv) increases, and the vessels become larger as the absolute intravascular pressure increases. Moving down the lung, in zone 3 where Ppa > Ppv > Palv, flow increases slowly as driving pressure does not change (because Ppa and Ppv are increasing by the same amount), however, the vessels become larger as the absolute intravascular pressure increases.

The effects of gravity on ventilation are due to the vertical variation in Ppl. At FRC, dependent alveoli are smaller than nondependent ones due to the weight of the lung above. Because the lung sits in the chest and is affected by gravity, the weight of the lung causes the pleural pressure to be more negative in nondependent regions and less negative in dependent regions. However, alveolar pressure is the same throughout the lung. Hence, dependent lung regions are exposed to a lower transmural pressure, the alveoli are smaller, and are on a more compliant part of their pressure–volume curve. Inspiration results in greater increases in volume (more ventilation) of dependent alveoli compared to the already relatively expanded and less compliant nondependent alveoli.

There is little doubt that gravity affects both ventilation and perfusion in the same direction, and thus contributes to $\dot{V}/\dot{Q}$ matching, but the magnitude of this effect remains a subject of debate (4).

Anatomic Effects

Higher resolution studies than those done by West reveal isogravitational heterogeneity in regional pulmonary $\dot{V}$ and $\dot{Q}$, in addition to the vertical heterogeneity described above (5). Within a horizontal plane the majority of ventilation and perfusion is located in the center of the lung with a decreasing gradient toward the periphery. Congruence between the geometry of the pulmonary arterial and bronchial arborizations likely contributes considerably to $\dot{V}/\dot{Q}$ matching.

Hypoxic Pulmonary Vasoconstriction

HPV is a physiologic response of the pulmonary arterioles to local alveolar hypoxia. HPV is only exhibited by the pulmonary circulation – other arterial beds dilate in response to hypoxemia.

The precise mechanism of HPV is still unknown. It is believed to be a phenomenon of smooth muscle cells in small (<500 μm) pulmonary resistance vessels, and involves hypoxia-triggered inhibition of voltage-gated potassium channels, membrane depolarization, and calcium release from sarcoplasmic reticulum. HPV is thought to function independently of endothelium but may be modulated at this level. Its onset occurs within seconds and has a time constant of about 150 s; 63% of the maximal effect will be reached within about 150 s and 95% in about 450 s (8 min) (6, 7).

The primary trigger to HPV is alveolar hypoxia; low mixed venous oxygen saturation acts as a secondary trigger. Pulmonary vascular resistance may increase up to three times baseline values due to widespread HPV. Regional or local HPV responses divert perfusion from hypoxic alveoli to better ventilated ones, powerfully fine tuning $\dot{V}/\dot{Q}$ matching.

The effects of HPV are decreased by beta agonists, calcium channel blockers, inhalational agents, and nitrodilators. The effects of HPV are augmented by cyclo-oxygenase inhibitors, beta blockers, and the drug almitrine.

These mechanisms (gravitational, anatomic, HPV) are normally the most important agents influencing $\dot{V}/\dot{Q}$ matching. Other influences impact the distribution of pulmonary perfusion and $\dot{V}/\dot{Q}$ matching, including, but not limited to:

- Cardiac output
- Pulmonary artery pressure
- Local autocrine/paracrine molecules
    - Nitric oxide
    - Endothelin
    - Prostaglandins

  - Thromboxane
  - Leukotrienes
- Neural effects (autonomic and nonautonomic)
- Humoral agents (catecholamines, etc.)

Pulmonary pathophysiology and the perturbations of anesthesia, thoracic surgery, and one-lung ventilation impose considerable disruption of this complex balance, and impact efficiency of gas exchange (see Chapters 3–5).

Gas Transport

Oxygen in the blood is carried both in a dissolved form and a more significant fraction that is bound to hemoglobin (Hb). Arterial oxygen content is calculated as:

$CaO_2 ml\ O_2/dl\ blood = (1.34\ ml\ O_2/gm\ Hb \times SaO_2 \times Hb) + (0.003 ml\ O_2/dl/torr \times PaO_2)$

PaO_2 = partial pressure of oxygen in arterial blood in mmHg;

SaO_2 = arterial oxygen saturation

Oxygen saturation and hemoglobin concentration are the primary determinants of arterial oxygen content.

Carbon dioxide is carried in blood as bicarbonate, in a dissolved form, and in combination with proteins, of which Hb is the most significant. Bicarbonate carries the majority of CO_2 although in venous blood it carries somewhat less than that in arterial blood. Bicarbonate formation from CO_2 and water is shown below; the first step of which requires carbonic anhydrase.

$$CO_2 + H_2O \leftrightarrow H_2CO_3 \leftrightarrow H + HCO_3$$

Selected References

1. Aubier M, Murciano D, Fournier M, et al. Central respiratory drive in acute respiratory failure of patients with chronic obstructive pulmonary disease. Am Rev Resp Dis. 1980;122:191–8.

2. Hanson CW, Marshall B, Frasch HF, Marshall C. Causes of hypercarbia with oxygen therapy in patients with chronic obstructive pulmonary disease. Crit Care Med. 1996;24(1):23–8.

3. Mead J. Mechanical properties of lungs. Physiol Rev. 1961;41(2):281–330.

4. Glenny RW, Lamm WJ, Bernard SL, An D, Chornuk M, Pool SL, et al. Selected contribution: redistribution of pulmonary perfusion during weightlessness and increased gravity. J Appl Physiol. 2000;89(3):1239–48.

5. Hakim TS, Lisbona R, Dean GW. Gravity-independent inequality in pulmonary blood flow in humans. J Appl Physiol. 1987;63(3):1114–21.

6. Jensen KS, Micco AJ, Czartolomna J, Latham L, Voelkel NF. Rapid onset of hypoxic vasoconstriction in isolated lungs. J Appl Physiol. 1992;72(5):2018–23.

7. Morrell NW, Nijran KS, Biggs T, Seed WA. Magnitude and time course of acute hypoxic pulmonary vasoconstriction in man. Respir Physiol. 1995;100(3):271–81.

Further Suggested Reading

Aubier M, Murciano D, Fournier M, et al. Central respiratory drive in acute respiratory failure of patients with chronic obstructive pulmonary disease. Am Rev Resp Dis. 1980;122:191–8.

Glenny RW, Lamm WJ, Bernard SL, An D, Chornuk M, Pool SL, et al. Selected contribution: redistribution of pulmonary perfusion during weightlessness and increased gravity. J Appl Physiol. 2000;89(3):1239–48.

Hakim TS, Lisbona R, Dean GW. Gravity-independent inequality in pulmonary blood flow in humans. J Appl Physiol. 1987;63(3):1114–21.

Hanson CW, Marshall B, Frasch HF, Marshall C. Causes of hypercarbia with oxygen therapy in patients with chronic obstructive pulmonary disease. Crit Care Med. 1996;24(1):23–8.

Hyatt RE. Expiratory flow limitation. J Appl Physiol: Resp Environ Exerc Physiol. 1983;55(1):1–8.

Jensen KS, Micco AJ, Czartolomna J, Latham L, Voelkel NF. Rapid onset of hypoxic vasoconstriction in isolated lungs. J Appl Physiol. 1992;72(5):2018–23.

Lumb AB. Nunn's applied respiratory physiology. 6th ed. Philadelphia: Elsevier Butterworth Heinemann; 2005.

Mead J. Mechanical properties of lungs. Physiol Rev. 1961;41(2):281–330.

Morrell NW, Nijran KS, Biggs T, Seed WA. Magnitude and time course of acute hypoxic pulmonary vasoconstriction in man. Respir Physiol. 1995;100(3): 271–81.

Wagner PD, Laravuso RB, Uhl RR, West JB. Continuous distributions of ventilation-perfusion ratios in normal subjects breathing air and 100 per cent O_2. J Clin Invest. 1974;54(1):54–68.

West JB. Respiratory physiology – the essentials. 7th ed. Philadelphia: Lippincott Williams & Wilkins; 2005.

Weibel ER. The pathway for oxygen: structure and function in the mammalian respiratory system. Cambridge: Harvard University Press; 1984.

Suggested Sources

Lumb AB. Nunn's applied respiratory physiology. 6th ed. Philadelphia: Elsevier Butterworth Heinemann; 2005.

West JB. Respiratory physiology – the essentials. 7th ed. Philadelphia: Lippincott Williams & Wilkins; 2005.

Chapter 3
Respiratory Pathophysiology

Shannon S. McKenna

Keywords Respiratory pathophysiology • Obstructive pulmonary disease • Restrictive pulmonary disease • Pulmonary vascular disease

Introduction

The enormous topic of respiratory disease may be functionally organized, for the purposes of this manual, into the following general categories:

- Obstructive pulmonary disease
- Restrictive pulmonary disease
- Pulmonary vascular disease

Obstructive Disease

Definition

The key feature of obstructive lung disease is increased resistance to air flow.

P.M. Hartigan (ed.), *Practical Handbook of Thoracic Anesthesia*,
DOI 10.1007/978-0-387-88493-6_3,

Etiology

Physically, increased resistance can occur as a result of changes in the lumen of the airways, the walls of the airways themselves, or the tissue surrounding and supporting the airways (Table 3-1).

The two most common obstructive diseases are asthma and chronic obstructive pulmonary disease (COPD). Asthma is a chronic inflammatory disorder that results increased airway reactivity. Airflow limitation is fully reversible between acute exacerbations. COPD is also a chronic inflammatory disease. It is, however, pathologically much more complex. Changes include airway inflammation, edema, fibrosis, secretion overproduction, and emphysema (see Figs 3-1 and 3-2). Elastin and collagen are destroyed leading to

Table 3-1 – Causes of obstructive lung disease
Obstruction of lumen
Excessive/inspissated secretions
Foreign body
Intraluminal tumor
Blood clots
Airway wall processes
Bronchospasm (asthma)
Hypertrophy/stenosis
Infiltrate
Edema
Tumor infiltration
Peribronchial processes
Loss of radial traction (emphysema)
Compression – mass effect
Edema

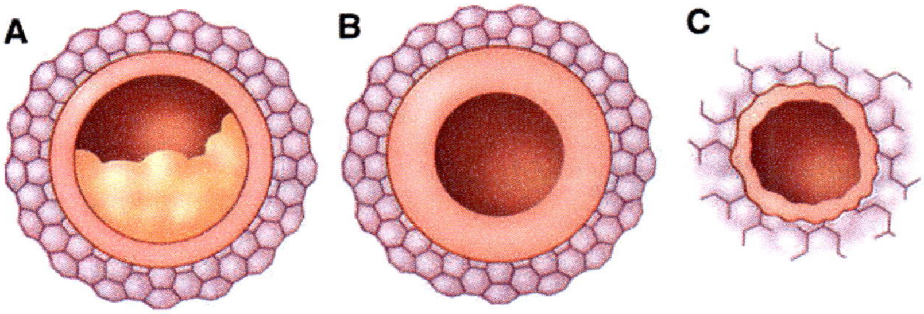

Figure 3-1 – Mechanisms of airway obstruction. (**A**) Luminal occlusion by secretions. (**B**) Airway wall thickening by edema, inflammation, fibrosis or smooth muscle hypertrophy. (**C**) Alveolar destruction leading to airway narrowing from loss of radial traction (from West JB. Obstructive Diseases. In: Pulmonary Pathophysiology. 7th ed. Philadelphia, PA. Lippincott Williams & Wilkins; 2008:52).

loss of tethering effect and elastic recoil. Patients have variable components of bronchitis and emphysema. Unlike asthma, the airflow limitation of COPD is never fully reversible. COPD is a progressive disease.

Clinical Presentation

Asthma frequently occurs in patients with a history of other atopic disease. Frequently, a trigger can be identified for a given exacerbation. Between exacerbations the patient will be asymptomatic. Dyspnea is the primary symptom during an exacerbation, but cough and increased secretions also occur. Accessory muscle use may be observed and wheezing is common on auscultation. The lungs are hyperinflated on CXR. Hyperinflation is typical in COPD as well (see Fig 1-13). COPD is a progressive disease. A chronic, productive cough is usually the first symptom of the disease. Dyspnea on exertion occurs with disease progression. Eventually, patients with the most severe forms of COPD progress to dyspnea at rest. Some patients will develop significant gas exchange abnormalities with chronic hypoxia, hypercarbia, or both, due to significant abnormalities in $\dot{V}/\dot{Q}$ matching

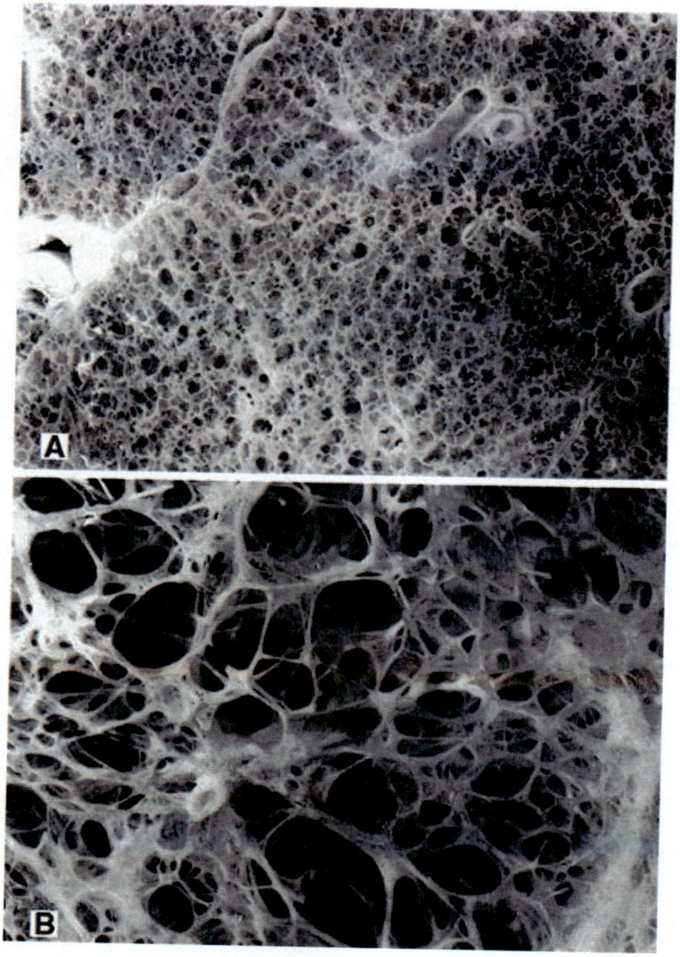

Figure 3-2 – Emphysematous lung compared to normal. Panacinar emphysematous changes (**B**) are shown in contrast to normal lung (**A**) (magnified 14×) (from West JB. Chronic Obstructive Pulmonary Diseases. In: Pulmonary Physiology and Pathophysiology: an Integrated, Case-Based Approach. 2nd ed. Philadelphia, PA. Lippincott Williams & Wilkins; 2007:33).

(see Fig 3-3). Cor pulmonale occurs in the most extreme cases. Clinical feature of COPD are detailed in Table 3-2.

Evaluation and Testing

Diagnosis of obstructive lung disease is made by spirometry. Both the FEV_1 and FEV_1/FVC ratio are reduced. An FEV_1/FVC ratio of

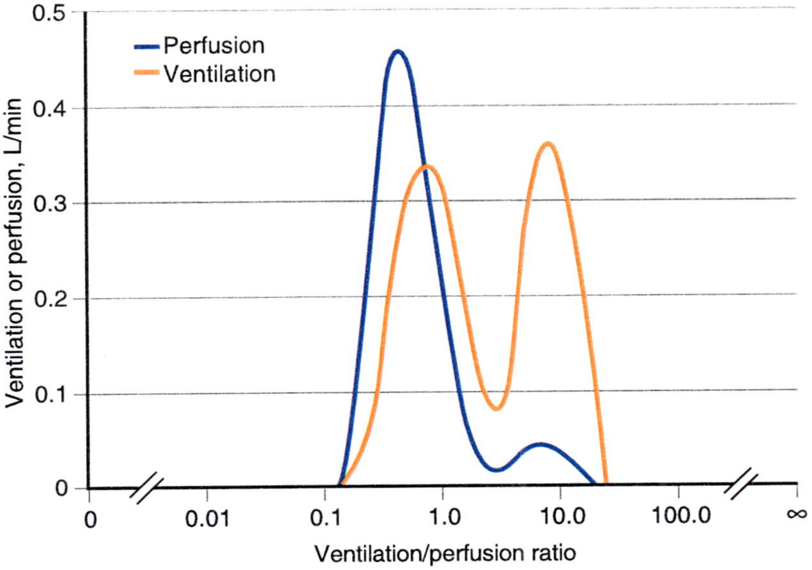

Figure 3-3 – Distribution of ventilation and perfusion in a patient with COPD. Multiple gas elimination technique depicts excessive ventilation to areas with minimal perfusion (high V/Q ratio) which represents increased physiologic dead space (from Wagner PD, Dantzker DR, Dueck R et al. Ventilation-perfusion inequality in chronic obstructive pulmonary disease. J Clin Invest 1977; 59:203–206).

0.7 or less is required for the diagnosis of an obstructive lung disease. Bronchodilator testing can be used to assess the degree of reversible obstruction. Increased FRC, RV, and TLC indicate hyperinflation and gas trapping. Staging of COPD is based on the FEV_1 (Table 3-3).

Management

Management is disease specific. Current recommendations for asthma focus on monitoring, symptom assessment, and controlling triggering factors. Patients with mild, intermittent asthma are treated with short acting B_2 agonists. Treatment of more severe disease incorporates inhaled steroids, long acting bronchodilators, leukotriene inhibitors, and if needed, oral glucocorticoids.

Table 3-2 – Clinical features of COPD

Increased mucous production
Chronic productive cough
Mucous plugging/impaction
Recurrent infections
Air flow obstruction
Wheezing or silent chest if minimal air movement
Accessory muscle use
Purse lip breathing
Barrel chest
Increased lung volumes on PFT's
CXR – hyperlucency and flat diaphragm
Increased work of breathing
Dyspnea
Limited exercise capacity
Respiratory muscle fatigue during exacerbations
Worsened V/Q matching
Hypoxia
Hypercarbia
Digital clubbing
Elevated hematocrit
Blebs and Bullae – spontaneous pneumothorax
Pulmonary hypertension and cor pulmonale

Management of COPD focuses on minimizing dyspnea and maximizing exercise capacity. The only interventions that effect the progression of disease are smoking cessation and oxygen therapy for hypoxemic patients. Vaccination against pulmonary pathogens is important to prevent life threatening exacerbations. Mild symptoms

Table 3-3 – Staging of COPD

STAGE	SPIROMETRY
I Mild	FEV1 >80% predicted
II Moderate	FEV1 50–80% predicted
III Severe	FEV1 30–50% predicted
IV Very severe	FEV1 <30% predicted

Table 3-4 – Management of secretions during general anesthesia

Endotracheal suctioning
Fiberoptic bronchoscopy
Humidification (passive or active)
Judicious hydration
Mucolytics (*n*-acetylcysteine, dornase alfa)

can be treated with short acting bronchodilators. Long acting bronchodilators and inhaled corticosteroids can be used for more symptomatic patients. Systemic corticosteroids, administered as a pulse and taper, along with antibiotics, may be needed to treat acute exacerbations. In very specific cases, end-stage disease may be treated with lung volume reduction surgery or lung transplantation.

Perioperative Pitfalls

Perioperative problems center around secretion management, bronchospasm, hyperinflation, and impaired gas exchange. Strategies for dealing with secretion management are listed in Table 3-4. Bronchospasm is dealt with via adequate anesthesia during airway manipulation, administration of short acting inhaled bronchodilators,

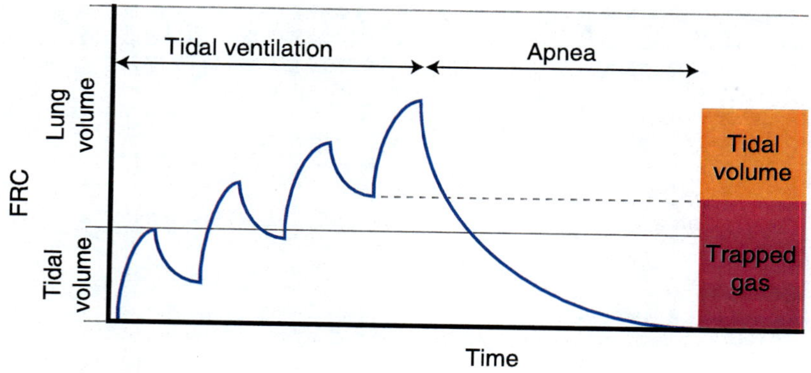

Figure 3-4 – The development of dynamic hyperinflation during positive pressure ventilation (from Myles PS et al. J Cardiothoracic and Vascular anesthesia. 11:100, 1997).

and rarely intravenous corticosteroids (delayed onset of action) or low dose intravenous epinephrine (0.25–0.5 mg/min).

Dynamic hyperinflation occurs when inspiration occurs before the entire prior tidal volume has been exhaled. It results in a progressive rise in intrathoracic volume (dynamic hyperinflation) and end-expiratory pressure (auto- or intrinsic PEEP) (Fig 3-4) until a new steady state is achieved. Lung compliance is decreased, alveolar rupture may occur, and venous return is markedly decreased. This can cause severe hypotension and even pulseless electrical activity. Induction of anesthesia is a high risk period for dynamic hyperinflation in the vulnerable patient. Several strategies help to avoid, or mitigate the effects of, dynamic hyperinflation (Table 3-5). If profound hypotension occurs, the most effective treatment is to transiently stop ventilating the patient while maintaining a patent airway and allowing the patient to completely exhale.

Timely emergence from general anesthesia can be a particular challenge in patients with severe and very severe obstructive lung disease. Residual postoperative respiratory depression and ineffective ventilation are significant postoperative concerns. Patients with COPD have increased sensitivity to the respiratory depressant effects of many medications routinely used during general anesthesia (Table 3-6). A number of strategies can help to promote timely emergence and adequate respiratory function in the postoperative period (Table 3-7).

Table 3-5 – Strategies to manage at risk for dynamic hyperinflation

Preinduction hydration (to prevent hypotension)
Preinduction bronchodilator administration
Use low respiratory rate (6–8 bmp)
Use short I:E ratio (1:3 or greater)
Use lowest tidal volume tolerated
Consider replacing 50–75% intrinsic PEEP with extrinsic PEEP

Table 3-6 – Agents causing respiratory depression in COPD patients

Benzodiazepines
Barbiturates
Opiates
Propofol
Volatile anesthetics

Table 3-7 – Strategies for timely emergence and maximal postoperative pulmonary function

Intraoperative	Postoperative
Bronchodilator use	Bronchodilator use
Regional analgesia	Regional analgesia
Avoid long acting neuromuscular blockers	Lung expansion maneuvers
Avoid unnecessary respiratory depressants	Early mobilization
TIVA for patients with severe/ very severe obstruction	Avoidance of sedatives and respiratory depressants

Restrictive Disease

Definition

Restrictive diseases impair lung expansion. They are characterized by decreased pulmonary compliance, reduced vital capacity, and low resting lung volumes.

Etiology

Restrictive disease can originate from the lung parenchyma, the pleural space or the chest wall (Table 3-8).

Clinical Presentation

The clinical presentation will vary greatly depending on the underlying disease process. Dyspnea and limited exercise tolerance are common, as is a rapid, shallow breathing pattern. Most of the parenchymal diseases are associated with a dry cough and fine crepitations on auscultation. Clubbing and cyanosis also occur with some frequency. Pulmonary hypertension occurs in many cases of long-standing restrictive disease. Signs of right heart dysfunction may be present.

Evaluation and Testing

Diagnosis of restrictive lung disease is typically made with pulmonary function testing. Additional evaluation includes a careful history to identify occupational, toxic and infectious etiologies, and chest imaging with a chest radiograph (see Fig 1-12) and CT scan. Arterial blood gas evaluation, serologic testing for autoimmune diseases, and analysis of pleural fluid may also be of use. In many instances, lung biopsy may be required to allow definitive diagnosis and appropriate treatment.

Management

Management is directed at treatment of the underlying disease. There are no general treatments for restrictive lung disease.

Table 3-8 – Causes of restrictive lung disease

Parenchymal disease
Primary lung diseases: idiopathic pulmonary fibrosis, sarcoidosis, BOOP, LAM, interstitial pneumonia
Pulmonary vasculitides
Hypersensitivity pneumonitis
Radiation pneumonitis
Drug toxicity (bleomycin, amiodarone, Busulfan, etc.)
Autoimmune diseases/collagen vascular diseases
ARDS
Chronic aspiration
Cardiogenic pulmonary edema
Lymphangitic carcinomatosis
Alveolar filling disorders: diffuse alveolar hemorrhage, PAP, Good Pasteur's
Inherited disorders: neurofibromatosis, tuberous sclerosis, Gaucher's disease
Pleural disease
Pneumothorax
Pleural effusion
Pleural thickening: infection, inflammation, tumor
Chest wall disease
Congenital: scoliosis, pectus excavatum
Ankylosing spondylitis
Obesity

Precautions in the Perioperative Setting

Low pulmonary compliance can make it difficult to both oxygenate and ventilate the patient effectively. Treatable contributors to impaired lung function should be sought out and addressed preoperatively. These may include pulmonary edema, acute infection, and large pleural effusions. If one-lung ventilation (OLV) is required and a significant contra-lateral effusion is present, consideration should be given to draining the effusion prior to commencement of OLV. Perioperative volume administration should be kept to the minimum needed to support organ function to prevent worsening of compliance and hypoxia.

These patients have a low FRC and will desaturate quickly during apneic periods. Intraoperative ventilation should utilize a strategy of smaller tidal volumes, higher rates, and PEEP titrated to maximize pulmonary compliance. OLV may be poorly tolerated secondary to hypoxia. CPAP applied to the operative lung may permit longer periods of lung isolation. In some instances, use of an ICU ventilator, combined with an intravenous anesthetic, may provide the best ventilation. Effective pain control is critical in the postoperative period if the patient is to be extubated. Postoperative atelectasis and hypoxia are common.

Pulmonary Vascular Disease

Definition

Pulmonary hypertension is generally defined by a mean pulmonary artery pressure greater than 25 mmHg at rest or 30 mmHg during exercise. If the elevated pressure originates from the precapillary arterioles, it is further classified as pulmonary arterial hypertension. Elevated pressure originating distal to the arterioles is classified as pulmonary venous hypertension, and is associated with increased pulmonary capillary wedge pressures.

Etiology

Fundamentally, pulmonary hypertension arises from one of three physiologic derangements: increased pulmonary vascular resistance (PVR), increased pulmonary blood flow, or increased left atrial pressure. Increased PVR can result from vasoconstrictive, obstructive, or obliterative processes (Table 3-9). Primary pulmonary

Table 3-9 – Causes of pulmonary hypertension

Diseases that increase PVR
Primary pulmonary HTN
COPD
Chronic hypoxia – any etiology
Thromboembolic disease
Pulmonary fibrosis
Pulmonary vasculitis
Collagen vascular disease
Interstitial lung diseases
Drugs/toxins
Chronic infections
Diseases associated with increased pulmonary blood flow
Atrial septal defects
Ventricular septal defects
Patent ductus arteriosus
Diseases associated with increased left atrial pressure
Left ventricular dysfunction
Valvular heart disease
Hypertrophic cardiomyopathy
Fibrosing mediastinitis
Extrinsic compression of pulmonary veins or left heart
Pulmonary veno-occlusive disease

hypertension, the most well studied form of pulmonary hypertension, occurs when both genetic and nongenetic factors lead to an imbalance in the proportion of endogenous vasodilators (prostacyclin and nitric oxide) to vasoconstrictors (thromboxane and endothelin-1). Fibrosing lung diseases destroy small blood vessels, decreasing the total cross-sectional area, and thereby increasing PVR.

Hypoxia is another common cause of pulmonary arterial hypertension. This response is initially adaptive to the extent that it improves V–Q matching. Chronic hypoxia leads to vascular remodeling with a permanent increase in PVR. Thromboembolic disease and pulmonary veno-occlusive disease increase PVR via both direct occlusion and reactive vasoconstriction.

Increased pulmonary circulation primarily elevates pulmonary pressures based on simple volume–pressure relationships. Chronic over circulation, such as occurs with intracardiac left to right shunts, leads to medial and intimal hypertrophy and ultimately, vascular fibrosis. The final result is a nonreversible increase in PVR.

Heart disease and total body volume overload both increase left atrial pressure and pulmonary capillary pressure, leading to pulmonary venous hypertension. Pulmonary hypertension in this setting is associated with pulmonary edema formation.

Clinical Presentation

Presenting symptoms are nonspecific and include dyspnea on exertion, fatigue, and syncope. Palpitations, angina, cough, and hemoptysis may also occur depending on the etiology of the pulmonary hypertension. As the disease progresses signs of right ventricular (RV) strain and failure may become evident on physical exam (Table 3-10).

Evaluation and Testing

Patients suspected of having pulmonary hypertension will require an extensive workup to confirm the disease, identify the underlying etiology, determine the severity of the disease, and evaluate various therapeutic modalities. Initial evaluation includes a chest radiograph, EKG, and transthoracic echocardiogram (TTE). The TTE can estimate pulmonary artery systolic pressures provided that tricuspid regurgitation is present. It can also allow assessment of the size and function of the both ventricles and identify structural lesions. Pulmonary function tests may help to identify the underlying pathologic condition. An arterial blood gas may also be helpful.

Table 3-10 – Signs of pulmonary HTN, RV Strain or RV Failure

Increased intensity of P_2 heart sound
Splitting of second heart sound
Pulmonic regurgitant murmur
Tricuspid regurgitant murmur with V wave in jugular venous pulse
RV heave
Prominent A wave in jugular venous pulse
Elevated jugular venous pulse or CVP
Hepatomegaly
Hepatojugular reflux
Ascites
Pedal edema

Most patients will also undergo a chest CT scan to evaluate for diseases causing pulmonary hypertension. Ultimately, right heart catheterization confirms the presence of elevated pulmonary pressure and allows for direct testing of vascular responsiveness against the various pulmonary vasodilators that can be used to treat pulmonary hypertension. Exercise testing may be used to help stage the disease and evaluate progression and response to therapy over time.

Management

Once identified, the underlying disease should be aggressively treated. Hypoxia, if present, should be treated with oxygen therapy. Diuretic therapy to control peripheral edema, anticoagulants to prevent secondary thromboembolism, and vaccination against common pulmonary pathogens are key adjuvants to treatment. Pulmonary rehabilitation can increase exercise capacity in many patients.

There are a number of pulmonary vasodilators that can be used as advanced therapy to decrease PVR and increase cardiac output

Table 3-11 – Agents for advanced therapy of pulmonary HTN

AGENT	ROUTE OF ADMINISTRATION
Calcium channel blockers	
Nifedipine	Oral
Diltiazem	Oral, i.v.
Amlodipine	Oral
Prostanoids	
Epoprostenol	i.v.
Treprostinil	s.q., i.v.
Iloprost	Inhaled
Endothelin receptor antagonists	
Bosentan	Oral
Ambrisentan	Oral
Sitaxsentan	Oral
PDE5 inhibitors	
Sildenafil	Oral

(Table 3-11). Choice of treatment is guided by acute vasoreactivity during right heart catheterization. It is important to note that pulmonary hypertension is a heterogenous disease. Vasodilator therapy has actually been found to be harmful in certain subsets of patients. This treatment should be initiated and monitored by physicians specializing in the long-term treatment of pulmonary hypertension. Ultimately, if the disease process cannot be stabilized, lung transplantation may be required.

Precautions in the Perioperative Setting

Perioperative considerations can be broken down into three parts: (1) avoiding triggers of sudden increases in pulmonary vascular pressures, (2) managing volume status and, (3) appropriate drug selection.

Hypoxia, hypercarbia, acidosis, pulmonary hyperinflation, and hypothermia all increase PVR. Additionally, any catecholamine surge will abruptly increase PVR. In the perioperative period, anxiety, pain, agitation, and light anesthesia are all likely causes of catecholamine surges. Arterial blood gas monitoring is the only way to accurately assess for hypercarbia or acidosis. These concepts apply equally to the postoperative period. Abrupt increases in PVR can decrease right heart cardiac output and lead to cardiogenic shock with systemic hypoperfusion.

Volume management is quite complex. Excessive fluid administration will lead to an increase in pulmonary pressures and can provoke decompensation. At the same time, chronic RV hypertrophy can decrease RV compliance, leading to the need for somewhat elevated central venous pressure to maintain adequate diastolic filling. Right ventricular ischemia can further compound this problem. Monitoring central venous pressure, being careful to note the baseline pressure at the time of line placement, can help guide volume management. In some instances, a pulmonary artery catheter may provide more useful information. Likewise, echocardiography can provide a real-time assessment of both pulmonary artery pressures and ventricular performance. It is limited by the fact that it provides a "brief clip" of time.

Anesthetic drug selection should be aimed at preventing postoperative respiratory depression and at the same time providing adequate analgesia. A further concern is the need to avoid severe systemic vasodilatation. Significant decreases in venous return will lead to a disproportionate decrease in cardiac output. Vasoconstrictors may be needed to treat systemic vasodilatation, but one must remember that most vasoconstrictors also raise PVR. Norepinephrine may be preferred to phenylephrine because the B_1 stimulation provides some inotropic support to the RV to help counter the increase in PVR. Low dose vasopressin ($<=0.04$ units/min) is the only vasoconstrictor that is thought to not increase PVR. This may be a first line choice for treating mild peripheral vasodilatation leading to hypotension. Decreased cardiac output in the setting of pulmonary hypertension is best treated with an inodilator such as dobutamine or milrinone. Both drugs have significant side effects, and skill and experience is needed for safe titration. Finally, inhaled nitric oxide is a locally acting vasodilator that may be very useful to treat acute exacerbations of pulmonary hypertension. It does not cause systemic vasodilatation.

Further Suggested Reading

Ali J, Summer W, Levitzky M. Pulmonary pathophysiology. 2nd ed. New York: Lange Medical Books/McGraw-Hill; 2005.

West J. Pulmonary pathophysiology: the essentials. 7th ed. Philadelphia: Lippincott Williams & Wilkins; 2008.

Seigne P, Hartigan P, Body S. Anesthetic considerations for patients with severe emphysematous lung disease. Int Anesthesiol Clin. 2000;38:1–23.

Chapter 4
Respiratory Effects of General Anesthesia

Philip M. Hartigan

Keywords Functional residual capacity • Respiratory mechanics • Airway resistance • Respiratory compliance • True shunt • VD/VT

Introduction

Respiratory function is impaired by general anesthesia on multiple fronts (Table 4-1). In addition to anesthesia per se, aspects related to general anesthesia (supine position, paralysis, mechanical ventilation) impact respiratory function and efficiency. While some effects are agent-specific, certain generalizations may be made, broadly categorized here as effects on FRC, respiratory mechanics, gas exchange, and control of breathing.

Functional Residual Capacity

Functional residual capacity (FRC) is the lung volume at end-expiration, determined by the apposing forces of the chest wall and the elastic recoil of the lungs. FRC declines significantly with induction of anesthesia compared to the awake, supine state. This impairs pulmonary mechanics and gas exchange, and may exacerbate mass effects within the chest (see Chapter 20). Collapse of small airways occurs if FRC falls below closing capacity. Table 4-2 summarizes generally accepted statements regarding FRC and anesthesia (1).

P.M. Hartigan (ed.), *Practical Handbook of Thoracic Anesthesia*,
DOI 10.1007/978-0-387-88493-6_4, © Springer Science+Business Media, LLC 2012

Table 4-1 – Adverse respiratory effects of anesthesia

- Impaired ventilatory response to hypercarbia and hypoxia
- Reduced tidal volume spontaneous ventilation
- Rapid and lingering reduction in FRC
- Dependent atelectasis
- Increased airflow resistance (minor)
- Decreased compliance
- Increased work of breathing
- Increased shunt
- Impaired V/Q matching
- Increased dead space
- Relaxation of pharyngeal muscles, predisposing to obstruction
- Potential inhibition of HPV (agent dependent)
- Altered surfactant function
- Vulnerability to anesthesia/surgery – associated adverse events; e.g.,
  - Apnea/airway obstruction
  - Bronchospasm/laryngospasm
  - Sputum retention/mucous plugging
  - Surgical disruption of ventilation or perfusion
  - Tension pneumothorax
  - Pulmonary embolus
  - Air trapping/auto-PEEP/dynamic hyperinflation
  - Barotrauma/volutrauma/ventilator associated lung injury
  - Pain-associated hypoventilation ("splinting")
  - Reflex diaphragm dysfunction related to surgery
  - Hemodynamic disruptions affecting V/Q matching, shunt, and dead space

Table 4-2 – FRC and anesthesia

- General anesthesia (supine) leads to a 16–20% decline in FRC (more in infants)
- Individual FRC reductions may be highly variable
- FRC reduction appears to be a nonspecific effect of anesthesia
  - Unrelated to the agents utilized (excepting ketamine which preserves FRC)
  - Unrelated to whether ventilation is spontaneous or controlled
  - Unrelated to the presence or absence of paralysis
- The decline in FRC occurs shortly after induction, plateaus, and persists for an ill defined period (hours-to-days) following emergence
- Anesthesia in the sitting position preserves FRC
- Postulated causes of anesthesia-related FRC reduction include
  - Decreased chest wall inspiratory muscle tone
  - Increased expiratory muscle tone
  - Cephalad shift in the diaphragm
  - Increased thoracic blood volume

Cause of the FRC Effect

Although recognized since the 1960s, the cause of the FRC reduction by anesthesia remains unclear. CT scan studies before and after induction reveal that the anterior–posterior chest dimensions decrease, the thoracic kyphosis increases, and the diaphragm's shape and position change (Fig 4-1). The simple explanation that the diaphragm becomes lax and shifts cephalad is inadequate. While the dorsal (dependent) diaphragm consistently shifts cephalad with anesthesia, the ventral portion shifts caudad in some subjects, neutralizing the net effect on thoracic volume by the diaphragm (2).

At rest (FRC), some muscle tone normally exists in inspiratory muscles to counter lung elastic recoil. The notion that the FRC effect of anesthesia is due to abolition of this basal inspiratory tone is not

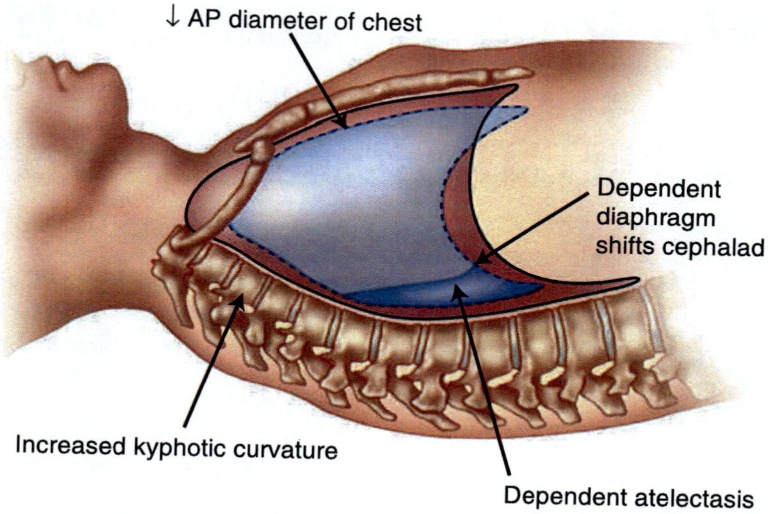

Figure 4-1 – Schematic lateral view of chest wall and diaphragm at functional residual capacity (FRC), supine, without (*red shaded*) and with (*blue shaded*) anesthesia. Anesthesia is associated with a decrease in FRC. The anterior–posterior diameter decreases, the spinal curvature increases, and the dorsal (dependent) diaphragm moves cephalad. The ventral diaphragm position is variable, but tends to move caudad. Dependent atelectasis (*dark shaded region*) is common.

cleanly supported by electromyographic (EMG) studies, though it is apparent that this may contribute (3).

Chest wall skeletal muscles functionally interconnect the spine, sternum, ribs, and diaphragm. This interconnectedness confounds attempts to attribute the FRC effect of anesthesia to a single change. Although increased thoracic blood volume may contribute to the FRC effect of anesthesia, it is likely a minor factor.

Respiratory Mechanics

Resistance

Airway *resistance* increases with anesthesia, as lower lung volumes reduce the caliber of airways. The supine position and general anesthesia combine to reduce lung volume and airway conductance (Fig 4-2). The bronchodilating effects of inhalational agents generally

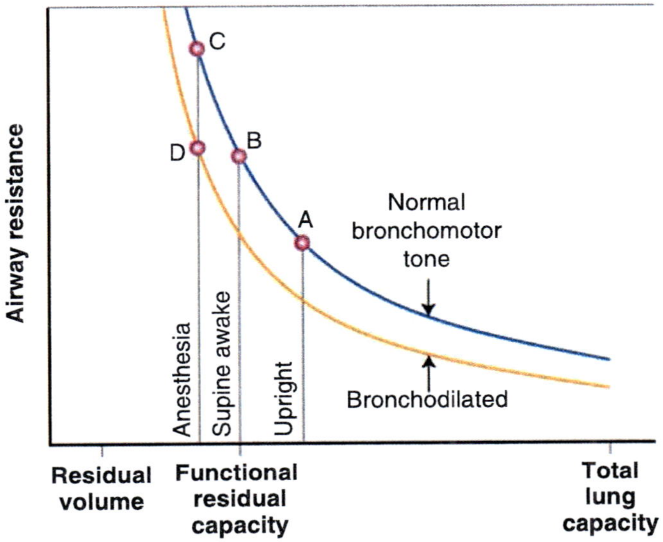

Figure 4-2 – Airway resistance as a function of lung volume with and without the degree of bronchodilation that typically occurs with anesthesia. A=Upright, awake. B=Supine, awake. C=Supine, anesthetized. D=Supine, anesthetized, with bronchodilation. Functional residual capacity (FRC) declines, and airway resistance increases with supine position, and further with anesthesia. Note that the FRC effect of anesthesia on airway resistance is negated by the bronchodilation effect of anesthesia (B vs. D). Reproduced with permission from Lumb AB. Nunn's Applied respiratory Physiology, 6th Edition, Elsevier Butterworth Heinmann, 2005.

offset the effects of anesthesia on resistance. Currently used inhalational anesthetics have comparable, dose-dependent bronchodilating effects. Mechanisms include suppression of vagal-mediated reflex bronchoconstriction, direct smooth muscle relaxation, and inhibition of bronchoconstrictor mediators. Intravenous anesthetics also counteract reflex bronchospasm by inhibition of vagal reflexes at sufficient depth. Airway resistance decreases with decreased flow rates and higher inflation lung volumes during anesthesia.

Anesthesia apparatus is another potential source of airflow resistance (small endotracheal tubes, valves, connectors, and breathing system). Airflow resistance from pharyngeal obstruction may also occur in the unintubated patient, as pharyngeal muscle relaxation from anesthesia predisposes to posterior displacement of the tongue, epiglottis, and soft palette. The anterior–posterior diameter of the pharynx decreases by over 50% at the level of the soft palette during anesthesia. In addition, the normal pharyngeal dilation by genioglossus muscles during inspiration is impaired or ablated by anesthesia. Supraglottic airway devices impose less resistance than tracheal tubes, and stent open pharyngeal tissue, but do not protect against laryngospasm.

Compliance

Respiratory *compliance* is reduced by anesthesia, primarily due to decreased compliance of the lung rather than the chest wall (4). Paralysis contributes insignificantly to this reduction in compliance. The cause of the compliance reduction is likely the reduction in lung volume. The work of breathing is increased during anesthesia with spontaneous ventilation, primarily due to decreased compliance rather than increased resistance, although mechanical ventilation obviates this issue.

Gas Exchange

The alveolar–arterial gradient for the partial pressure of oxygen (A-aPO_2 gradient) increases variably during anesthesia due to increased shunt, and increased perfusion of regions of poor ventilation (increased scatter of V/Q ratios) (Fig 4-3). Because the metabolic rate declines by 15% during anesthesia, and because higher fractions of inspired oxygen (FiO_2) are frequently utilized, hypoxemia during two-lung ventilation is rare. Dead space also increases during anesthesia, making CO_2 removal less efficient, but decreased CO_2 production and the capacity to adjust minute ventilation allow compensation.

Shunt

True shunt (regions of perfusion with zero ventilation) increases during anesthesia due to airways closure and dependent atelectasis as FRC falls below closing capacity. This effect is variable; more

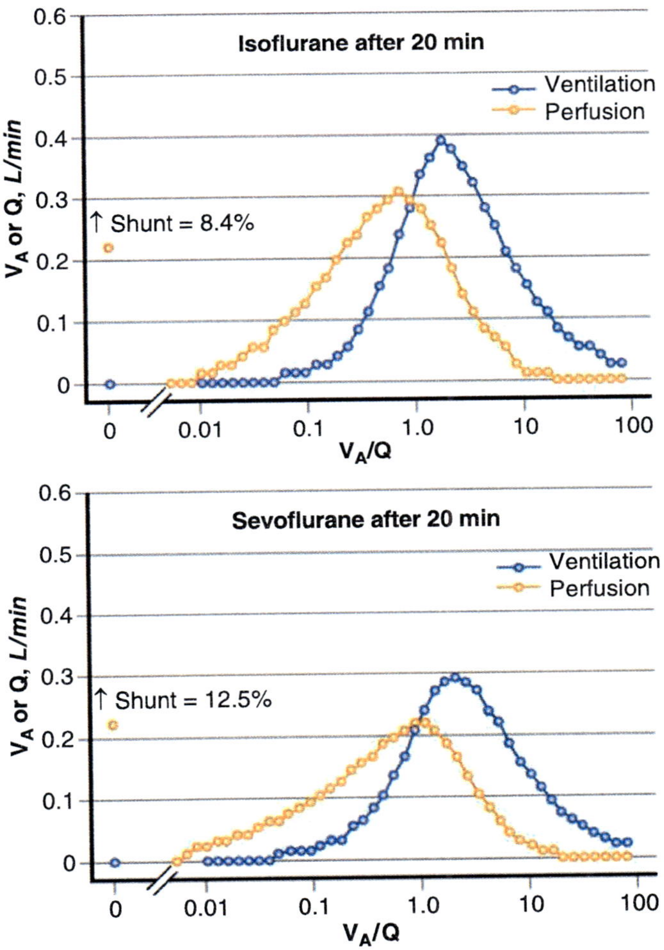

Figure 4-3 – Multiple inert gas elimination technique (MIGET) diagrams of the distribution of pulmonary ventilation and perfusion, as a function of V/Q ratios during anesthesia with 1 MAC of inhalational anesthetic. Contrast this with normal MIGET diagrams in awake healthy patients (Chapter 2, Fig 2.8). Anesthesia is associated with more shunt, more perfusion of regions of low V/Q, and greater dispersion between the distributions of ventilation and perfusion. Modified with permission from Loeckinger A, Keller C, Lindner K, Kleinsasser A. Pulmonary gas exchange in coronary artery surgery patients during sevoflurane and isoflurane anesthesia. Anesth Analg 2002; 94:1107–12.

prominent in elderly and obese patients, and less prevalent in patients with COPD. In lung-healthy patients, the A-a PO_2 difference corresponds to an average shunt of 10% during anesthesia, compared to <2% awake. Approximately half of this venous admixture is attributable to true shunt (1). This correlates closely to the amount of dependent atelectasis by CT scan (5). Atelectasis during anesthesia may also result from absorption of high inspired oxygen concentrations (absorption atelectasis), or by compression (e.g., by mass, retractor, packing, surgical manipulation, etc.). Increasing FiO_2 is ineffective in overcoming hypoxia from true shunt, or in the presence a large total shunt (Fig 4-4). Recruitment maneuvers and PEEP are more effective, but must be balanced against the potential for lung injury or adverse hemodynamic effects.

Ventilation: Perfusion Matching

True shunt is not the sole cause of an increased A-a PO_2 gradient during anesthesia. Some of the venous admixture observed during anesthesia is attributable to dispersion of the V/Q distribution, and

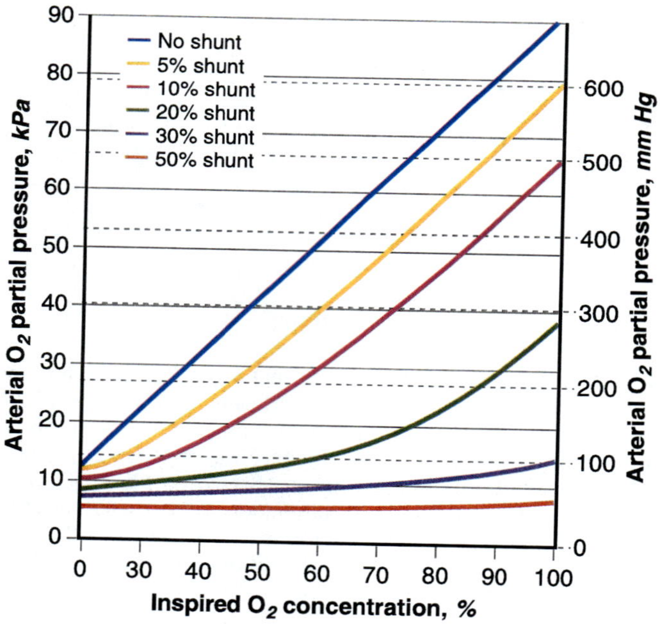

Figure 4-4 – Effect of shunt on arterial oxygenation. Note that in the presence of a large shunt, increasing inspired oxygen concentration has little effect on arterial oxygenation. Modified with permission from Benetar SR, Hewlett AM, Nunn JF. The use of isoshunt lines for control of oxygen therapy. Br J Anaesth 1973;45:711.

to perfusion of areas of low ventilation–perfusion ratios (0.005–0.1). The relative contribution of true shunt vs. broadened V/Q distribution is variable between patients (6) (Fig 4-5). While COPD protects against atelectasis (auto-PEEP), it is associated with greater perfusion to regions of low V/Q ratio (7).

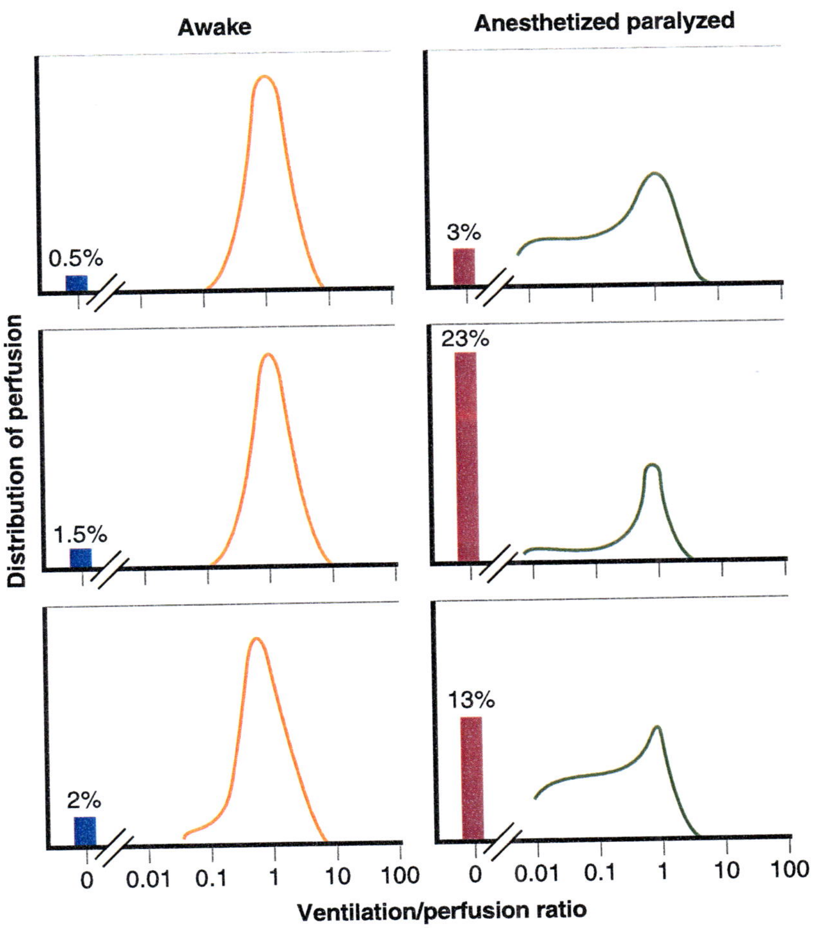

Figure 4-5 – The distribution of pulmonary perfusion as a function of different V/Q ratios by the MIGET before and after anesthesia in three different subjects. Note the variability. In response to anesthesia; subject "A" displays increased perfusion of regions of low V/Q, with little increase in shunt. Subject "B" principally increases shunt, and subject "C" displays a combination of the two. Reproduced with permission from Nunn JF. Oxygen – friend or foe. J Roy Soc Med 1985; 78:618–22.

Dead Space

Dead space relative to tidal volume (VD/VT) increases during anesthesia, reducing the efficiency of CO_2 elimination. Physiologic dead space (sum of anatomical plus alveolar dead space) increases during anesthesia principally due to increased alveolar dead space. The cause of anesthesia-related increased alveolar dead space is uncertain, but thought to be due to increased distribution of ventilation to regions of relatively poor perfusion. If systemic and pulmonary hypotension accompanies anesthesia, this may increase West Zone 1, further increasing dead space.

Anesthesia apparatus also increases VD/VT by two mechanisms. First, all anesthesia breathing circuits (excluding Mapleson E [Ayre's T-Piece]) cause rebreathing of expired gas, which is equivalent to dead space ventilation. Second, the apparatus capacity itself imposes additional dead space. While endotracheal tubes reduce dead space within the airway, the added external dead space (between Y-connector and mouth) results in a net increase in VD/VT from roughly 33 to 45%. Patients breathing through a mask have even greater VD/VT (62%), while those with an LMA are similar to intubated patients.

The manner of ventilation during anesthesia will also affect VD/VT. Mechanical ventilation with increased airway pressures (PEEP) increases alveolar dead space. Breathing patterns with rapid, short inspirations favor dead space ventilation because they fail to distribute to long time constant, compliant, better perfused alveoli. Anesthesia with spontaneous ventilation frequently results in hypercapnea due to the effects of anesthetics on the drive to breathe, rather than due to greater VD/VT relative to mechanical ventilation at similar breathing patterns.

Control of Breathing

General anesthesia depresses central and peripheral chemoreceptors which control the drive to breathe. The net effect is dose-dependent: light levels cause rapid, shallow, irregular breathing with relative preservation of minute ventilation, while deeper levels depress both RR and minute ventilation. Surgical stimulation may partially counteract this. Despite reduced CO_2 production, arterial CO_2 tends to be elevated during spontaneously breathing general anesthetics.

The PCO_2 ventilation–response curve is progressively flattened and right-shifted by increasing doses of inhalational anesthetics (Fig 4-6), as well as most intravenous agents. Inhalation agents also increase the apneic threshold to CO_2. Although not free of controversy, it is commonly stated that the ventilatory response to hypoxia is inhibited by even subanesthetic concentrations (0.1 MAC) of currently used inhalational agents (8) as well as subhypnotic levels of propofol (9). Since such concentrations extend into the recovery room, this has obvious management implications.

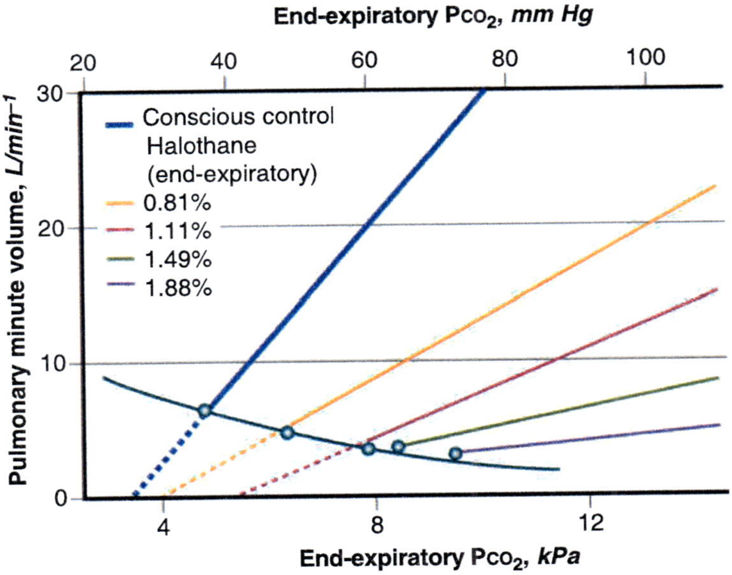

Figure 4-6 – The effect of halothane on the ventilatory response to CO_2. Increasing concentrations of halothane right-shifts, and flattens out the CO_2 – ventilatory response curve, and increases the PCO_2 threshold for apnea (extrapolated intersection with abscissa). The *blue curve* represents end-expired PCO_2/Minute Ventilation without addition of exogenous CO_2. Reproduced with permission from Lumb AB. Nunn's Applied Respiratory Physiology, 6th Edition. Elsevier, Butterworth, Heinmann, 2005.

Selected References

1. Lumb AB. Anaesthesia. In: Lumb AB, editor. Nunn's applied respiratory physiology. 6th ed. Philadelphia: Elsevier, Butterworth-Heinemann; 2005. p. 297–326.

2. Warner DO. Diaphragm function during anesthesia: still crazy after all these years. Anesthesiology. 2002;97:295–7.

3. Warner DO, Warner MA, Ritman EL. Human chest wall function while awake and during halothane anesthesia. 1. Quiet breathing. Anesthesiology. 1995;82:6–10.

4. Westbrook PR, Stubbs SE, Sessler AD, et al. Effects of anesthesia and muscle paralysis on respiratory mechanics in normal man. J Appl Physiol. 1973;34:81–6.

5. Warner DO, Warner MA, Ritman EL. Atelectasis and chest wall shape during halothane anesthesia. Anesthesiology. 1996;85:49–59.

6. Dueck R, Young I, Clausen J, Wagner PD. Altered distribution of pulmonary ventilation and blood flow following induction of inhalational anesthesia. Anesthesiology. 1980;52:113–25.

7. Hedenstierna G. Gas exchange during anesthesia. Acta Anaesthesiol Scand. 1990;94:27–31.

8. Dahan A, Sarton E, van den Elsen M, et al. Ventilatory response to hypoxia in humans: influence of subanesthetic dsesflurane. Anesthesiology. 1996;85:60–8.

9. Nagyova B, Dorrington KL, Gill EW, Robbins PA. Comparison of the effects of sub-hypnotic concentrations of propofol and halothane on the acute ventilatory response to hypoxia. Br J Anaesth. 1995;75:713–18.

Chapter 5
Physiology of One-Lung Ventilation

Philip M. Hartigan

Keywords One-lung ventilation • Hypoxic pulmonary vasoconstriction • Multiple inert gas elimination technique • Perfusion • Ventilation • Hypoxemia • Continuous positive airway pressure • Positive end-expiratory pressure • High-frequency jet ventilation • Air insufflation

Introduction

Published estimates of the incidence of hypoxemia during one-lung ventilation (OLV) have decreased from 25% in the 1970s to currently less than 10% (1, 2). Technical improvements (fiberoptic bronchoscopy, DLT design, etc.) account for some of this progress (Chapter 8). Improved understanding of the physiology of OLV has also contributed importantly and is the topic of this chapter.

Operational Definition of OLV

For the purposes of this discussion, the term one-lung ventilation (OLV) refers to all of the following, unless otherwise specified:

- Single (dependent) lung ventilation.
- Lateral decubitus position.
- Open chest (nondependent).
- General anesthesia, with paralysis and positive pressure, controlled ventilation.

P.M. Hartigan (ed.), *Practical Handbook of Thoracic Anesthesia*,
DOI 10.1007/978-0-387-88493-6_5, © Springer Science+Business Media, LLC 2012

Collectively, these conditions severely disrupt gas exchange. A practical approach to the pathophysiology of OLV is presented here as a foundation to clinical management decisions. Beyond CPAP and PEEP, other variables are considered with respect to their impact on oxygenation during OLV. Consideration of such variables provides insights into the complexity of OLV physiology.

Note that this chapter focuses primarily on optimization of gas exchange during OLV. Ultimately, ventilatory strategies must balance optimal gas exchange against risk of lung injury (Chapter 6).

Pathophysiology of OLV

At its essence, efficient gas exchange in the OR largely depends on (is most frequently limited by) the spatial approximation of pulmonary perfusion and ventilation. Such "*V/Q* matching" in the upright healthy spontaneously breathing subject is achieved to a remarkable degree by multiple factors (Chapter 2), including but not limited to the following:

- Gravity.
- Hypoxic pulmonary vasoconstriction (HPV).
- Anatomical congruence of the pulmonary arterial and airway arborizations.

The OLV situation disrupts this efficiency. At FiO_2 of 1.0, the PaO_2 during OLV typically decreases from over 400 mmHg to an average range of 100–200 mmHg. Individual responses can be highly variable.

Figure 5-1 provides a simplified visual way to think of OLV and illustrates the central point emphasized in Box 5-1.

The multiple inert gas elimination technique (MIGET) provides a visual of the distribution of pulmonary ventilation and perfusion with respect to regions of the lung functionally divided into areas of different *V/Q* ratios (see Chapter 2). Figure 5-2 depicts MIGET diagrams of a patient under anesthesia during lateral OLV, compared to lateral two-lung ventilation. Markedly increased are the magnitudes

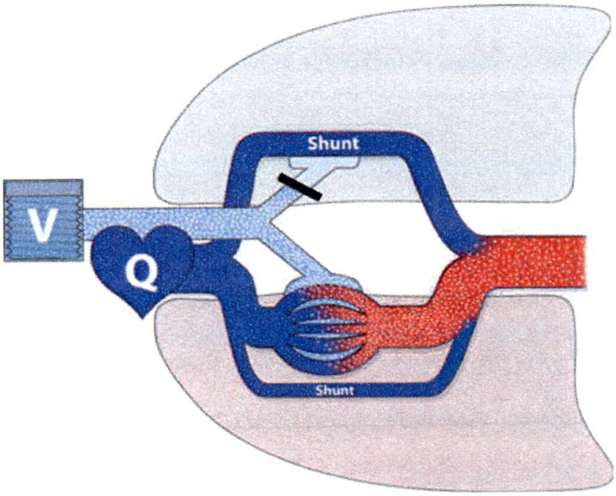

Figure 5-1 – Schematic depiction of the one-lung ventilation (OLV) situation, to emphasize the three physiologic causes of hypoxemia during OLV: (1) shunt in the nondependent lung, (2) shunt in the dependent lung, and (3) imperfect *V*/*Q* matching in the dependent lung. *V* ventilation, *Q* perfusion. Illustration by Marcia Williams.

Box 5-1 – Physiologic Causes* of Hypoxemia During OLV Include

- Shunt in the nondependent lung.
- Shunt in the dependent lung.
- *V*/*Q* mismatch in the dependent lung.

*Excludes technical issues such as malpositioned DLT, secretions, inappropriate ventilator settings, etc.

of shunt and dead space, and the proportion of perfusion directed to regions of low ventilation–perfusion ratio. Note that intrapulmonary shunt here is the sum of dependent and nondependent lung shunt. The elevated perfusion of areas of low *V*/*Q* emphasizes that the region of dependent lung gas exchange in Fig 5-1 represents a spectrum of different, and frequently suboptimal, zones of *V*/*Q* matching (Figs 5-1 and 5-3).

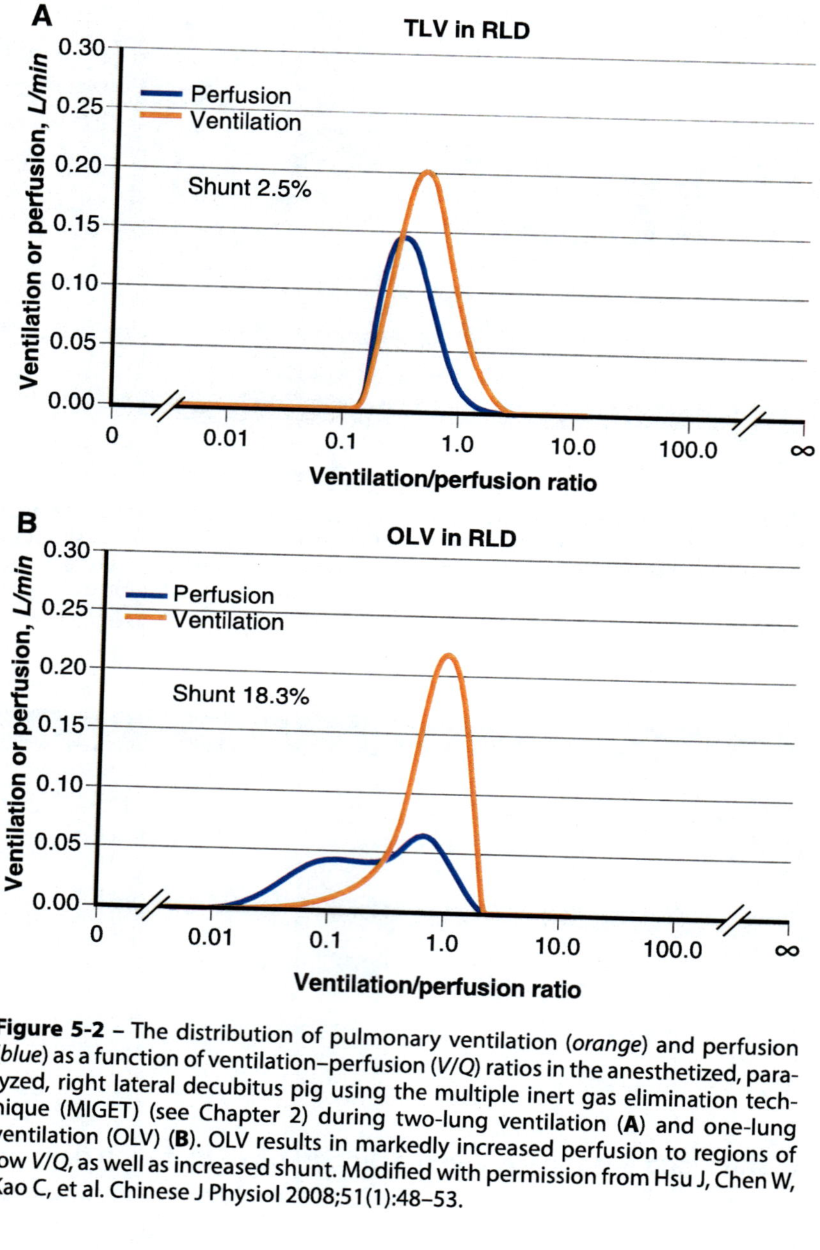

Figure 5-2 – The distribution of pulmonary ventilation (*orange*) and perfusion (*blue*) as a function of ventilation–perfusion (*V/Q*) ratios in the anesthetized, paralyzed, right lateral decubitus pig using the multiple inert gas elimination technique (MIGET) (see Chapter 2) during two-lung ventilation (**A**) and one-lung ventilation (OLV) (**B**). OLV results in markedly increased perfusion to regions of low *V/Q*, as well as increased shunt. Modified with permission from Hsu J, Chen W, Kao C, et al. Chinese J Physiol 2008;51(1):48–53.

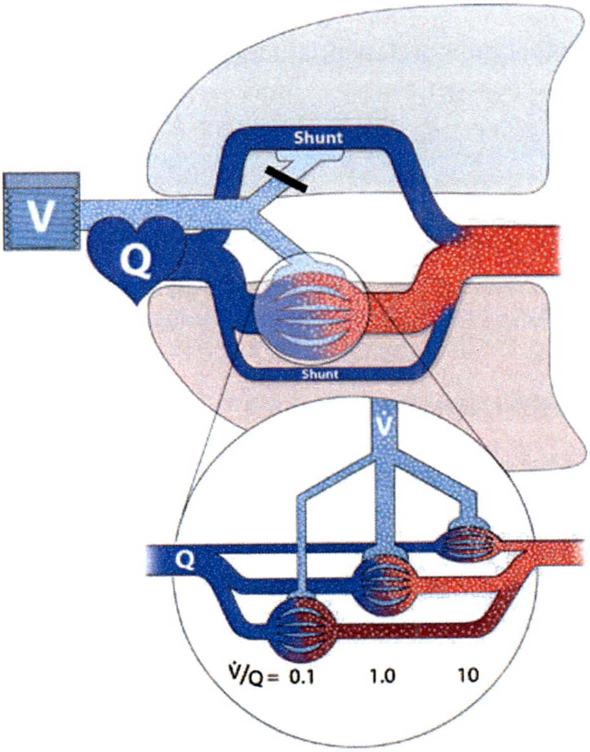

Figure 5-3 – Schematic of the OLV situation emphasizing that the *V/Q* matching in the dependent lung takes place within a range of different functional units of different *V/Q* ratios. Illustration by Marcia Williams.

Physiology of the Nondependent-Lung

Perfusion

All blood flow to the nondependent, unventilated lung is true shunt. This wasted perfusion of the nondependent lung is typically reduced from approximately 50% of cardiac output (CO) to roughly 25%. Individual variability can be substantial. Hypoxic pulmonary vasoconstriction (HPV), and Gravity account for most of this reduction. Preexisting disease-related alterations of perfusion also impact. Surgical manipulation may either enhance (via prostaglandin release), or reduce blood flow (by kinking, clamping, and compressing vessels), to the nondependent lung. Pharmacologic agents inhibiting HPV may effect the nondependent lung shunt fraction, but the net effect on oxygenation is more complex (see below).

Ventilation

By definition, there is no ventilation of the nondependent lung during OLV. The existing air in that lung gradually exits by egress through the DLT/BB, and by absorption atelectasis.

Physiology of the Dependent-Lung

Perfusion

During OLV, the dependent lung is hyperperfused with approximately 75% of CO, due to the effects of gravity and HPV on the nondependent lung as described above. The distribution of perfusion within the dependent lung during OLV is not well defined. There is recruitment of pulmonary vascular beds with less precise linkage to ventilation. MIGET studies reveal increased perfusion of regions of low *V/Q* ratio, as well as true shunt (Fig 5-2). Barring significant preexisting pathophysiology, pulmonary arterial pressures do not generally increase during OLV.

Ventilation

The FRC (volume at end-expiration) of the dependent lung is reduced in the LDP during OLV. Circumferential restrictive forces are exerted from the cephalad shift of the dependent hemidiaphragm, the weight of the mediastinum, the anterior/posterior stabilizers, and the table underneath. Ventilation is accordingly maldistributed, with a predilection for dependent atelectasis and nondependent hyperaeration of the ventilated lung (3). A high FiO_2 likely contributes to (absorption) atelectasis in the dependent lung (4). These forces contribute to dependent lung *V/Q* mismatch and frequently increase dependent lung shunt in atelectatic regions. PEEP (intrinsic or extrinsic), recruitment maneuvers, lung disease, and the pattern of ventilation may modify this.

Clinical Application: Optimizing Gas Exchange During OLV

Overview

Predictors, treatment algorithms, and specific effects of selected variables on hypoxemia during OLV are considered here. Specific ventilator management decisions must integrate gas exchange considerations with competing concerns regarding lung injury, discussed in the following chapter.

Predicters of Hypoxemia During OLV

The list of factors associated with desaturation during OLV is of limited clinical utility because so few are modifiable (Table 5-1). If available, split-lung perfusion data is often the most predictive. The probability and degree of OLV desaturation is correlated to the amount of blood flow to the operative lung (5). Intuitively, one would expect this to predict the amount of nondependent lung shunt.

Table 5-1 – Factors associated with desaturation during OLV

- High preoperative perfusion of the operative lung
- Low preoperative PaO_2
- Right-sided surgery
- Restrictive, or normal spirometry pattern
- Supine position
- Significant pathology of the dependent (nonoperative) lung:
  - Pneumonia
  - Bronchospasm
  - Pleural effusion
  - Pneumothorax
  - Interstitial pulmonary edema, etc.

Less intuitively, the presence of obstructive lung disease tends to protect against desaturation, possibly due to intrinsic (auto) PEEP in the dependent lung, and/or slow collapse of the operative lung, in contrast to patients with normal elastic recoil or restrictive physiology (6).

Treatment of Hypoxemia During OLV

The traditional prioritized list of maneuvers to improve one-lung oxygenation (Table 5-2) combines technical with physiologic maneuvers. Certainly, technical issues are the most common causes and should be addressed first, time permitting. This discussion will presume that the technical issues have been addressed (i.e., the DLT is perfectly positioned, secretions have been removed, and 100% oxygen is being effectively delivered to the dependent lung with each tidal volume).

The Clinical Scenario Should Dictate Which Maneuver(s) Should Be Employed, and in What Order

Reinflation

When desaturation is abrupt, severe, or the patient is intolerant (EKG changes, etc.), reinflation of the operative lung will most rapidly

Table 5-2 – Treatment of hypoxemia during OLV

- Confirm $FiO_2 = 1.0$
- Bronchoscopy to rule out malposition, obstruction, secretions, etc.
- Reinflation of nondependent lung
- CPAP to nondependent lung
- Recruitment maneuver/PEEP to dependent lung
- Combined CPAP/PEEP
- PA cross-clamp
- Insufflation or jet ventilation to the nondependent lung

and reliably restore saturation. Communication and coordination with the surgeon is obviously imperative. Technical issues (misplaced DLT, secretions, etc.) are the most likely cause of rapid desaturation and are best addressed by bronchoscopy *after* the patient is stabilized. *Recruitment maneuvers* require an extended (3–5 s) positive pressure hold at 25–35 cmH_2O to expand slow time constant lung units. Attention to hemodynamics during recruitment is essential. Visual inspection of the lung acts as a guide to the required pressure and time course for recruitment.

CPAP to the Nondependent Lung

Continuous positive airway pressure (CPAP) may be delivered to the operative lung by a variety of mechanisms (Chapter 10) to effectively deliver oxygen to the nondependent lung, and thus reduce nondependent lung shunt. Between 3 and 10 cmH_2O are generally effective after partial recruitment of the operative lung. Without prerecruitment, CPAP is less effective. Importantly, the use of CPAP maintains a degree of inflation of the operative lung, and may not be suitable during minimally invasive surgery. Formerly considered a first-line maneuver, CPAP is now uncommonly performed because of the prevalence of minimally invasive surgical approaches.

PEEP to the Dependent Lung

Positive end-expiratory pressure (PEEP) delivered to the dependent lung may reduce the alveolar collapse (shunt) in that lung. Dependent lung PEEP has a point of diminishing returns. Excessive PEEP increases airway pressures, thereby exerting pressure on the transalveolar vessels traversing those alveoli, and redirecting blood flow to the nondependent lung (increasing nondependent lung shunt). The "optimal PEEP" for any given patient is determined by the compliance characteristics of their respiratory system during OLV (Fig 5-4) (7). In general, patients are likely to benefit from a degree of PEEP (5–15 cmH_2O) if they have restrictive lung disease, obesity, or mechanical reasons to suspect atelectasis in the dependent lung. Patients with young healthy lungs (normal elastic recoil) generally

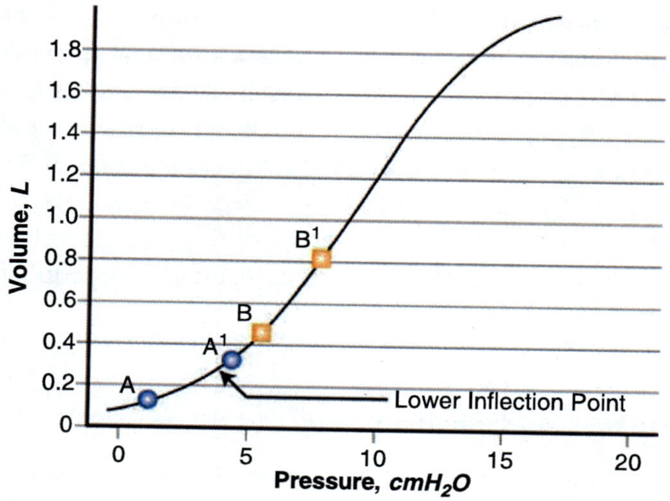

Figure 5-4 – Hypothetical static compliance curve during OLV. *LIP* lower inflection point. A = end-expiratory pressure for patient "A". B = end-expiratory pressure for patient "B". Increasing PEEP in patient A shifts the end-expiratory position toward a more favorable position on the compliance curve (A^1), and reduces dependent lung atelectasis. Increasing PEEP to patient B shifts to position B^1, simply increasing airway pressures within a relatively fully recruited dependent lung. Adapted from data of Slinger et al. Relation of the static compliance curve and positive end-expiratory pressure to oxygenation during one-lung anesthesia. Anesthesiology 2001; 95(5):1098–2006.

benefit. By contrast, patients with significant obstructive physiology tend to have unavoidable auto-PEEP in excess of optimal PEEP, and would be unlikely to improve oxygenation with extrinsic PEEP. A dependent lung recruitment maneuver prior to instituting PEEP may allow use of lower levels of PEEP.

Combined CPAP–PEEP

When CPAP is employed to the nondependent lung and oxygenation remains unsatisfactory, the addition of PEEP to the dependent lung may be more effective than PEEP alone. This is because blood redirected to the nondependent lung by PEEP will be more likely to pick up oxygen due to CPAP.

PA Cross-Clamp

Surgical cross-clamp of all or part of the pulmonary artery effectively reduces or eliminates nondependent lung shunt, and reliably improves oxygenation. When this is surgically imminent, it may be appropriate to transiently tolerate marginal oxygenation rather than disrupt surgery with reinflation during critical hilar dissection.

High-Frequency Jet Ventilation to the Nondependent Lung

High-frequency jet ventilation to the nondependent lung (HFJV) resembles CPAP in that it delivers oxygen to the otherwise unventilated lung. The low tidal volumes and high frequency result in a relatively immobile surgical field. As with CPAP, HFJV results in improved oxygenation and partial reinflation (8). Concerns of barotrauma, as well as expense and lack of familiarity of the equipment, have prevented its widespread use.

Air Insufflation

Insufflation of 100% oxygen via a catheter in the DLT lumen to the nondependent lung has been widely trialed informally. Clinical experience suggests that it is only effective in improving oxygenation when performed in such a manner, and with sufficient flows to effectively induce CPAP. It is, therefore, not currently recommended over CPAP.

Other Variables: Effects on Oxygenation During OLV

Ventilator Settings

FiO_2

A high initial FiO_2 provides a margin of safety. The improvement of PaO_2 from a high FiO_2 outweighs the negative of absorption atelectasis (4). Collapse of the operative lung is faster when a high

FiO_2 is used prior to lung isolation (9). Thereafter, FiO_2 may be titrated down as tolerated for a $SpO_2 \geq 90\%$. Drugs such as Bleomycin, Mitomycin, and Amiodarone have been associated with oxygen toxicity and should prompt the lowest tolerated FiO_2.

When recruiting the operative lung following a period of collapse, oxygen radical mediated ischemia reperfusion injury may theoretically be ameliorated by use of a lower FiO_2. This is probably most important during lung transplantation.

Tidal Volume

Selection of tidal volume reflects a trade-off between optimizing dependent lung recruitment, oxygen delivery and CO_2 elimination versus lung injury (see Chapter 6). In this trade-off, adequate oxygenation trumps, and may require more aggressive tidal volumes if hypoxemia cannot be reversed by other maneuvers (CPAP, PEEP, bronchoscopy, etc.). Generally, lung-protective OLV (TV=6 ml/kg) results in satisfactory oxygen saturation. With severe obstructive disease, CO_2 elimination must be balanced against perceived risk of lung injury. In this setting, "permissive hypercapnea" is often preferable for the limited duration of OLV rather than risking lung injury with more aggressive ventilation. Individual exceptions may apply (e.g., pulmonary hypertension).

Respiratory Rate and I:E Ratio

Respiratory rate (RR) and *I:E* ratio interact to effect inspiratory and expiratory durations. Longer expiratory times and higher minute ventilation help eliminate CO_2 in the presence of low (protective) tidal volumes, up to a point. Dead space ventilation increases at high respiratory rates, impairing CO_2 elimination. High respiratory rates and long expiratory times also shorten the inspiratory phase, and may result in failure to recruit lung units of long time constants. Patients with obstructive lung disease are prone to air trapping (auto PEEP) during OLV, (10) an effect which is exacerbated by the short expiratory phase of high respiratory rates.

PEEP

Optimal PEEP for purposes of oxygenation during OLV seeks a compromise between maintaining patency of atelectasis-prone dependent lung alveoli, and redirection of perfusion to the nondependent lung due to elevated airway pressures (see "Treatment of Hypoxemia During OLV" above).

Some degree of PEEP (≤5 cmH_2O) is generally recommended during OLV. Low TV (protective) ventilatory strategies predispose to atelectasis in the dependent lung. PEEP helps maintain alveolar recruitment, thus potentially improving oxygenation and compliance, and reducing atelectrauma. Excessive PEEP increases shunt due to increased dependent lung airway pressures. Patients with obstructive lung disease have unavoidable auto-PEEP during OLV, (10) but the addition of low levels of extrinsic PEEP in such patients (<70% of auto PEEP) does not increase airway pressures or total PEEP (11).

Ventilator Mode

Volume controlled ventilation (VC) delivers a set tidal volume at a constant flow rate. Pressure-controlled ventilation (PC) delivers a high initial flow up to a preset peak ceiling pressure, followed by a rapidly decelerating flow rate, maintaining the preset peak pressure throughout inspiration. The tidal volume delivered by PC depends on the resistance and compliance of the respiratory system. It is unclear whether one or the other is advantageous during OLV.

One study found that PC ventilation provided improved oxygenation during OLV compared to VC ventilation (12). This was attributed to more homogeneous distribution of ventilation, and was more beneficial to those with restrictive physiology. In a more recent study, in patients with normal lung function, PC offered no oxygenation advantage over VC during OLV (13).

Whether ventilation mode affects the risk of lung injury is controversial. It is difficult to make an "apples-to-apples" comparison between PC and VC. During scenarios of changing lung compliance, if PC is employed, one must be attentive to avoid overdistention of the lung. Although peak airway pressure (PIP) is lower with PC, PIP correlates poorly with lung injury. Plateau airway pressures (P_{PL}), which are more likely to predict lung injury, were not different in the most recent comparison (13). Although animal data exists to suggest that the high flow rates of PC ventilation may potentially be injurious, there is no consensus in human studies.

At this writing, evidence is insufficient to recommend one over the other from the standpoint of gas exchange or lung injury. Attention to tidal volumes and air trapping is the best defense against volutrauma in either mode.

Recruitment Maneuvers

Recruitment maneuver (RM) is a vaguely defined inspiratory hold at an elevated positive pressure. A RM is most commonly delivered manually with 25–35 cmH_2O positive pressure for >5 s. Longer durations, or repeated maneuvers, are needed to reinflate a collapsed operative lung. When employed to the dependent lung during OLV, recruitment maneuvers reinflate atelectatic alveoli and may improve oxygenation, compliance, and dead space (14, 15). PEEP following a RM is necessary to sustain the benefits. The increased airway pressure of a RM impairs cardiac output, and attention to hemodynamics is imperative. Multiple brief maneuvers are safer than a prolonged RM. The risk of lung injury by RM is undefined. In theory, sustained recruitment by a RM followed by PEEP reduces atelectrauma. Intermittent gentle recruitment maneuvers are widely employed and recommended, particularly when low tidal volumes are employed, or when the patient is particularly prone to atelectasis (restrictive physiology).

Permissive Hypercapnea

The term permissive hypercapnea implies deliberate hypoventilation, when in fact some patients (especially those with severe obstructive disease) may be impossible to ventilate to normocapnea with one lung because of parenchymal destruction, and long time constants for exhalation. Relative contraindications to permissive hypercapnea include pulmonary hypertension, right ventricular dysfunction, fragile coronary artery disease, and increased intracranial pressure. The limits of permissive hypercapnea are not well defined. Excessive CO_2 burden acquired in the one-lung phase may take time to correct, and the acidosis may result in cognitive and diaphragmatic dysfunction, delaying emergence and extubation. Generally, however, permissive hypercapnea with lung-protective tidal volumes is well tolerated for the limited duration of OLV.

Position (Gravity Effect)

Gravity helps redirect pulmonary perfusion from the nondependent lung to the dependent lung during OLV. This effect may be counteracted by other factors, such as high airway pressures in the dependent lung. However, other things being equal, oxygenation is improved by gravity when patients are lateral decubitus. OLV in the supine position results in lower oxygenation than OLV in the lateral position, with the deflated lung on top (16).

Hypoxic Pulmonary Vasoconstriction

Recall that HPV is an exquisitely local phenomenon peculiar to small pulmonary arteries which serves to fine tune *V*/*Q* matching (Chapter 2). The primary trigger is low alveolar oxygen tension (P_AO_2); the secondary trigger is low mixed venous oxygen tension (P_VO_2). HPV is inhibited by most vasodilators (including inhalational anesthetics), beta adrenergic agonists, alpha adrenergic and calcium channel blockers, alkalosis, hypocapnea, and prostaglandin E_1. In addition to low P_AO_2 and P_VO_2, HPV is enhanced by most vasoconstrictors, acidosis, hypercapnea, and almitrine.

During OLV, HPV reduces the shunt perfusion of the nondependent lung by roughly 40% (4). It is also essential to *V*/*Q* matching in the dependent lung. HPV is often focused on as the most important variable effecting one-lung oxygenation, but in practice, it is difficult to assess or manipulate in isolation. Direct effects on HPV may be counteracted by indirect, secondary effects; the net effect on one-lung oxygenation is usually difficult to predict.

Vasoconstrictors

Vasoconstricting drugs directly enhance HPV. However, if they also result in elevated cardiac output, and redistribution of more pulmonary perfusion to the nondependent lung, the elevated flow and intraluminal pressure within nondependent pulmonary arteries may counteract HPV there. Oxygenation will depend on the net effect on the distribution of pulmonary perfusion within and between each lung, and may be complicated by effects on cardiac output and mixed venous oxygen saturation. Almitrine, which has a relatively specific constrictor effect on pulmonary vessels, has been shown to improve oxygenation during OLV.

Mixed Venous Oxygen Tension

The effect of *mixed venous oxygen tension* (P_VO_2) is complex. HPV is said to be maximal at normal P_VO_2. High P_VO_2 delivers more oxygen to the nondependent lung potentially inhibiting HPV there. Low P_VO_2 enhances HPV in the dependent lung resulting in competing vasoconstriction in that lung (4). The greater the total shunt, the greater the negative impact of a low P_VO_2 on arterial oxygenation (17).

Acid–Base Status

While *alkalosis* inhibits, and *acidosis* enhances HPV directly, the net clinical effect depends on the magnitude of other variables. Often alkalosis results from hyperventilation, and acidosis from relative hypoventilation. Such changes in the pattern of ventilation alter airway pressures, and may redirect perfusion within and between lungs during OLV. Moderate respiratory alkalosis and moderate permissive hypercapnea generally have little net impact on oxygenation during OLV.

Other Variables Affecting HPV

Diseased lung may have an impaired HPV response, possibly due to a fixed reduction in pulmonary vascular cross sectional area. Patients with COPD during OLV exhibit a lower increase in shunt when administered nitrodilators, compared to patients with normal lungs (18). The HPV response also depends on the baseline tone of the vessels. When >70% of the pulmonary vascular tree is hypoxic, the HPV response is impaired because there is no place to redirect the blood.

The notion that manipulation of HPV is the solution to hypoxemia during OLV is a widespread misconception. Nonetheless, one-lung oxygenation will likely improve if major, obvious offenders of HPV (e.g., high-dose intravenous nitroglycerine infusion) are avoided.

Bronchodilators

With sufficient anesthetic depth, bronchospasm is an unusual cause of hypoxemia during OLV, particularly when inhalational anesthetics are employed. When bronchospasm does occur, it disrupts *V/Q* matching and oxygen delivery in the dependent lung, and may lead to air trapping, elevated airway pressures, and redirection of blood to the nondependent lung (increasing shunt). Although bronchodilating agents are often inhibitors of HPV, their salutary effects outweigh their negatives in the presence of bronchospasm.

Inhaled Nitric Oxide

Delivery of inhaled nitric oxide (NO) to the dependent lung might be expected to selectively vasodilate that lung in favor of reduced shunt perfusion in the nondependent lung. Multiple studies of inhaled NO during OLV have failed to demonstrate an oxygenation benefit (19). Recently, Sticher et al. (20) found a moderate increase in PaO_2 during OLV in the instrumented porcine model. The advantage was seen at a dose of 4 ppm, but not at the higher doses as used in prior studies. Others have demonstrated an oxygenation improvement when NO was coadministered with the selective pulmonary vasoconstrictor, almitrine (21) which exceeded that produced by almitrine alone. Presumably the almitrine enhanced HPV in the nondependent lung while NO increased capacity in the dependent lung. These findings reinforce our understanding of the physiology, but the expense of NO and unavailability of almitrine in the USA makes this an impractical option.

Choice of Anesthetic

Because inhalational anesthetic agents inhibit HPV, some practitioners attempt to limit the dose, or avoid such agents altogether (TIVA), to optimize oxygenation during OLV. The numerous studies on this topic (22–27) may be summarized as follows:

- All inhalational anesthetics inhibit HPV in a dose-dependent fashion in vitro.
- There is no difference in oxygenation during OLV when the dose of an inhalational agent is increased from 0.5 to 1.5 MAC.
- There are no differences between current agents (isoflurane, sevoflurane, and desflurane) on oxygenation during OLV in vivo within clinically relevant dosage ranges.
- TIVA agents (propofol and narcotics) do not inhibit HPV in vitro.
- There is no conclusive evidence that TIVA is superior to inhalation agent-based anesthetics in terms of oxygenation during OLV in vivo. At the time of writing this chapter, there are conflicting studies and opinions on this question.
- It is apparent that despite undeniable evidence that inhalational agents inhibit HPV in vitro, the secondary effects on CO, and P_VO_2 counteract those effects on oxygenation during OLV.
- *Conclusion*: Altering anesthetic agent selection or dose (within clinically relevant range) is unlikely to improve oxygenation during OLV.

Use of Thoracic Epidural

Use of a thoracic epidural during OLV has no direct effect on HPV, and generally should not impact oxygenation during OLV. The HPV response is independent of the somatic and autonomic nervous system. In extreme circumstances, sympathetic blockade may effect one-lung oxygenation through effects on cardiac output and P_VO_2.

Hemoglobin Concentration

Acute isovolemic hemodilution with removal of 500 ml of blood during OLV had no adverse effect on oxygenation in normal patients, whereas those with COPD suffered significant reductions in PaO_2 (28).

Manipulation of Cardiac Output

Boosting cardiac output (CO) with inotropes or vasopressors may occasionally result in improved oxygenation during OLV. This is most likely to occur in patients who have very low CO. The complex interactions between the agents' direct and indirect effects, as well as secondary effects on P_VO_2, oxygen extraction, HPV, PA pressures, and shunt fraction and distribution, make this a fascinatingly complex question. A mathematical model, derived from a combination of the shunt and Fick equations supports the clinical impression that little is gained by boosting CO unless the CO is already very low, or the shunt is very large (Fig 5-5) (29). Among the agents utilized to

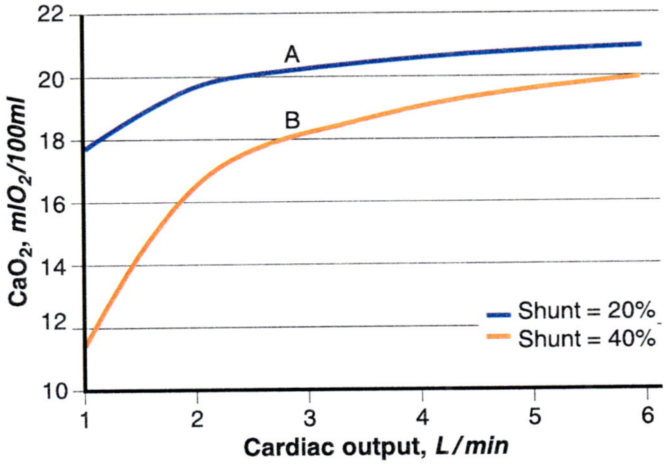

Figure 5-5 – The effect of cardiac output on oxygen content during OLV for hypothetical patient A (who has a 20% shunt) (*blue curve*), and patient B (who has a 40% shunt) (*orange curve*). See text for explanation. Both curves assume that hemoglobin = 15 g/dl, and oxygen consumption = 150 ml/min. Adapted with permission from Levin AI, Coetzee JF, Coetzee A. Arterial oxygenation during one-lung anesthesia. Current Opin Anesthesiol 2008;21(1):28–36.

augment CO in human trials, dobutamine has the most favorable effects, but available studies are poorly controlled and results are inconsistent.

Summary

Barring technical difficulties (misplaced DLT, etc.) excessive shunt in the dependent and/or nondependent lungs is the cause and should be the target of therapy for hypoxemia during OLV. Despite intriguing recent investigations, little value results from manipulation of variables other than the familiar use of CPAP, PEEP, recruitment maneuvers, or reinflation. Nonetheless, consideration of those minor variables provides insights into the physiology of OLV.

Clinical attempts to improve one-lung oxygenation by manipulation of HPV have been relatively ineffective or impractical. Examples include use of inhaled nitric oxide and choice of anesthetics (see above).

Clinical one-lung ventilatory management decisions should also take into account the risk of lung injury, discussed in the following chapter.

Selected References

1. Karzai W, Schwarzkopf K. Hypoxemia during one-lung ventilation. Anesthesiology. 2009;110:1402–11.

2. Brodsky JB, Lemmens HJ. Left double-lumen tubes:clinical experience with 1170 patients. J Cardiothorac Vasc Anesth. 2003;17:289–98.

3. Kozian A, Schilling T, Schutze H, Hachenberg T, Hedenstierna G. Lung computed tomography density distribution in a porcine model of one-lung ventilation. Br J Anaesth. 2009;102(4):551–60.

4. Lohser J. Evidence-based management of one-lung ventilation. Anesthesiol Clin. 2008;26:241–72.

5. Hurford W, Kolker AC, Strauss HW. The use of ventilation/perfusion lung scans to predict oxygenation during one-lung anesthesia. Anesthesiology. 1987;67:841–44.

6. Slinger P, Suissa S, Triolet W. Predicting arterial desaturation during one-lung anaesthesia. Can J Anaesth. 1992;39:1030–5.

7. Slinger P, Kruger M, McRae K, et al. Relation of the static compliance curve and positive end-expiratory pressure to oxygenation during one-lung ventilation. Anesthesiology. 2001;95(5):1098–2006.

8. Nakatsuka M, Wetstein L, Keenan RL. Unilateral high-frequency jet ventilation during one-lung ventilation for thoracotomy. Ann Thorac Surg. 1995;59(6): 1610–4.

9. Ko R, McRae K, Darling G, et al. The use of air in the inspired gas mixture during two-lung ventilation delays lung collapse during one-lung ventilation. Anesth Analg. 2009;108(4):10926.

10. Ducros L, Moutafis M, Castelain M, et al. Pulmonary air trapping during two-lung and one-lung ventilation. J Cardiothorac Vasc Anesth. 1999;13(1):35–9.

11. Gay G, Rodarte J, Hubmayer R, et al. The effects of positive end-expiratory pressure on isovolemic flow and dynamic hyperinflation in patients receiving mechanical ventilation. Am Rev Resp Dis. 1989;139:621–6.

12. Tugrul M, Camci E, Karadeniz H, et al. Comparison of volume controlled with pressure controlled ventilation during one-lung anesthesia. Br J Anaesth. 1997; 79:306–10.

13. Unzueta MC, Casa JI, Moral MV. Pressure-controlled versus volume-controlled ventilation during one-lung ventilation for thoracic surgery. Anesth Analg. 2007; 104:1029–33.

14. Tusman G, Bohm SH, Sipman FS, Maisch S. Lung recruitment improves the efficiency of ventilation and gas exchange during one-lung anesthesia. Anesth Analg. 2004;98(6):1604–9.

15. Cinnella G, Grasso S, Natale C, et al. Physiologic effects of a lung-recruiting strategy applied during one-lung ventilation. Acta Anasthesiol Scand. 2008; 52(6):766–75.

16. Bardoczky G, Szegedi L, d'Hollander A, et al. Two-lung and one-lung ventilation in patients with chronic obstructive pulmonary disease: the effects of position and FiO_2. Anesth Analg 2000;90(1):35–41.

17. Dennehy KC, Dupuis JY, Nathan HJ, Wynands JE. Profound hypoxemia during treatment of low cardiac output after cardiopulmonarty bypass. Can J Anaesth. 1999;46:56–60.

18. Casthely PA, Lear F, Cottrell JE, Lear E. Intrapulmonary shunting during induced hypotension. Anesth Analg. 1982;61:231–5.

19. Hartigan P, Formanek V, Shernan S, et al. Inhaled nitric oxide fails to improve gas exchange during one-lung ventilation. Anesthesiology. 1996;A1165.

20. Sticher J, Scholz S, Boning O, et al. Small dose nitric oxide improves oxygenation during one-lung ventilation: An experimental study. Anesth Analg. 2002; 95:1557–62.

21. Moutafis M, Dalibon N, Liu N, et al. The effects of intravenous almitrine on oxygenation and hemodynamics during one-lung ventilation. Anesth Analg. 2002;94:830–4.

22. Schwarzkopf K, Schreiber T, Bauer R, et al. The effects of increasing doses of isoflurane and desflurane on pulmonary perfusion and systemic oxygenation during one-lung ventilation in pigs. Anesth Analg. 2001;93:1434–38.

23. Slinger P, Scott W. Arterial oxygenation during one-lung ventilation. A comparison of isoflurane and enflurane Anesthesiology. 1995;82(4):940–46.

24. Wang J, Russell G, Page R, et al. Comparison of the effects of desflurane and isoflurane on arterial oxygenation during one-lung ventilation. Br J Anaesth. 1998;81(6):850–3.

25. Wang J, Russell G, Page R, et al. A comparison of the effects of desflurane and isoflurane on arterial oxygenation during one-lung ventilation. Anaesthesia. 2000;55(2):167–73.

26. Abe K, Shimizu T, Takashina M, et al. The effects of propofol, isoflurane, and sevoflurane on oxygenation and shunt fraction during one-lung ventilation. Anesth Analg. 1998;87:1164–9.

27. Schwarzkopf K, Schreiber T, Preussler N-P, et al. Lung perfusion, shunt fraction, and oxygenation during one-lung ventilation in pigs: the effects of desflurane, isoflurane, and propofol. J Cardiothorac Vasc Anesth. 2003;17(1):73–5.

28. Szegedi LL, Van der Linden P, Ducart A, et al. The effects of acute hypovolemic hemodilution on oxygenation during one-lung ventilation. Anesth Analg. 2005; 100:15–20.

29. Levin AI, Coetzee JF. Arterial oxygenation during one-lung anesthesia. Anesth Analg. 2005;100(1):12–4.

Chapter 6
Idiopathic Acute Lung Injury Following Thoracic Surgery

Philip M. Hartigan

Keywords ALI • Acute lung injury • Postpneumonectomy pulmonary edema • Idiopathic ALI following thoracic surgery • Balanced drainage system

Introduction

This controversial and evolving topic deserves a brief discussion here as a dedicated chapter for two reasons. First, acute lung injury (ALI) is a leading cause of death following pulmonary resection, particularly pneumonectomy (1, 2). Second, putative causes have important direct implications to anesthetic management on two fronts:

(1) Intravascular fluid management

(2) Ventilator management during OLV

ALI is defined by the American-European Consensus Conference on the acute respiratory distress syndrome (ARDS) (3) as acute hypoxemic respiratory failure characterized by

- Bilateral pulmonary infiltrates on chest X-ray

P.M. Hartigan (ed.), *Practical Handbook of Thoracic Anesthesia*,
DOI 10.1007/978-0-387-88493-6_6,

- Pulmonary capillary wedge pressure <18 mmHg
- PaO_2/FiO_2 <300 mmHg

In addition, ALI is characterized by low lung volumes (widespread airway collapse), surfactant deficiency, and reduced lung compliance. Several causes of ALI are well recognized, including gastric acid aspiration, pneumonia, extrapulmonary sepsis, pulmonary embolic events, transfusion-related acute lung injury (TRALI), and ventilator-associated lung injury (VALI).

A subset of patients following thoracic surgery (particularly pneumonectomy) develops postoperative pulmonary edema and ALI *in the apparent absence of any known causes.*

This subset was previously termed "postpneumonectomy pulmonary edema" (PPE) because of an early focus on interstitial fluid in the lungs. Recognition that PPE is histologically and pathophysiologically a form of ALI has lead to a shift in semantics, as well as thinking. Licker introduced the term "Primary ALI following thoracic surgery" to highlight the distinction of this entity from ALI secondary to recognized etiologies (4). As a diagnosis of exclusion, this entity should perhaps more properly be termed "Idiopathic ALI following thoracic surgery" (Fig 6-1).

Characteristics of this entity are summarized in Table 6-1.

Progress in understanding this problem has been hampered by the relative rarity of its incidence, by confusion related to its definition, and by a paucity of data. Much of what is known about the entity (Table 6-1) is derived from retrospective studies in which it is difficult to rigorously exclude known etiologies. In addition, low/normal pulmonary artery occlusion pressures, typically used to exclude cardiogenic pulmonary edema, may be unreliable in pneumonectomy patients (5).

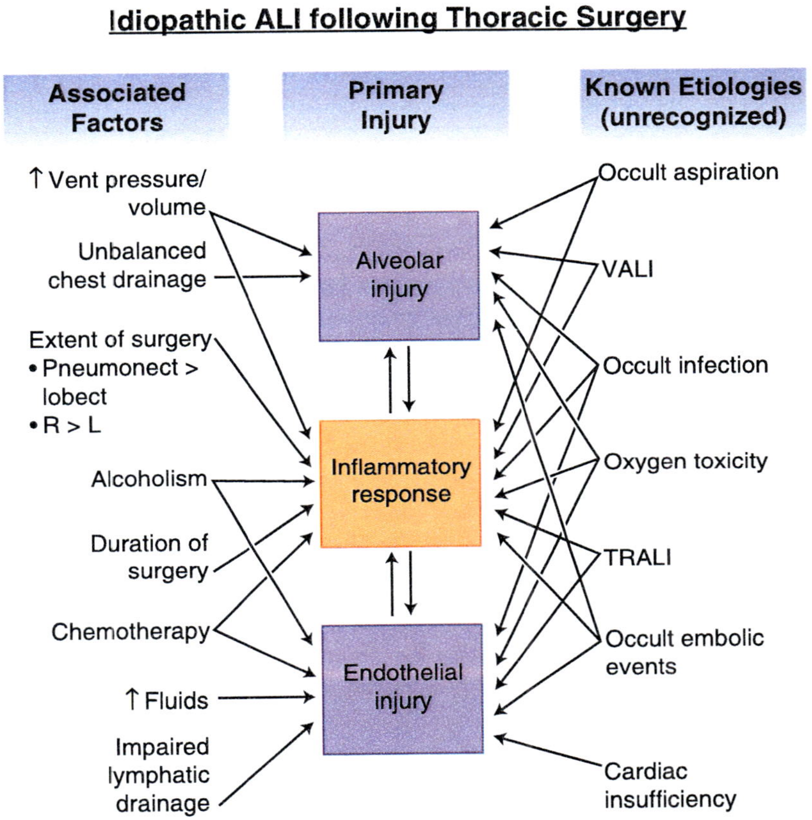

Figure 6-1 – Postulated mechanisms of idiopathic ALI following thoracic surgery may be broadly bundled by the site if primary injury; either the alveoli or endothelium. Factors associated with idiopathic ALI following thoracic surgery (*left-hand column*) lend support to either an endothelial or alveolar primary injury (or both). The inflammatory response may link the two, or be the mechanism of primary injury to either. Known causes of ALI (*right-hand column*) which may not be recognized in retrospective studies, may be potential causes or contributing factors.

Clinical Presentation

The presentation and clinical course of idiopathic ALI following thoracic surgery are relatively nonspecific (Table 6-2). Treatment is largely supportive (Table 6-3). A role for steroids is not supported by evidence. Inhaled nitric oxide is widely employed but not clearly evidence-based.

Table 6-1 – Idiopathic acute lung injury following thoracic surgery

- Incidence: 2–9% of pneumonectomy patients
- Lower incidence and better outcomes following lobectomy and lesser resections
- Diagnosis of exclusion
- 25–50% Mortality
- Onset postoperative day # 1–3
- Low pulmonary capillary wedge pressure (noncardiogenic edema)
- High-protein content in alveolar lavage fluid (capillary leak)
- Impaired lymphatic drainage is likely a contributing factor
- Incidence after right pneumonectomy > left
- Histologically resembles ALI. May progress to ARDS
- Associated with larger fluid administration in some studies (see below)
- Associated with alcoholism in one study4
- Associated with higher ventilation pressures in several retrospective studies (see below)
- Possible association with chemotherapy
- Unknown etiology. Postulated causes include:
  - Ventilator-associated lung injury, possibly during OLV
  - Hyperexpansion from unbalanced chest drainage following pulmonary resection
  - Endovascular injury from hyperperfusion, shear stress, altered flow, and pressure
  - Inflammatory response to surgery
  - Oxygen toxicity
  - Unrecognized, known causes of ALI
    - Transfusion-related lung injury (TRALI)
    - Occult aspiration
- Occult infection
- Unrecognized microemboli

Table 6-2 – Clinical presentation and course of idiopathic ALI following thoracic surgery

- Onset postoperative day #1–3
- Pulmonary infiltrates on CXR (Fig 6-2)
- Dyspnea (12–24 h following radiographic appearance of infiltrates)
- Tachycardia, tachypnea, rales, and hypoxemia
- Normal or low pulmonary artery occlusion pressures (PAOP)
- Normal or low central venous pressures (CVP)
- Absence of cardiac insufficiency
- Negative blood cultures for sepsis
- Absence of evidence of aspiration
- Absence of evidence of pneumonia
- Absence of evidence of bronchopleural fistula
- Poor response to conventional treatments for pulmonary edema
- Variable clinical course: may progress to respiratory failure, ARDS, and death
- Autopsy histologic results resemble ARDS

Table 6-3 – Treatment of ALI following thoracic surgery

- Respiratory support
  - Mechanical ventilation
  - Low (protective) tidal volumes
  - PEEP
  - Minimal FiO_2 tolerated
- Fluid restriction
- Diuresis
- Invasive hemodynamic monitoring
- Hemodynamic support if indicated

(continued)

Table 6-3 – (continued)

- Search for, and address, known potential causes:
  - Infection
  - Aspiration
  - Cardiac failure
  - Bronchopleural fistula
  - Pulmonary embolic events
  - Etc.
- Inhaled nitric oxide
- Empiric antibiotics

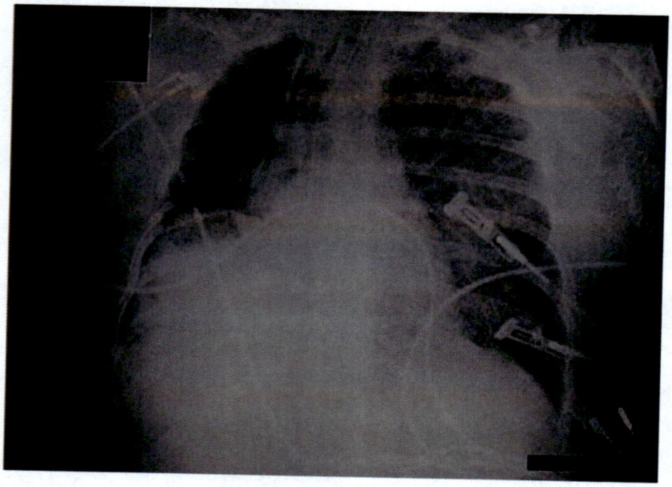

Figure 6-2 – Chest radiograph of a patient demonstrating acute pulmonary edema of the remaining lung following right pneumonectomy (postoperative day # 2).

Impact

In a review of 180 pulmonary resections at one institution, Alvarez reported that all in-hospital deaths following pneumonectomy were attributed to ALI/PPE (6). Slinger has speculated that ALI is emerging as the most prominent cause of perioperative mortality following pulmonary resection, as other complications have become better controlled (7). There is no clear evidence that the incidence of ALI following thoracic surgery is declining.

Endovascular Lesion

Increased permeability of the pulmonary capillary barrier is recognized as integral to the definition of ALI. Evidence for this in PPE is supported by early findings that patients had low/normal pulmonary artery wedge pressures, elevated alveolar edema protein, and resistance to diuretic therapy (8, 9). Waller demonstrated an increased distribution of technetium 99m-labeled albumin to the nonoperative lung following pneumonectomy, but not lobectomy (10). Alternative early nomenclature for PPE included "permeability pulmonary edema," "noncardiogenic pulmonary edema," and "low-pressure pulmonary edema." There is little doubt that vascular permeability is increased, but the mechanism of this lesion is controversial, and likely multifactorial.

Implications for Fluid Management During Thoracic Surgery

The practice of restrictive fluid management for pulmonary resection patients is deeply entrenched. Perspective on this issue is essential for rational patient management.

Early retrospective observational studies reported an association between ALI and increased intraoperative fluid administration (8, 11). Subsequent reports contradicted this association (10, 12). Elevated fluid balance nonetheless, continues to crop up as a persistent factor associated with ALI following thoracic surgery (4). When fluid balance was limited to under 20 ml/kg in the first 24 h, it is difficult to demonstrate such an association. Notably, such restrictive fluid management reduces, but does not eliminate ALI. Cause and effect have not been established, and the limitations of retrospective methods must be acknowledged.

The postulated mechanism by which excessive fluid administration might cause idiopathic ALI has not been well articulated. Within a given patient, whether fluid excess is the root cause, or an exacerbating factor of ALI is unknowable and irrelevant with regard to clinical management. If lung injury is established by any mechanism, the extra hydrostatic pressure of excessive intravascular fluid will exacerbate the pulmonary edema and complicate subsequent management. The greater the pulmonary edema, the greater the deterioration in gas exchange, compliance, and work of breathing. Moreover, pulmonary resection, particularly, pneumonectomy, leaves patients with impaired lymphatic drainage, increased right heart stress, and reduced cardiopulmonary reserve to recover from these problems.

On this basis, relatively restrictive intraoperative fluid management is widely recommended and practiced in anesthesia for pulmonary resection, not because excessive fluid is a proven cause of ALI, but because it is generally unnecessary and may complicate management of patients, should they develop ALI following thoracic surgery.

The appropriate perspective acknowledges the substantial degree of uncertainty of the evidence and recognizes that rigid or overzealous fluid restriction may create more problems than it solves. Fluid administration must be tailored to blood loss and third space losses. Fluid requirements for extrapleural pneumonectomy and esophagectomy will be substantially higher than for standard pneumonectomy. Patients are not well served by fluid restriction which impairs end-organ perfusion or results in intolerance of an epidural block. There is no evidence or logic to suggest an advantage of colloid over crystalloid in the setting of ALI following thoracic surgery.

Implications for Ventilation During OLV

Ventilator-induced lung injury due to conventional OLV is another postulated mechanism for idiopathic ALI following thoracic surgery. The possibility that traditional methods of OLV might be a cause or contributing factor to ALI and that modification of practice may reduce the risk, has lead to a shift in practice toward smaller tidal volume ventilation with PEEP ["lung-protective ventilation (LPV)"].

Traditional recommendations for OLV called for tidal volumes of 10 ml/kg without PEEP (13). These stemmed from the 1970s when hyoxemia during OLV was common. The rationale was to aggressively recruit the atelectasis-prone dependent lung to counteract the effects of nondependent lung shunt on PaO_2. PEEP was avoided for fear that further increased airway pressures would only redirect perfusion to the unventilated nondependent lung.

LPV, with decreased tidal volumes/airway pressures (with PEEP), has now become widely adopted for OLV. The precise *parameters of lung-protective OLV* are not consistently defined. Published ranges include tidal volumes of *5–7 ml/kg predicted body weight*, with low levels of *PEEP (5 cm H_2O)*. The reduced tidal volumes with increased respiratory rates generally result in tolerable oxygenation ($SpO_2 > 90\%$) and acceptable or "permissive" hypercapnea for the limited period of OLV. PEEP is employed to reduce cyclic derecruitment/recruitment (*atelectrauma*) that would otherwise occur with low volume ventilation in the restrictive environment of the dependent lung.

The current evidence basis for lung-protective OLV may be summarized as follows:

- Several retrospective observational human reports of an association between elevated intraoperative ventilatory pressures and the occurrence of ALI (4, 14, 15).
- Limited animal experimental findings that protective one-lung ventilatory patterns are associated with reduced stigmata of ALI compared to traditional OLV (16).
- Extrapolation of the general body of literature on VALI and LPV in ARDS patients (3) to the OLV situation during thoracic surgery.
- Recent findings that inflammatory markers associated with ALI are elevated more markedly with traditional OLV compared to lung-protective OLV (17).

Criticisms of this evidence include, but are not limited to the following:

- Retrospective studies may have failed to separate idiopathic ALI from ALI of known causes.
- Important details of ventilatory mechanics (inspiratory plateau pressures, timing and duration of elevated pressures, etc.) are not easily culled with accuracy in retrospective studies.
- It may be invalid to extrapolate conclusions from animal studies (16) or from the critical care setting (3) to the relatively brief, human OLV situation that occurs during thoracic surgery.
- The inflammatory events leading to ALI are extremely complex and incompletely understood. Substantial inconsistencies exist in studies looking at inflammatory mediators and traditional vs. protective ventilation (18). Cause–effect conclusions are premature.

Protective OLV is not currently a standard of care and is not without dissenting opinion (19). At this writing, the rationale in favor of protective OLV is compelling while the body of evidence is still developing. The finding that OLV is associated with the elaboration of inflammatory mediators and that protective OLV may reduce this effect (17) provides a plausible mechanism.

The consequences of ALI are potentially severe, while the consequences of LPV are generally benign. However, those with conditions such as pulmonary hypertension, right ventricular dysfunction, or fragile coronary disease may be intolerant of the relative hypercapnea or marginal oxygenation which sometimes results from low tidal volume ventilation.

Thus, LPV should be employed as the general default setting for OLV, but it need not be rigidly adhered to in patients with relative contraindications, or those who appear intolerant of such settings.

Balanced Chest Drainage

Hyperexpansion and injury of the remaining lung following pneumonectomy can occur postoperatively due to mediastinal shift (20). The techniques for surgical management of the empty hemithorax are variable and may impact this. Three methods are commonly employed:

- No drain
- Pleural drainage tube which is clamped and intermittently released to underwater seal
- Balanced underwater seal system (limits the amount of negative pressure in the empty hemithorax)

In the absence of a balanced drainage system, coughing and straining can lead to air egress from the operative empty hemithorax, and negative pressure which draws the mediastinum and hyperexpands the remaining lung. Remarkably, Alvarez has reported the elimination of idiopathic ALI/PPE since their institution of balanced chest drainage system in 1996 (6). A potential downside of balanced drainage systems is the ingress of air into the hemithorax as a route for infection.

The extent to which postoperative drainage management contributes to ALI is presently unclear.

Inflammatory Response to Thoracic Surgery

There is no debate that a potent inflammatory response typically accompanies thoracic surgery, as it does for all major surgery and trauma. ALI may represent the pulmonary manifestation of a local or panendothelial inflammatory vascular injury. The players and temporal sequence of this complex cascade are not completely characterized. Broad agreement exists that proinflammatory cytokines (IL-8, IL-1Beta, TNF-alpha, etc.), chemokines, neutrophils, reactive oxygen, and reactive nitrogen species are involved, among others. Oxidative stress and ischemia–reperfusion injury may contribute to the injurious response. This overall shift in the balance of proinflammatory vs. antiinflammatory forces may be viewed as a common pathway potentially leading to a systemic inflammatory response syndrome (SIRS), ALI, and ARDS in response to a variety of insults. The precise nature and magnitude of the inflammatory response is almost certainly subject to modification based on the original insult, patient factors (genetic and pathologic), and iatrogenic factors.

What is it about major thoracic surgery, and pneumonectomy in particular that leads to such a high incidence of, and poor outcome from ALI and ARDS? Postulated contributing factors include:

- Lung manipulation/dissection/contusion (known inciting factors)
- Preexisting lung disease
- Lung collapse/single-lung ventilation
- Possible mechanical endothelial injury (shear stress due to abrupt hyperperfusion of contralateral lung during crossclamp of pulmonary artery)
- Possible mechanical alveolar injury (volutrauma/atelectrauma during OLV, hyperexpansion due to postoperative mediastinal shift)
- Oxidative stress (high FiO_2 to offset effect of OLV)
- Possible ischemia–reperfusion injury
- Impaired lymphatic drainage

It is probably the case that the typical inflammatory response to pulmonary resection is necessary, but rarely sufficient by itself to cause ALI. Exacerbating factors are likely involved in the majority of cases ("second hit hypothesis"). Certain factors are beyond the control of the anesthesiologist (Table 6-4). The extent to which idiopathic ALI can be prevented by avoiding injurious ventilation, oxygen toxicity, volume overload, and mediastinal shift postoperatively is unclear. At the current juncture, however, that appears to be all that can be done.

Table 6-4 – Prevention of ALI during thoracic surgery

Anesthetic factors

Minimize injurious mechanical ventilation (as tolerated):

- Tidal volumes = 6 ml/kg ideal body weight
- PEEP = 5 cm H_2O
- Monitor and avoid excessive intrinsic PEEP
- Intermittent recruitment maneuvers
- Consider decreasing FiO_2 to target $SpO_2 > 90\%$

Restrictive fluid management (24 h fluid balance = 20 ml/kg)

Surgical factors

- Minimally invasive surgical approach
- Balanced pleural drainage postoperative
- Minimize lung contusion

Immutable factors

- Side of surgery
- Extent of resection
- Extent of lymphatic compromise
- Genetic predisposition
- Alcoholism
- Chemotherapy
- Preexisting pulmonary or immunologic pathology
- Unrecognized other triggers of ALI

Perspective

The pathophysiology of ALI following thoracic surgery is multifactorial. Whether "idiopathic ALI" is truly an entity of novel etiology is uncertain (as opposed to known triggers such as occult infection/aspiration, etc. (21) exacerbating the inflammatory response to surgery).

The search for causes and modifiable factors has yielded a short list (Table 6-4). The extent to which LPV and fluid restriction will limit ALI or improve outcome is unknown. Therefore, implementation of these maneuvers should be employed with some flexibility. Ventilatory strategies must ultimately be balanced against the need to oxygenate and remove CO_2, as well as avoid lung injury. Fluid management must be balanced against the requirement for a safe margin of reserve to ensure end-organ perfusion and tolerance of epidural analgesia. In the future, as the cascade of events responsible for ALI is characterized, pharmacologic protection against ALI (including anesthetic choices) (22, 23) may be possible.

Selected References

1. Alam N, Park BJ, Wilton A, et al. Incidence and risk factors for lung injury after lung cancer resection. Ann Thorac Surg. 2007;84:1085–91.

2. Licker M, Widikker I, Robert J, et al. Operative mortality and respiratory complications after lung resection for cancer: impact of chronic obstructive pulmonary disease and time trends. Ann Thorac Surg. 2006;81:1830–7.

3. The Acute Respiratory Distress Syndrome Network. Ventilation with lower tidal volumes as compared to traditional tidal volumes for acute lung injury and the acute respiratory distress syndrome. N Engl J Med. 2000;342:1301–8.

4. Licker M, de Perrot M, Spiliopoulos A, et al. Risk factors for acute lung injury after thoracic surgery for lung cancer. Anesth Analg. 2003;97:1558–65.

5. Wittnich C, Trudel J, Zidulka A, Chiu R. Misleading "pulmonary wedge pressure"after pneumonectomy. Its importance in postoperative fluid therapy. Ann Thorac Surg. 1986;42:192.

6. Alvarez JM, Tan J, Kejriwal N, Ghanim K, et al. Idiopathic postpneumonectomy pulmonary edema: hyperinflation of the remaining lung is a potential etiologic factor, but the condition can be averted by balanced pleural drainage. J Thorac Cardiovasc Surg. 2007;133(6):1439–47.

7. Slinger P. Postpneumonectomy pulmonary edema. Good news, bad news. Anesthesiology. 2006;105(1):2–5.

8. Zeldin RA, Normandin D, Landtwing D, Peters RM. Postpneumonectomy pulmonary edema. J Thorac Cardiovasc Surg. 1984;87:359–65.

9. Mathru M, Blakeman B, Dries D, Kleinman B, Kumar P. Permiability pulmonary edema following lung resection. Chest. 1990;98:1216–8.

10. Waller D, Gebitekin C, Saunders N, Walker D. Noncardiogenic pulmonary edema complicating lung resection. Ann Thorac Surg. 1993;55:140–3.

11. Verheijan-Breemhaar L, Bogaard JM, van den Berg B, Hilvering C. Postpneumonectomy pulmonary oedema. Thorax. 1988;43:323–6.

12. Turnage WS, Lunn JL. Postpneumonectomy pulmonary edema. A retrospective analysis of associated variables. Chest. 1993;103:1646–50.

13. Benumof JL. Anesthesia for thoracic surgery. 2nd ed. Philadelphia: W.B. Saunders; 1995. p. 410.

14. Fernandez-Perez ER, Keegan MT, Brown DR, et al. Intraoperative tidal volume as a risk factor for respiratory failure after pneumonectomy. Anesthesiology. 2006;105:14–8.

15. Licker M, Diaper J, Villiger Y, et al. Impact of intraoperative lung protection interventions in patients undergoing lung cancer surgery. Crit Care. 2009;13(2): R41–51.

16. De Abreu M, Heintz M, Heller A, et al. One-lung ventilation with high tidal volumes and zero PEEP is injurious in the isolated rabbit lung model. Anesth Analg. 2003;96:220–8.

17. Schilling T, Kozain A, Huth C, Buhling F, et al. The pulmonary immune effects of mechanical ventilation in patients undergoing thoracic surgery. Anesth Analg. 2005;101:957–65.

18. Dreyfuss D, Rouby J. Mechanical ventilation-induced release of cytokines. A key for the future or Pandora's box? Anesthesiology. 2004;101:1–3.

19. Gal TJ. Con: low tidal volumes are indicated during one-lung ventilation. Anesth Analg. 2006;103(2):271–3.

20. Deslauriers J, Aucoin A, Gregoire J. Postpneumonectomy pulmonary edema. Chest Surg Clin N Am. 1998;8:611–31.

21. Agnew N, Kendall J, Akrofi M, Tran J, et al. Gastroesophageal reflux and tracheal aspiration in the thoracotomy position: should ranitidine premedication be routine? Anesth Analg. 2002;95:1645–9.

22. Schilling T, Kozian A, Kretzschmar M, Huth C, et al. Effects of propofol and desflurane anaesthesia on the alveolar inflammatory response to one-lung ventilation. Br J Anaesth. 2007;99(3):368–75.

23. De Conno E, Streurer M, Wittlinger M, et al. Anesthetic-induced improvement of the inflammatory response to one-lung ventilation. Anesthesiology. 2009;110: 1316–26.

Further Reading

Alvarez J. Postpneumonectomy pulmonary edema. Chapter 9. In: Slinger PD, editor. Progress in thoracic anesthesia. Baltimore: Lippincott, Williams & Wilkins; 2004. p. 187–219.

Jordan S, Mitchell JA, Quinlan GJ, Goldstraw P, Evans TW. The pathogenesis of lung injury following pulmonary resection. Eur Respir J. 2000;15:790–9.

II

Essential Technical Aspects

Chapter 7
Thoracic Positioning and Incisions

Teresa M. Bean

Keywords Lateral decubitus position • Standard supine postioning • Semisupine position • Lithotomy position • Thoracosternotomy position • Posterolateral thoracotomy • Video-assisted thoracoscopic surgery • Axillary thoracotomies • Anterior thoracotomy • Transverse thoracosternotomy • Thoracoabdominal incision • Median sternotomy

Introduction

This chapter reviews major categories of positions and incisions for thoracic surgery. Specific procedures (see Section IV) and surgeons' preferences may dictate minor variants. Understanding of surgical positions and incisions helps to avoid complications, improve surgical exposure, and anticipate events.

Thoracic Positions

Lateral Decubitus Position

The lateral decubitus position (LDP, Fig 7-1) is employed for most procedures requiring access to the ipsilateral contents of the hemithorax. It is used for posterolateral thoracotomy, some variants of muscle-sparing thoracotomies, and video-assisted thoracoscopic surgery (VATS).

P.M. Hartigan (ed.), *Practical Handbook of Thoracic Anesthesia*,
DOI 10.1007/978-0-387-88493-6_7,

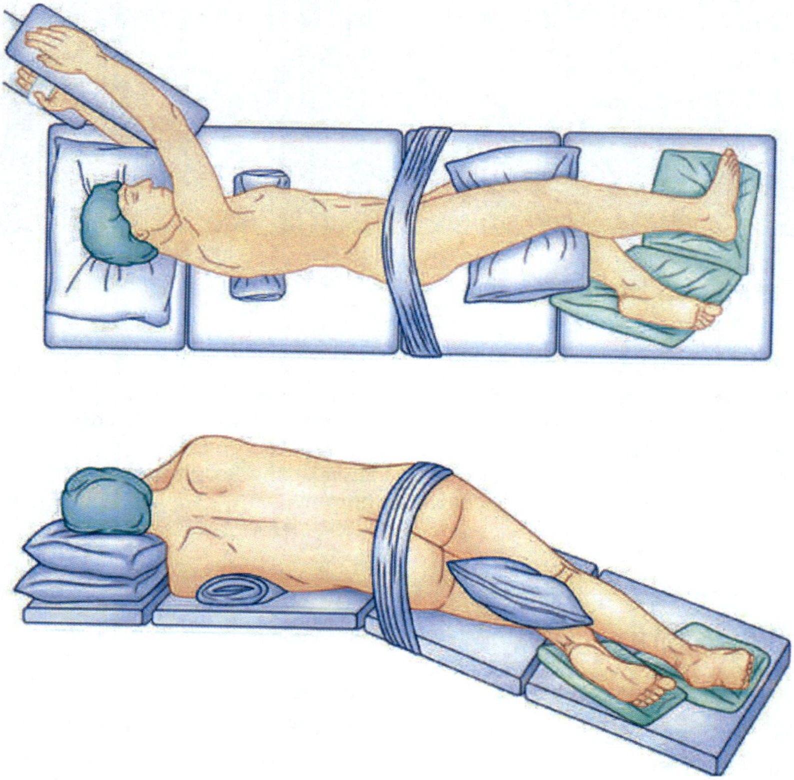

Figure 7-1 – Lateral decubitus position.

Box 7-1 highlights aspects of the LDP requiring attention to prevent nerve or pressure injuries.

Box 7-1 – Lateral Decubitus Position	
Head	▪ Support with stabilizing pillow
	▪ Avoid pressure on the eye and ear pinnae
Neck	▪ Axial alignment of cervical and thoracic spine
	▪ Avoid excessive lateral neck flexion (*suprascapular nerve stretch injury*)

(continued)

Box 7-1 – (continued)

Dependent arm	▪ Extend on armrest, pad elbow at ulnar groove (*ulnar nerve injury*) ▪ Bend <90° at shoulder and elbow
Dependent axilla	▪ Place "axillary" roll under upper thorax to prevent *brachial plexus compression injury* by humeral head. *Note*: if placed high within axilla, the roll itself may compress plexus
Nondependent arm	▪ Support on padded armrest. ▪ Keep angles of shoulder and elbow <90°
Chest/hips	▪ Anterior-posterior support with bolsters or sandbag ▪ Avoid compression of breasts and genitals ▪ Tape spanning the table across patient's hips helps secure lateral position ▪ Attention to avoid *sciatic nerve* compression by tape ▪ Attention to avoid pressure injuries to skin by EKG leads, bolsters, etc.
Legs	▪ Bend dependent leg for stability ▪ Pad lateral knees to prevent *peroneal nerve* compression injury ▪ Extend the nondependent leg ▪ Pillow between legs
Ankles	▪ Pad malleoli

The last adjustment is to flex the bed to open the interspaces between the ribs, followed by reverse Trendelenberg to level the chest cavity.

Box 7-2 – Variants of Lateral Decubitus Position

VARIANT INDICATION	PURPOSE	POSITION CHANGE
"Swimmer's position" for high axillary incisions, VATS procedures	Exposure of nondependent axilla	Nondependent arm just <90° to torso at the shoulder, elbow bent just <90°
Surgeon preference	Removal of the lower armrest; surgeon can move more freely	Dependent arm rests fully on surgical bed; elbow bent just <90°
"Lazy" or "Sloppy" lateral	Expose the upper abdomen; expose groin for cannulation	Tilt nondependent hip toward supine
First rib resection	Modify abduction of nondependent arm throughout case	Nondependent arm prepped into surgical field, suspended on a traction pulley

Supine and Semisupine Positions

Standard supine postioning (Fig 7-2) is employed for rigid bronchoscopy, cervical and anterior mediastinoscopy, and median sternotomy.

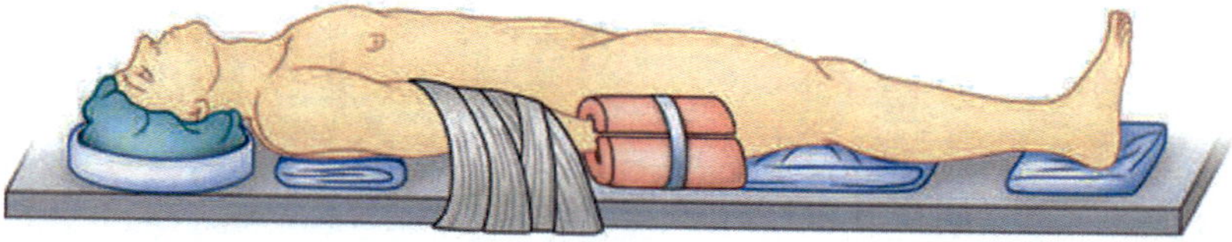

Figure 7-2 – Supine position.

Box 7-3 – Supine Position

Head/neck	▪ Maximally extend, without hyperextension, support with doughnut-shaped pillow
Shoulders	▪ Transverse roll underneath
Arms	▪ Tuck bilaterally; elbows padded at ulnar groove
	▪ Hands protected and padded
	▪ Pad between vertical retractor holder and arm if applicable
Knees	▪ Pillow underneath knees to reduce lordosis of lumbar spine
Heels	▪ Pad pressure points

A *semisupine* position (Fig 7-3) is utilized for many procedures including anterior thoracotomy, pleurex catheter, and chest tube placements.

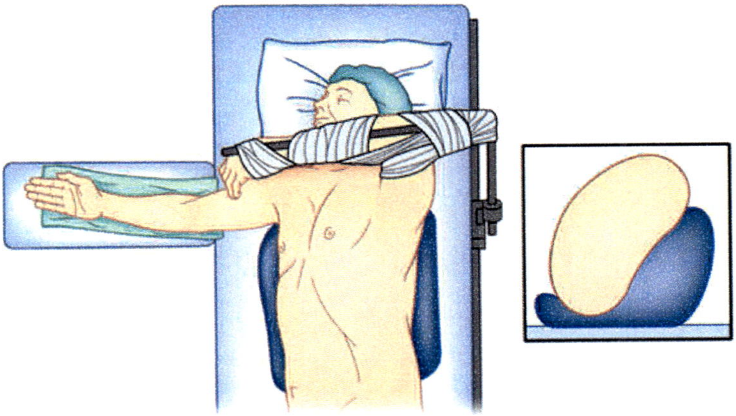

Figure 7-3 – Semisupine position.

Box 7-4 – Semisupine Position

Head	▪ Neutral position, support with doughnut-shaped pillow
Ipsilateral hemithorax	▪ Prop 30–45° lateral with rolled blanket(s)
Ipsilateral arm	▪ Supported and tucked along posterior axillary line, or overhead as depicted in Figure 7-3 ▪ Pad ulnar groove and hand ▪ Attention to avoid posterior abduction stretch of shoulder
Knees/heels	▪ Pressure points padded as per supine positioning

A variant of supine positioning is employed for thoracosternotomy (Fig 7-4), an incision commonly used for double lung transplantation and selected large central mediastinal or bilateral surgical resections.

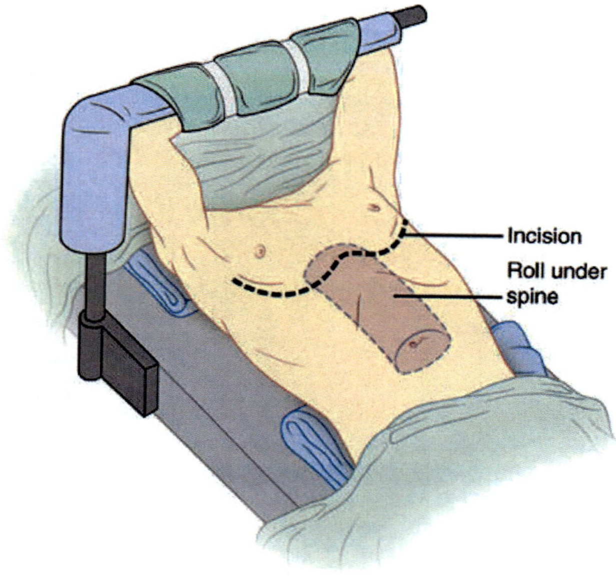

Figure 7-4 – Thoracosternotomy position and transverse thoracosternotomy incision.

Box 7-5 – Thoracosternotomy Position

Head and neck	▪ Extend slightly, support with doughnut-shaped pillow
	▪ Avoid neck hyperextension as above
Arms	▪ Pad and secure against an ether screen above the patient's head
	▪ Alternatively, tuck at sides as per supine position
Shoulders	▪ Place a roll horizontally underneath
Spine	▪ Place a roll vertically midline underneath
Hips	▪ Place a roll horizontally underneath
Knees/heels	▪ Pad pressure points as per supine position

Lithotomy

Lithotomy position (Fig 7-5) is employed for the abdominal portion of minimally invasive esophagectomies and laparoscopic Nissen fundoplications.

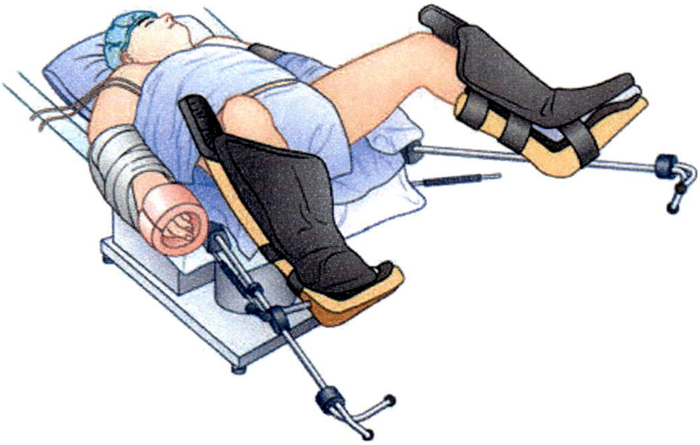

Figure 7-5 – Lithotomy position.

Box 7-6 – Lithotomy Position

Head	▪ Support with doughnut-shaped pillow
Arms	▪ Tuck bilaterally, elbows padded
	▪ Be sure hands, especially fingers won't be pinched by table or stirrups
Legs	▪ Rest in stirrup supports, slightly flexed, and abducted at the hips
	▪ Bend 90° at knees
	▪ Pad between stirrups/leg holders and patient's legs
	▪ Avoid popliteal fossa or peroneal nerve compression by leg holders

Thoracic Incisions

Posterolateral Thoracotomy

The posterolateral thoracotomy is a large incision (Fig 7-6) that provides excellent exposure of the chest contents including hilum. The main disadvantage of the incision is the time it takes for the multiple layers of tissue to be dissected and the obvious injury to those layers. Previously regarded as the standard approach for lobectomy and pneumonectomy, full posterolateral incisions are now reserved for select situations where less traumatic incisions are inadequate.

With the patient in LDP, the incision travels from the anterior axillary line, curves up to 4 cm under the tip of the scapula, and extends vertically between the midline vertebral column and the medial edge of the scapula. The lower portion of the trapezius, the latissimus dorsi, the lower portion of the rhomboid, and, if necessary, the serratus anterior muscles are divided.

The interspace (usually fourth or fifth) is identified by counting the ribs coming off the spinal column under the scapula. This scapular retraction has been implicated as contributing to postoperative

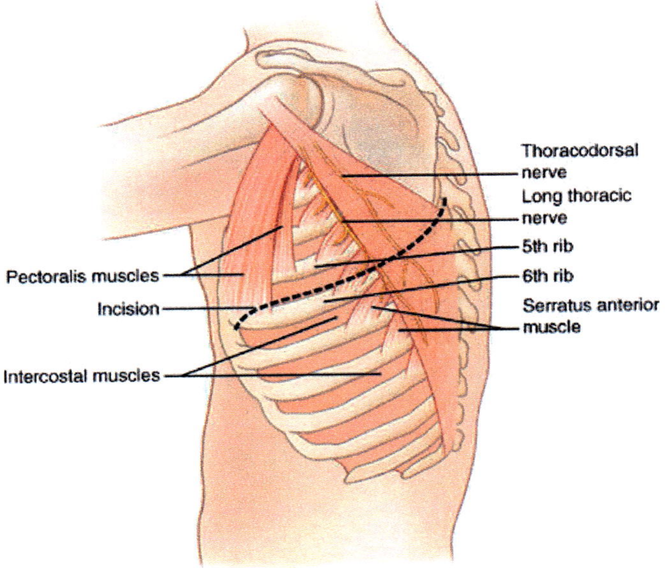

Figure 7-6 – Posterolateral thoracotomy incision.

shoulder pain. The pleural space can be entered by making an incision in the rib bed of a subperiosteally excised ("shingled") rib; or an intercostal muscle incision can be made in the lower portion of the interspace to avoid injury to the neurovascular bundle. A rib spreading retractor, opened slowly and in stages, avoids rib fracture and exposes the chest contents. Some trauma to intercostal nerves is inevitable through division, stretch, or crush between retractor and rib. Closure requires reapproximation of divided muscles and ribs. Midshaft rib fractures are less painful if the jagged section of rib is removed.

Limited Variants of Posterolateral Thoracotomy

The terminology is imprecise for this family of incisions. The common denominators are that the length of the incision is more limited, and division of major muscles is avoided. Terms utilized include: "muscle-sparing thoracotomy," "mini-thoracotomy," or "lateral or anterolateral thoracotomy." Depending on the target, the incision is usually made along the posterolateral thoracotomy incision line (Fig 7-7). Generally, no ribs are removed.

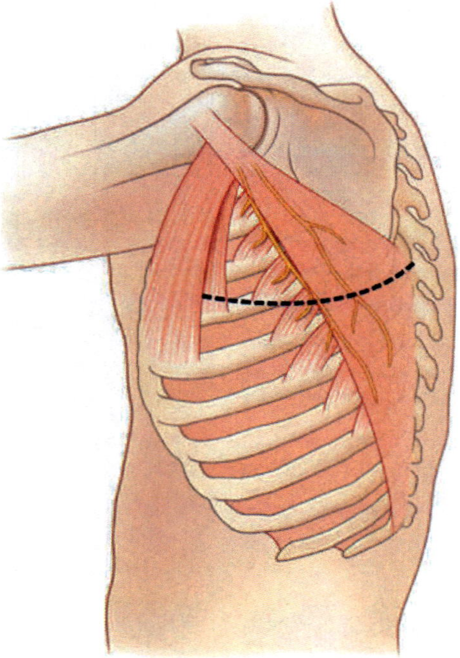

Figure 7-7 – Limited lateral thoracotomy incision.

The latissumus dorsi is mobilized posteriorly and the long thoracic nerve is carefully avoided. The serratus anterior is split in the direction of its fibers over the desired interspace. The intercostal muscle is divided at its inferior border and the pleural space is entered as described above.

These incisions are widely employed for pneumonectomy, lobectomy, segmentectomy, or technically challenging lesser resections.

Video-Assisted Thoracoscopic Surgery

Thoracoscopic procedures utilize three to four small 2–3 cm incisions that serve as ports of entry for video cameras, surgical retractors, and stapling devices. Through these small incisions, wedge resections, lung and pleural biopsies, and drainage of effusions can be performed. To remove larger specimens, like lobes, or for necessary surgical exposure, a larger "utility port" may be required to remove the specimen.

The placement of the incisions varies depending on surgical target and the patient's pathology, but is often on the anterior and posterior axillary line. The larger incision for VATS procedures is usually made high in the axilla, in between the third and fourth interspace and is usually made just large enough to pass the specimen.

Axillary Thoracotomy

Axillary thoracotomies (Fig 7-8) are performed for first rib resections, sympathectomies, apical bullectomies, and greater exposure

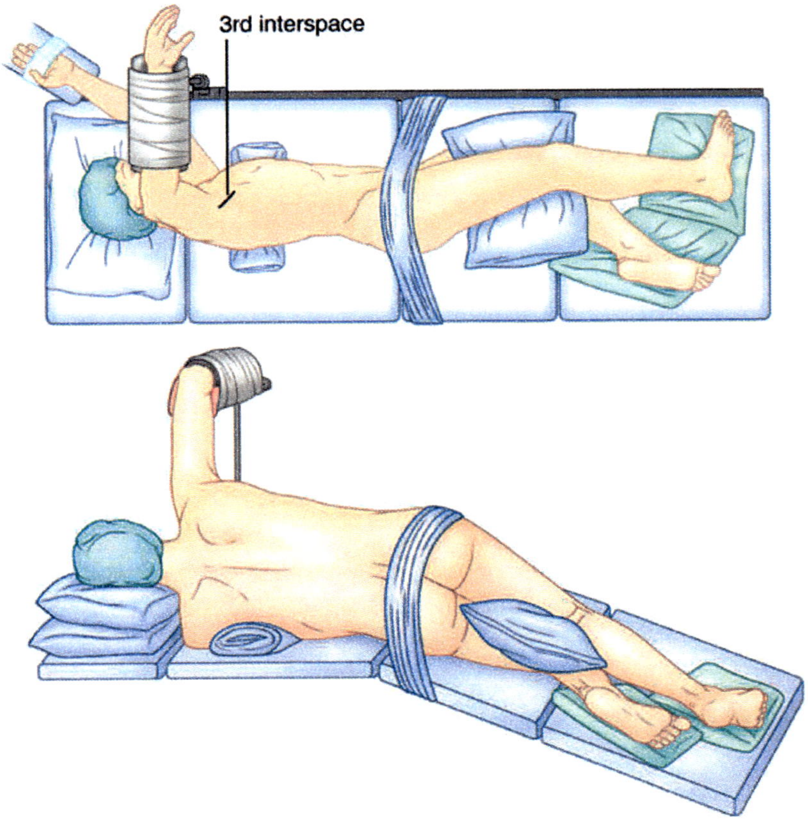

Figure 7-8 – Axillary thoracotomy incision and variant lateral decubitus position. Notice the change in nondependent arm position to improve axillary exposure.

during VATS. With the patient in LDP, an incision is made at the base of the axillary hair line from the pectoralis major anteriorly to the latissimus dorsi posteriorly. The thorax is entered at the third intercostal space, anterior to the long thoracic nerve, which may be gently mobilized posteriorly to allow rib distraction. The interspace can be opened widely under both the pectoralis major and latissimus dorsi muscles to improve surgical exposure. The superior portion of the serratus anterior muscle can be cut in the direction of its fibers, if needed, to improve surgical exposure.

Anterior Thoracotomy

The anterior thoracotomy (Fig 7-9), also known as the "hemi-clamshell incision," is probably most commonly performed for open lung biopsy; however, this incision provides good exposure for right middle lobe procedures and partial pericardectomy as well.

The semisupine patient will have an incision that extends from the fourth or fifth interspace at the sternal edge, curving under the

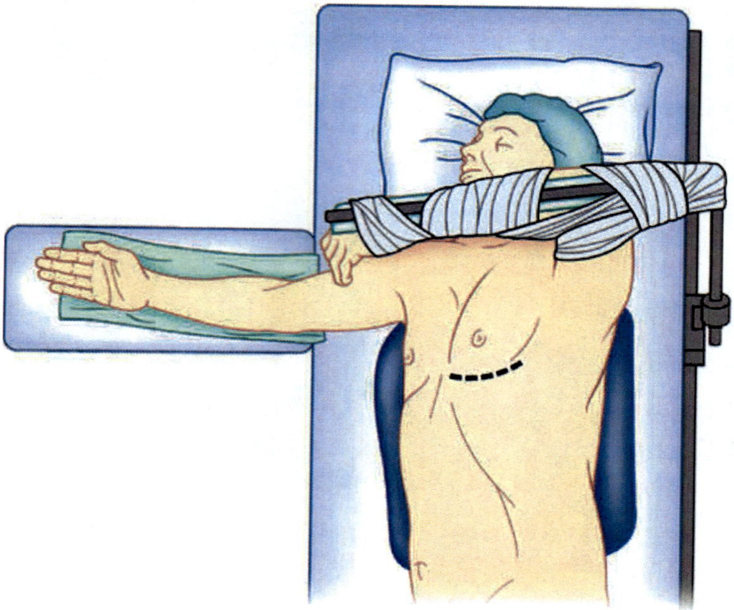

Figure 7-9 – Anterior thoracotomy incision.

inframammary crease to the mid-axillary line. Pectoralis major and minor are divided and, laterally, serratus anterior may be split along the course of its fibers. The pleural space is entered at the desired interspace by incising the intercostal muscle at its inferior attachment to the ribs. Caution must be made when extending the incision posteriorly as the intercostal neurovascular bundle lies toward the middle of the intercostal space close to midline. Extending the incision midline may require the internal mammary artery be ligated and would threaten any ipsilateral internal mammary coronary graft.

Transverse Thoracosternotomy

The transverse thoracosternotomy is also known as "bilateral anterior thoracotomy," "clamshell," or "crossbow" incision. This large incision is often employed for double lung transplants or large central masses, and has the longest recovery time.

The skin incision follows the inframammary crease bilaterally, rising to the anterior axillary line at each side. The thorax is usually entered in the fourth intercostal space bilaterally. Both internal mammary arteries are sacrificed. After the retrosternal space is bluntly dissected, the sternum is transected horizontally with a saw at or above the nipple level. Exposure of the chest is achieved with rib spreaders which lift the ribs like a trap door.

Thoracoabdominal Incision

The thoracoabdominal incision (Fig 7-10) provides exposure for surgery in both the hemithorax and abdomen. Dissection on the left side is frequently required for lower esophageal procedures. With the patient in a "lazy" LDP, a traditional posterolateral thoracotomy incision is made, and extended obliquely over the upper abdominal quadrant toward midline. After the latissimus dorsi and serratus anterior muscles are divided, the hemithorax is entered between the sixth through eighth interspace, depending on the surgical exposure desired. The costal margin is cut and the diaphragm is divided with care not to damage the phrenic nerve. Thus, the contents of the thorax and upper abdomen are exposed.

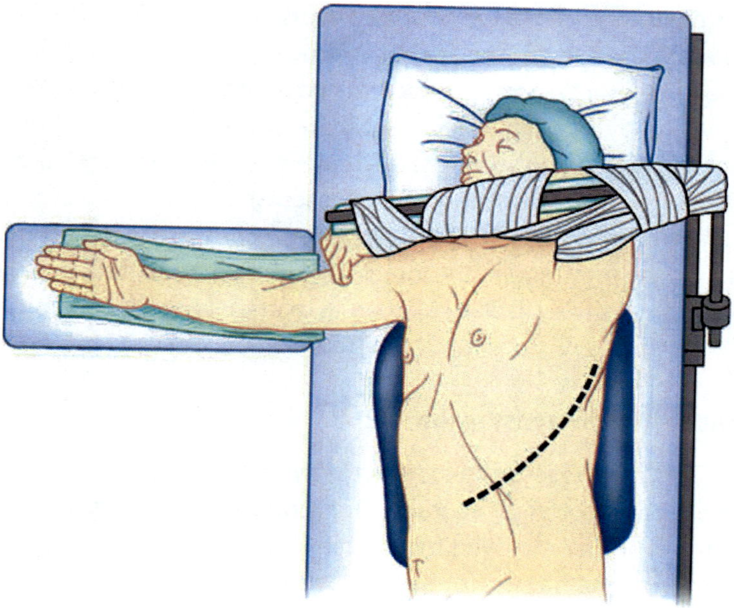

Figure 7-10 – Thoracoabdominal incision.

Sternotomy

Besides open heart surgery, median sternotomy (Fig 7-11) can be employed for thymectomy, anterior mediastinal mass resection, tracheal resection, and lung volume reduction surgery. The standard incision is made from the suprasternal notch to just below the xiphoid process through the skin and pectoralis fascia down to the linea alba. The superior end of the incision is retracted to expose the manubrium. The interclavicular ligament is divided with care to avoid the inominate artery and vein. Blunt dissection is used to open the retrosternal space superiorly and inferiorly before splitting the sternum with a saw. Also, immediately prior to sawing the sternum, the lungs are deflated. Periosteal bleeding is controlled with gauze, packing and electrocautery; marrow bleeding can be controlled with bone wax.

Sternal spreaders used to maintain exposure are best placed more inferiorly to avoid rib fracture and brachial plexus injury.

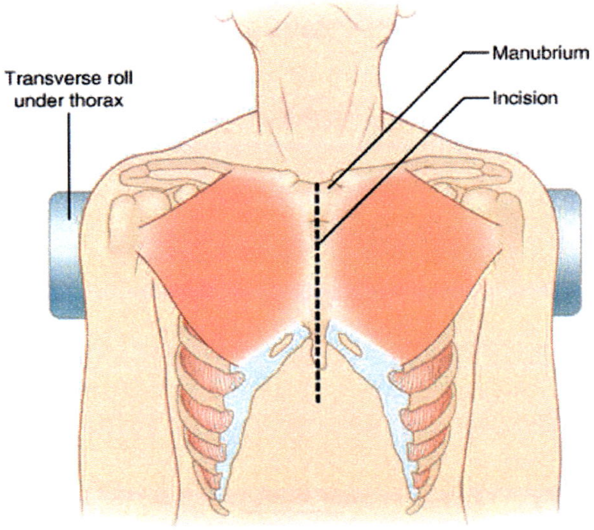

Figure 7-11 – Sternotomy.

Sternal retraction is also limited by traction placed on the innominate vein.

For cosmetic reasons, full sternotomy can be performed through a more limited incision by raising subcutaneous flaps. Partial sternotomy may also be employed or combined with another incision.

Tracheal surgery, mediastinal tumors, thymectomy, substernal goiter, upper esophageal surgery or surgery on the great vessels may be approached through a partial sternotomy which extends like a "T" to an anterior thoracotomy, resulting in an anterior "trap door-like" exposure. Apical tumors, such as those of the superior sulcus (Pancoast), may be approached by high posterolateral or hemi-clamshell incisions, or anteriorly as shown below with the Dartevelle approach (Fig 7-12). Access may require resection of part of the clavicle or partial sternotomy with foreword retraction of the clavicle and first rib.

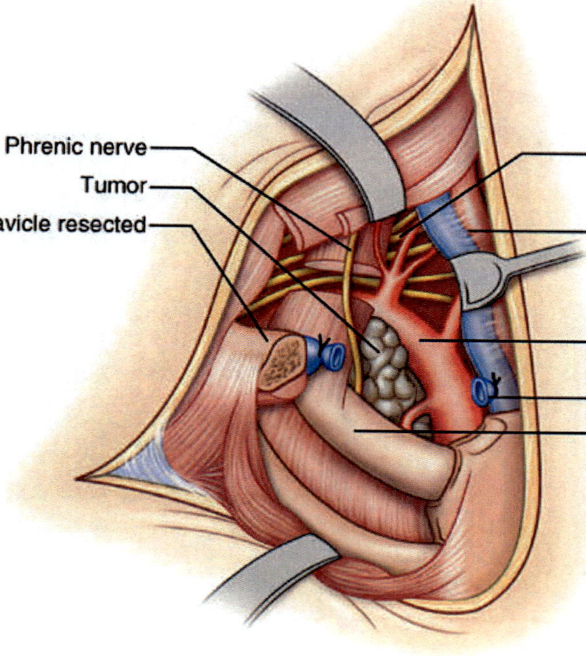

Figure 7-12 – Dartevelle incision for pancoast tumor.

Further Suggested Reading

Fry WA. Thoracic incisions. In: Shields TW, LoCicero III J, Ponn RB, editors. General thoracic surgery. 5th ed. Philadelphia, PA: Lippincott Williams & Wilkins; 2000. p. 367–74.

Martin LW, Krasna M. Pancoast's syndrome: anterior approach to Pancoast tumor (chapter 68). In: Sugarbaker DJ, Krasna MJ, Mentzer SJ, Zellos L, editors. Adult Chest Surgery. New York: McGraw-Hill; 2009. p. 584–93.

McRae KM, Bussieres JS, Campos JH, Slinger PD. Anesthesia for general thoracic surgery. In: Patterson GA, Cooper JD, Deslauriers J, Lerut AEMR, Luketich JD, Rice TW, editors. Pearson's thoracic & esophageal surgery. 3rd ed. Philadelphia, PA: Churchill Livingstone Elsevier; 2008. p. 119–35.

Murthy SC. Thoracic incisions. In: Patterson GA, Cooper JD, Deslauriers J, Lerut AEMR, Luketich JD, Rice TW, editors. Pearson's thoracic & esophageal surgery. 3rd ed. Philadelphia, PA: Churchill Livingstone Elsevier; 2008. p. 39–67.

Warner MA, Martin JT. Patient positioning. In: Barash PG, Cullen BF, Stoelting RK, editors. Clinical anesthesia. 4th ed. Philadelphia, PA: Lippincott Williams & Wilkins; 2001. p. 639–65.

Chapter 8
Bronchoscopic Anatomy

Thomas Edrich

Keywords Fiber-optic bronchoscopy • Left mainstem bronchus • Bronchoscopic view • Anomalous RUL Anatomy • Extrinsic Tracheal Compression • Intrinsic Tracheal Obstruction • Tracheomalacia • Lobar Torsion

Fiber-optic bronchoscopy has become increasingly available to anesthesiologists. When combined with videoscopic capabilities and display to the entire surgical team, the bronchoscopist can contribute significantly to the surgical team as listed in Table 8-1.

Normal Anatomy

When navigating the tracheobronchial tree with a bronchoscope the lungs are approached from the medial side, i.e., from the "inside-out." Thus, it is useful to maintain a mental image of the bronchopulmonary segments as viewed from the medial (hilar) perspective (Fig 8-1) while searching for visual landmarks (Fig 8-2).

When performing bronchoscopy from the head of the bed, the tracheal rings appear above (12 o'clock), while the membranous

P.M. Hartigan (ed.), *Practical Handbook of Thoracic Anesthesia*,
DOI 10.1007/978-0-387-88493-6_8, © Springer Science+Business Media, LLC 2012

Table 8-1 – Common indications for bronchoscopy during thoracic surgery

Lung Isolation	▪ Enable and intermittently monitor correct placement of DLT or BB, as well as cuff inflation relative to carina and RUL
Bronchial toilette	▪ Clear secretions to maintain adequate single-lung ventilation ▪ Facilitate deflation of the lung on the operative side
Guidance for surgical management	▪ Display stump to surgical team before definitive stapling of bronchus ▪ Display/guide anastomoses during sleeve resection or lung transplantation ▪ Detect airway injuries due to surgery/trauma (e.g. membranous tracheal injury during esophagectomy) ▪ Recognize anomalies pertinent to planned resection or lung isolation ▪ Display obstructive lesions in trachea and mainstem bronchi for surgical team during mechanical and laser debridement ▪ Confirm patency of adjacent lobes during lobectomy ▪ Early detection of lobar torsion ▪ Transillumination of bronchial segments to aid surgeon's identification of anatomy ▪ Definitively confirm absence of apparatus (nasogastric tube, temp probe, blocker, etc.) in target lung prior to surgical cross clamp

trachea appears below (6 o'clock). It is essential to orient oneself by this internal anatomy. Confusion can easily result from rotation of the bronchoscope, twisting of the fiber-optic fibers, or changes in patient position. To the right and left of the primary carina lie the right and left mainstem bronchi, respectively (Fig 8-2A).

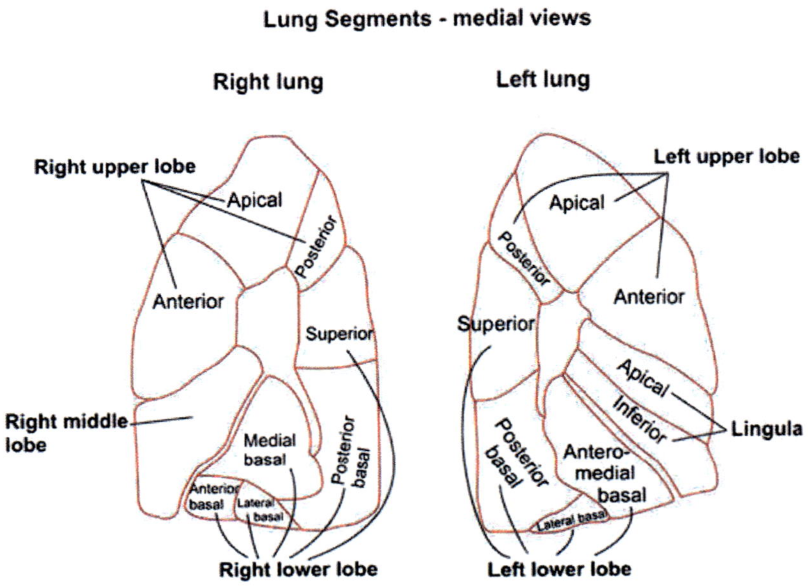

Figure 8-1 – Medial views of the bronchopulmonary segments (from vantage point of the carina).

Less commonly, the anesthesiologist will perform bronchoscopy while positioned next to and facing the patient. It this case, all the images in Fig 8-2 will appear upside down, reinforcing the importance of orienting oneself by the internal anatomy.

The thoracic anesthesiologist must have knowledge of bronchial anatomy at least to the lobar level to perform the functions described in Table 8-1. Too often, anesthesiologists are only comfortable with the primary carina and right upper lobe. Often, the double lumen tube is initially in too deep, precluding a view of the primary carina. Also, the right upper lobe is the most frequently anomalous of all lobes. Recognition of secondary carinas and lower/middle lobe anatomy provides great comfort and guidance in such situations.

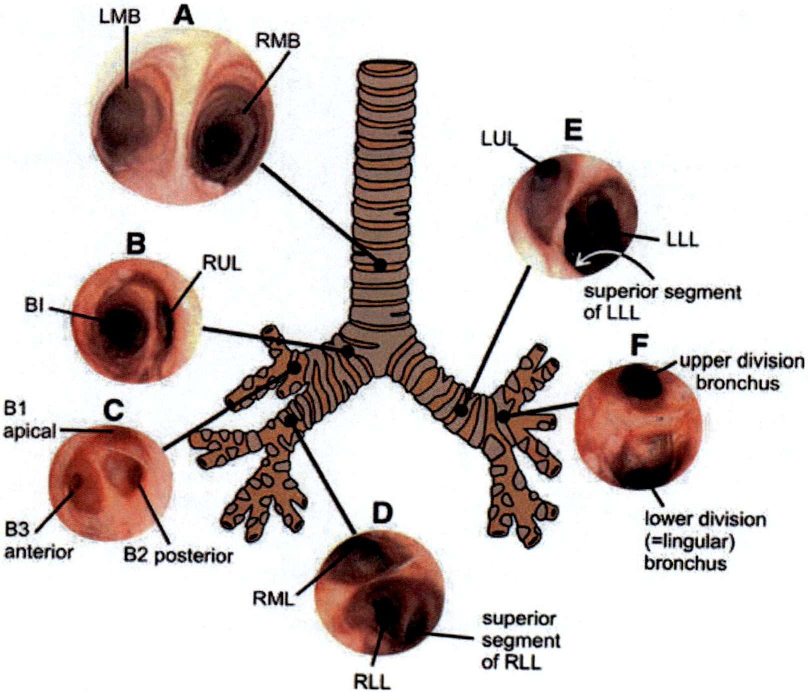

Figure 8-2 – Typical bronchoscopic views from different vantage points within the tracheobronchial tree. Abbreviations: *LMB and RMB* right and left mainstem bronchi, *LUL* left upper lobe, *LLL* left lower lobe, *RLL* right lower lobe, *RML* right middle lobe, B1, B2 and B3 are segmental bronchi, *BI* bronchus intermedius, *RUL* right upper lobe.

Right Lung

The right mainstem bronchus (RMB) is wider and more vertical (axial) than the left mainstem bronchus (LMB). It averages 1.8 cm in length, but can be <1 cm long in 10% of the population (1). The right upper lobe (RUL) bronchus is a significant landmark for anesthesiologists. It departs at a sharp angle to the right (Fig 8-2B). After entering the RUL bronchus, the trifurcation between the apical, anterior, and posterior segmental bronchi is visible. The configuration of the trifurcation can be quite variable. Considering that the RUL bronchus is entered by rotating the scope to the right and flexing, the view obtained (Fig 8-2C) corresponds to the upright medial view of the right lung in Fig 8-1. Thus, the anterior segmental bronchus typically lies to the left, the posterior to the right and the apical lies above.

When advancing into the bronchus intermedius (BI), the scope is directed toward the diaphragm. As expected from the segmental anatomy in Fig 8-1, the right middle lobe (RML) departs superiorly and medially while the right lower lobe bronchus (RLL) continues straight ahead (Fig 8-2D). The bronchus leading to the superior segment of the RLL is often visible at the same level as the RML exit but is directed posteriorly (Fig 8-2D). As an additional aid to distinguish the RML from the RLL, the bronchoscopist can follow the membranous part of the bronchial tree; most often it leads to the RLL as visible also in Fig 8-2D. Recognizing the BI anatomy is very useful. Note that the three main divisions (RML, Basilar RLL, and Superior Segment of the RLL) are typically arranged in a straight line, in contrast to the three segments of the RUL, which are typically arranged in a triangular configuration.

Left Lung

The left mainstem bronchus (LMB) has a smaller caliber than the RMB and is longer (4–5 cm). The left upper lobe (LUL) bronchus can be entered by rotating the scope to the left and flexing. This bronchoscopic view (Fig 8-2F) is comparable to the upright view of the medial aspect of the left lung as shown in Fig 8-1. Thus, the upper division bronchus leading to the *apicoposterior and anterior segments* appears above, and the lower division bronchus (*lingular bronchus*) appears below. After withdrawing back to the mainstem bronchus, the left lower lobe (LLL) is visible below with the superior segment of the LLL departing most posteriorly (Fig 8-2E). Similar to the right lung, the membranous part of the bronchus leads to the lower lobe and can help distinguish it from the LUL.

Note the differences between the secondary carina on the left (Fig 8-2E) and the BI (Fig 8-2D). This will be useful when one is unsure whether the DLT is in the right or left because it is too deep for a view of the primary carina.

Abnormal Bronchoscopic Findings with Anesthetic Implications

Anomalous RUL Anatomy

The RUL is subject to anomaly more frequently than any of the other lobes, with estimates as high as 10%. Not uncommonly, the RUL appears bifurcated rather than trifurcated. The average distance from carina to RUL takeoff is 1.8 cm in adults, but a shorter right mainstem bronchus is common. When the RUL or a segment thereof departs from the trachea (above the carina), it is referred to as a *tracheal bronchus* or pig bronchus (Fig 8-3) (2). A tracheal bronchus (or segment) may be displaced, or supernumerary (Fig 9-8). Both a short right mainstem and a tracheal bronchus are problematic for fitting a right-sided DLT and should be noted during initial bronchoscopy (See Chapter 9). Abnormal bifurcation of the RUL should be noted so as to avoid confusion when confirming position of any DLT.

Extrinsic Tracheal Compression

Stenosis from extrinsic compression of the trachea may take several forms. Anterior mediastinal masses tend to flatten out the trachea (Fig 8-4). Posterior mediastinal masses or general increased intrathoracic pressure (massive obesity) tends to cause anterior bowing of the membranous trachea (Fig 8-5). Both tend to produce

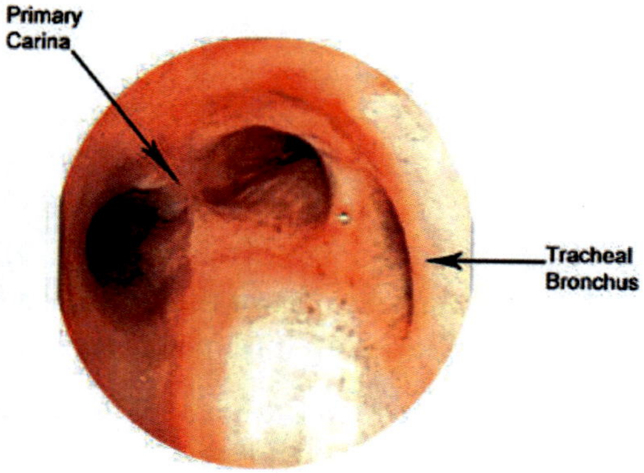

Figure 8-3 – Bronchoscopic image of a tracheal bronchus. Note that the tracheal bronchus exits the trachea directly, above the carina.

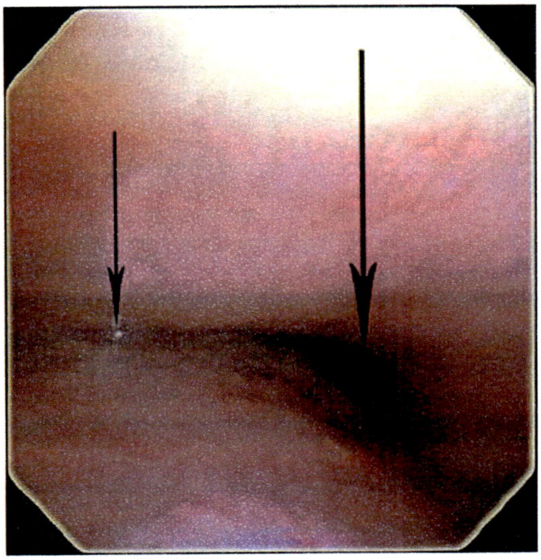

Figure 8-4 – Compression of the distal trachea at the carina due to an anterior mediastinal mass. The left mainstem bronchus (*short arrow*) is compressed more than the right mainstem bronchus (*long arrow*).

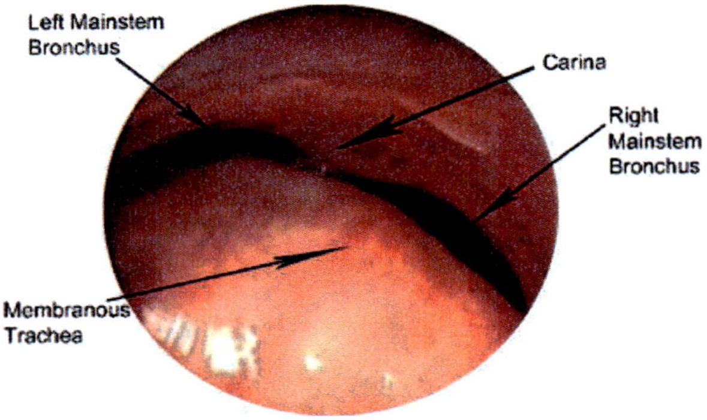

Figure 8-5 – Primary carina with anterior bowing of the membranous trachea.

variable tracheal obstruction which can be exacerbated by position and induction of anesthesia (Chapter 20). A "saber-sheath trachea" (Fig 8-6) is sometimes seen in association with COPD and may be a consequence of abnormal remodeling of cartilaginous rings in the presence of hyperexpanded lungs. Saber-sheath tracheas may obstruct the tracheal lumen of a DLT (Chapter 9).

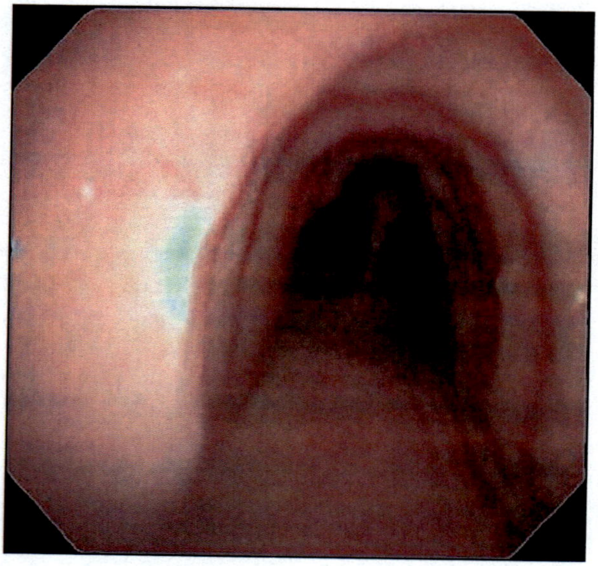

Figure 8-6 – Saber-sheath trachea associated with hyperexpanded lungs. The tracheal wall may obstruct the tracheal lumen of a DLT.

Intrinsic Tracheal Obstruction

Narrowing of the tracheal (or bronchial) lumen due to fixed strictures such as scarring at an anastomosis, or from a cuff injury, (Fig 8-7) may alter intubation or lung isolation plans. Intraluminal tumors (Fig 8-8) or foreign bodies such as stents may become disrupted by intubation. Intubation should be directly guided by bronchoscopy to avoid disruption, bleeding, or exacerbation of obstruction. Carcinoid tumors in particular may bleed and release mediators when disrupted.

Tracheomalacia

Weakening or loss of tracheal cartilaginous support results in a floppy trachea which tends to collapse during expiration (Fig 8-9). Airways with malacia can easily be injured by indelicate instrumentation or intubation. Intubation distal to the area of malacia safely

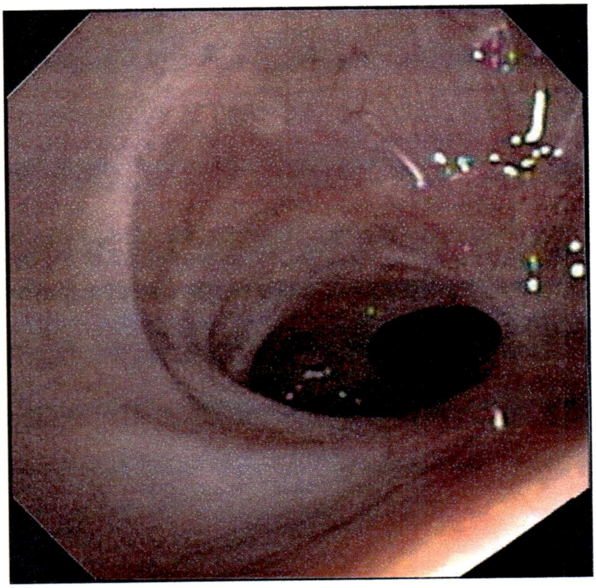

Figure 8-7 – Tracheal stricture due to scarring after a cuff injury. It may impede ETT placement or lung isolation plans.

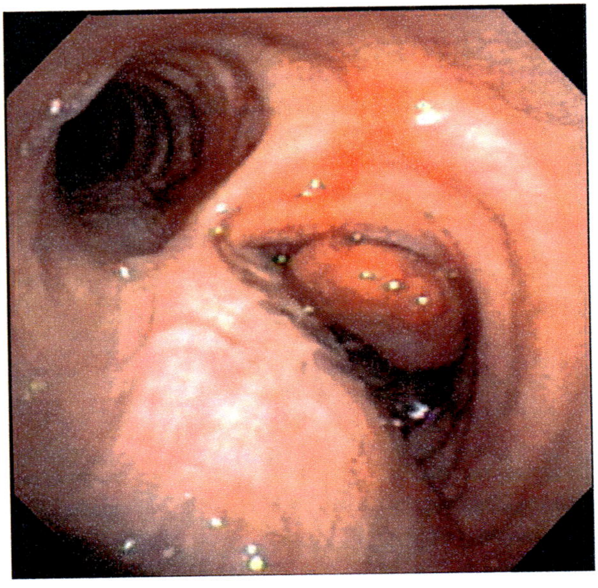

Figure 8-8 – Intraluminal tumor protruding from right mainstem bronchus. Risk of bleeding from inadvertent right mainstem intubation and difficulty ventilating or isolating the right lung may result.

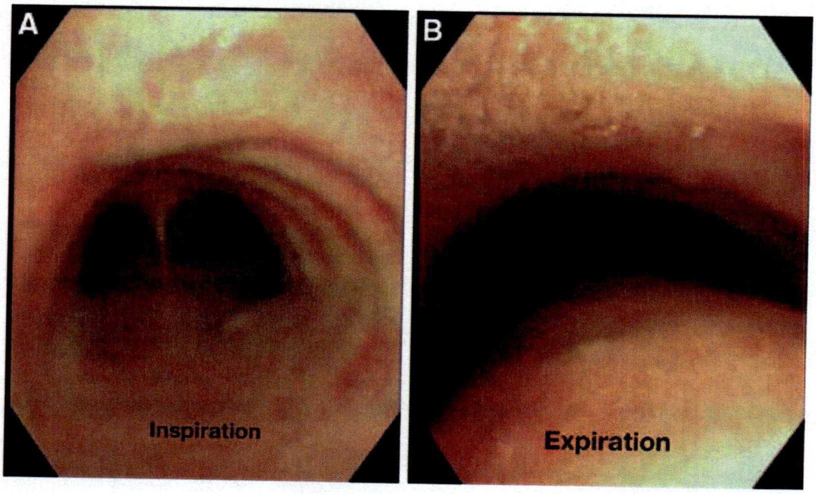

Figure 8-9 – *Tracheomalacia.* Legend: Bronchoscopic view of a patient with tracheomalacia and dynamic obstruction due to chronic infections. Obstruction is relieved during inspiration (**A**), but exacerbated during expiration (**B**) with broadening of the lateral dimensions, and relative shortening of the anterior–posterior dimensions due to loss of cartilaginous rigidity. (Images courtesy of Armin Ernst, MD, PhD).

Table 8-2 – Causes of tracheomalacia
Congenital such as polychrondritis
Post-traumatic after prolonged intubation or tracheostomy
Emphysema and chronic bronchitis
Chronic external compression, e.g., by mediastinal goiter, aortic aneurysm or malignancy

stents the trachea open, but patients tend to obstruct postoperatively. Causes of tracheomalacia are listed in Table 8-2.

Fistulae

Congenital or acquired fistulae between the airway and the esophagus (tracheoesophageal fistula – TEF)(Fig 8-10), pleura (bronchopleural fistula – BPF), or other structures should be noted

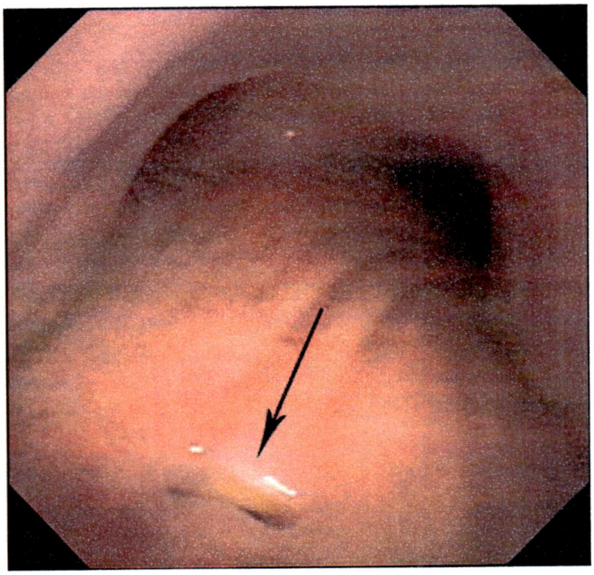

Figure 8-10 – Tracheoesophageal fistula (TEF) in the membranous part of the distal trachea.

because of their implications with regard to air leak and soilage of the airway, as well as strategies for lung isolation and positive pressure ventilation (Chapter 31).

Stents

Airway stents are increasingly common (Fig 8-11) (Chapter 28). Blind intubation may disrupt or fold over the edge of a stent resulting in airway obstruction. Smaller endotracheal tubes should be guided by bronchoscopy to prevent this. A bronchial blocker may be preferable to a DLT for lung isolation if a stent is present.

Lobar Torsion

Rarely, pulmonary resection may result in torsion of a remaining lobe due to rotation of that lobe (Fig 8-12). Prompt recognition by the anesthesiologist allows for immediate surgical correction (and placement of a pexy stitch to prevent recurrence). Failure to recognize this may result in lobar infarction.

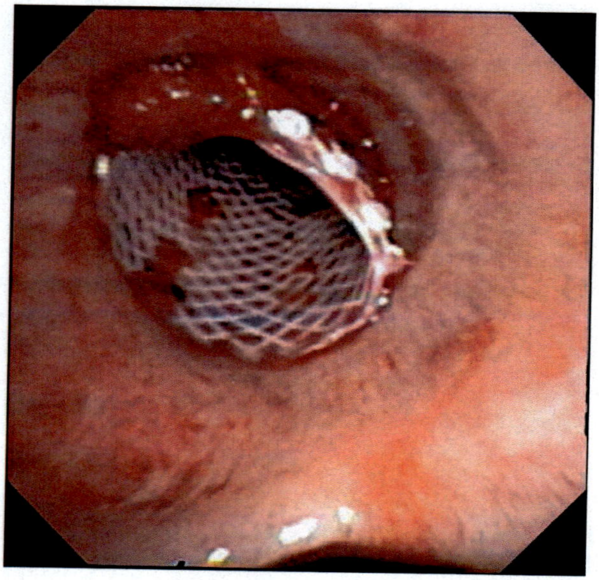

Figure 8-11 – Stent in the left mainstem bronchus. Note that the lip of the stent is exposed, raising the risk of malpositioning if manipulated with an ETT or a bronchial blocker.

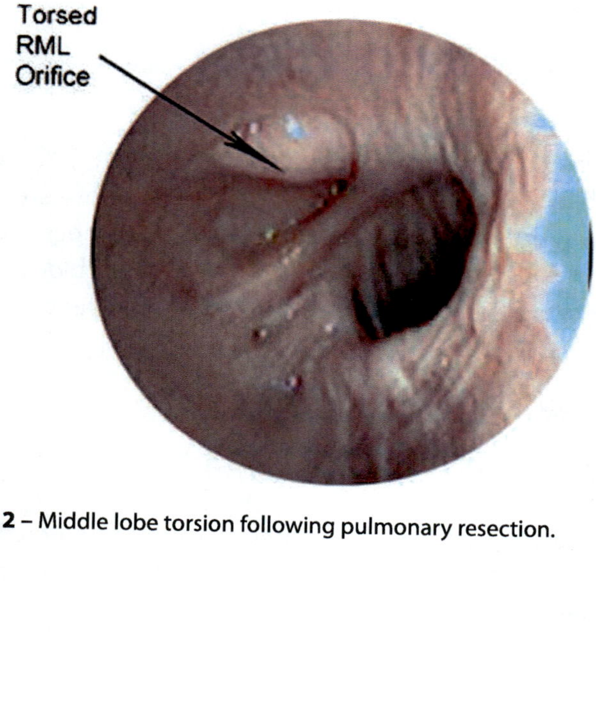

Figure 8-12 – Middle lobe torsion following pulmonary resection.

Selected References

1. Nino M, Body SC, Hartigan PM. The use of a bronchial blocker to rescue an ill-fitting double-lumen endotracheal tube. Anesth Analg. 2000;91:1370–1. TOC.

2. Ikeno S, Mitsuhata H, Saito K, Hirabayashi Y, Akazawa S, Kasuda H, et al. Airway management for patients with a tracheal bronchus. Br J Anaesth. 1996;76: 573–5.

Chapter 9
Technical Aspects of Lung Isolation

Sarah H. Wiser

Keywords Lung isolation • Double lumen tubes • Bronchial blockers • Endobronchial intubation • Resting cuff volume • Auscultation technique

Introduction

Lung isolation is the cornerstone of thoracic anesthesia. The indications for lung isolation vary according to procedure- and patient-related factors (Box 9-1). This chapter focuses on the technical aspects of lung isolation.

The three methods for achieving lung separation are (1) double-lumen tubes (DLTs), (2) bronchial blockers (BBs), and (3) endobronchial intubation. Regardless of the technique of lung isolation, it is imperative that the user is knowledgeable of tracheo-bronchial anatomy at least to the lobar level (Chapter 8).

Double-Lumen Tubes

DLTs are the most commonly employed device for lung isolation. Advantages and disadvantages of DLTs compared to bronchial blockers are listed in Box 9-2A, B.

P.M. Hartigan (ed.), *Practical Handbook of Thoracic Anesthesia*,
DOI 10.1007/978-0-387-88493-6_9,

Box 9-1 – Indications for Lung Isolation

Surgical indications	Procedures on the pulmonary tree
	Pneumonectomy
	Lobectomy
	Sleeve resections
	Segmentecomy or lesser resections
	Lung transplantation
	Unilateral broncho-alveolar lavage
	Procedures requiring enhanced surgical exposure
	Thoracoscopy for any reason
	Mediastinal exposure
	Esophagectomy
	Thoracic spine surgery via the anterior approach
	Repair of a thoracic aortic aneurysm
Patient pathology	Protection against contralateral lung soilage
	Unilateral hemoptysis
	Unilateral infection
	Control of the distribution of ventilation
	Tracheobronchial disruption
	Bronchopleural fistula
	Bronchocutaneous fistula
	Unilateral lung disease
	Large cyst
	Large bullae
	Severe hypoxemia due to unilateral lung disease

Box 9-2A, B – Advantages and Disadvantages of DLTs Compared to Bronchial Blockers

A: Advantages of DLT

Provides superior lung isolation (controversial).

Easy conversion from one-lung ventilation to two-lung ventilation.

Large lumen facilitates deflation/suctioning of the nondependent lung.

Allows for access to either lung:

- Selective ventilation/collapse of either lung.
- Easy application of CPAP.
- Bronchoscopic visualization of bronchial/lobar clamping during resection.

B: Disadvantages of DLT

Large size and fixed anatomic design:

Increased difficulty with tracheal intubation.

Unable to accommodate anomalous anatomy.

Potential trauma to airway.

Unavailable in small pediatric sizes.

Risk of tracheal cuff tear on the patients' teeth during intubation.

Can be difficult to predict correct tube size.

Inability to provide selective lobar blockade.

Necessitates ETT exchange if postoperative ventilation is required.

Design of the Double-Lumen Tube

The most common DLT design is the Robert-Shaw. The DLT comes in left- and right-sided configurations (see Box 9-3 for indications for left- versus right-sided DLT). General features of a DLT are depicted in Fig 9-1A, B.

Box 9-3 – Indications for Left Versus Right DLT

Left DLT	Any left- or right-sided procedure that does not require left bronchial resection
	Absence of any of the indications for a right DLT (see below)
	Inability to place a right-sided DLT
	Short, right mainstem bronchus (<10 mm)
	Tracheal bronchus (aka "pig trachea")
Right DLT	Procedures that require resection or division of left mainstem bronchus
	Left lung transplantation
	Left pneumonectomy
	Left sleeve resections
	Patient pathology
	Exophytic or stenotic lesion involving the left mainstem bronchus
	Left mainstem bronchial disruption
	Distortion of the left mainstem due to external compression (e.g., descending thoracic aortic aneurysm)
	Inability to place a left DLT
	Sharp angle on the left mainstem bronchus
	Shifted carina
	Other
	Left mainstem stent in situ

DLT = Double-lumen tube.

Resting Cuff Volume of DLTs

The *resting volume* for a cuff is the volume at which the cuff maintains its low pressure characteristics. Exceeding this volume results in a high-pressure cuff. The resting volume for the bronchial cuff varies according to the DLT manufacturer and size (1) (Table 9-1). The tracheal cuff has a resting cuff volume = 10 cc of air.

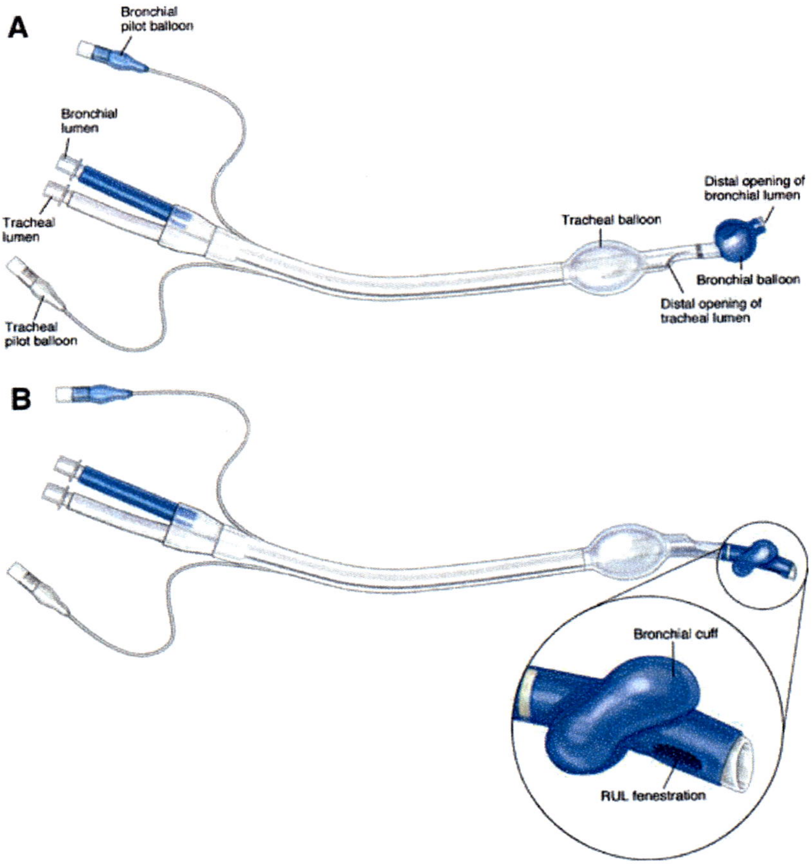

Figure 9-1 – Anatomy of: **A**. Left-sided DLT **B**. Right-sided DLT.

Table 9-1 – Resting bronchial cuff volumes of left-sided double-lumen tubes

	35 Fr	37 Fr	39 Fr	41 Fr
Mallinckrodt (cc)	3.7	2.5	2.0	2.0
Sheridan (cc)	2.5	2.0	2.0	2.0
Rusch (cc)	1.5	1.5	1.4	2.1
Portex (cc)	2.5	2.5	4.8	4.2

From Hannallah et al. (1) (used with permission).

Overinflation of either cuff or placement of a tube that is too large for the patient's bronchus can create a cuff pressure greater than 25 cm H_2O. Elevated cuff pressures increase the risk of mucosal ischemia or trauma

DLT Sizes

By convention, the size of a DLT is based on the French Catheter Scale. The outer diameter can be determined by dividing the French size by 3:

$$\text{OD(mm)} = \frac{\text{French}}{3}.$$

Typical adult sizes are 35, 37, 39, and 41 French. Smaller sizes, down to 26 Fr, are available from some manufacturers.

The increasing size of the DLT reflects an increase in:

1. Diameter of the tube as a whole
2. Diameter of the bronchial tube
3. Length from the opening of the tracheal lumen to the tip of the bronchial lumen

Despite their length, airflow resistance profiles for modern DLTs are favorable. Generally speaking, a 37 Fr DLT imposes less flow resistance than a 7.5-mm OD single-lumen tube (SLT). Notably, all four sizes of the Mallinkrodt tubes have higher flow resistances than a 7.5-mm OD SLT. This increased resistance is due to the specific design of the Y-connector on the Mallinkrodt DLT, not due to the tube itself (2).

Size Selection

The appropriate size of DLT is one which:

- Passes atraumatically through the glottis, trachea, and bronchus.

- The ventilation lumens align with the appropriate bronchi.
- An adequate seal is obtained when the cuffs are inflated at their appropriate volumes.

Many studies have looked at how to best size select a DLT for an individual patient. Studies have looked at the size of DLT and (1) the correlation between gender and height, (2) the size of the left mainstem bronchus on the CXR, (3) the size of tracheal diameter on the CXR, and (4) measurement of the left mainstem bronchus on CT scan. No single predictor is perfect, and there is no consensus on the best indicator.

The authors of this text have adopted a simplified system, based on the patient's height and gender to determine the size of DLT (Table 9-2A, B). Essentially, the first choice for an average-sized female or male would be a 37 or 39 Fr, respectively (sizing up or down for patients who are tall or short for their gender). We recognize that this is an imperfect method for size selection, especially for small individuals or persons of Asian descent, but it provides a reasonable starting point.

It is important to recognize an inappropriately sized DLT:

- Tight at glottis or bronchus.
- Requires extremes of depths of insertion (in too deep or out too far).
- Requires more or less than the appropriate resting cuff volume for air seal.

Table 9-2 – Simplified double-lumen tubes (DLTs) size selection based on height and gender (A, female and B, male)

(A) Female			
Height (ft)	<5.3	5.3–5.11	>6.0
DLT size (French)	35	37	39
(B) Male			
Height (ft)	<5.6	5.6–5.11	>6.0
DLT size (French)	37	39	41

If an inappropriately sized tube is recognized, it should be exchanged accordingly. A DLT that is too small leads either to inadequate lung isolation or cuff overinflation, both may lead to a mucosal ischemia. A DLT that is too large is more likely to cause airway trauma or may occlude lobar airways.

Insertion of a DLT

Recommended steps for placement of a DLT are listed in the box below (Box 9-4).

Box 9-4 – Recommended Steps for DLT Placement

Recommended Steps for Placement of a DLT

- Preparation:
  - Test and confirm competence of cuffs.
  - Lubricate tip with water-based lubricant.
  - Ensure that stylet does not protrude beyond bronchial tip.
- Direct Laryngoscopy with Macintosh blade[1].
- Advance bronchial cuff through glottis with convex curvature-oriented anteriorly.
- Remove stylet[2].
- Rotate 90° counterclockwise (clockwise for right-sided DLT).
- Advance DLT until gentle resistance is encountered.
- Inflate tracheal cuff only.
- Attach Y-connector and circuit, ventilate.
  - Confirm $ETCO_2$, chest rise, and breath sounds.
- Note the depth of insertion of the DLT[3].
- Perform bronchoscopy initially via tracheal lumen.
  - Confirm correct side and depth of DLT.
  - Inflate bronchial cuff under visualization.
  - Bronchial cuff should be just visible at the carina.

(continued)

Box 9-4 – (continued)

- Perform bronchoscopy via bronchial lumen.
  - For left DLT – ensure that secondary carina is unobstructed.
  - For right DLT – ensure that fenestration aligns with right upper lobe and that the middle and lower lobes are unobstructed.

[1–3]**Clinical Pearls**

1. Use of a MacIntosh blade for direct laryngoscopy may allow more space in the pharynx for DLT placement through the glottis.
2. Removing the stylet prior to rotating and advancing the DLT may reduce stylet-induced tracheobronchial injury.
3. The depth of insertion of a DLT in the adult is 29 ± 1 cm for every 10-cm difference in patient height from 170 cm.

DLT = Double-lumen tube.

An Alternative Method of Placement

- Intubate trachea with DLT.
- Remove stylet.
- Drive a bronchoscope through the bronchial lumen, and advance it in the desired bronchus.
- Advance the DLT over the bronchoscope into the bronchus.
- Confirm correct placement by bronchoscopy via the tracheal lumen.

Confirmation of DLT Placement

Visual inspection of chest rise, auscultation, and bronchoscopy are the most frequently employed techniques to confirm DLT position. Of these, bronchoscopy is sufficiently superior that its status approaches that of "standard of practice." In modern practice, visual inspection and auscultation should be regarded as adjuncts to bronchoscopy, as they have limitations.

- Visual inspection of chest rise may be subtle and be confounded by pulmonary pathology.

- The *auscultation technique* is summarized in Fig 9-2. It requires auscultation over each chest with sequential occlusion of each lumen of the DLT. Lung pathology may confound results. Studies have shown that the validity of auscultation alone is insufficient to identify up to 80% of major and minor malpositions (3).

Below describes the desired view when viewed from either the tracheal or bronchial lumen.

- Left-Sided DLT
    - Tracheal lumen (Fig 9-3A): Minimally visible inflated blue bronchial cuff in the left mainstem at the level of the carina; patent right bronchus.
    - Bronchial lumen: A clear view of the left secondary carina.
- Right-Sided DLT
    - Tracheal lumen: Minimally visible blue bronchial cuff in the right mainstem bronchus at the level of the carina; patent left mainstem.

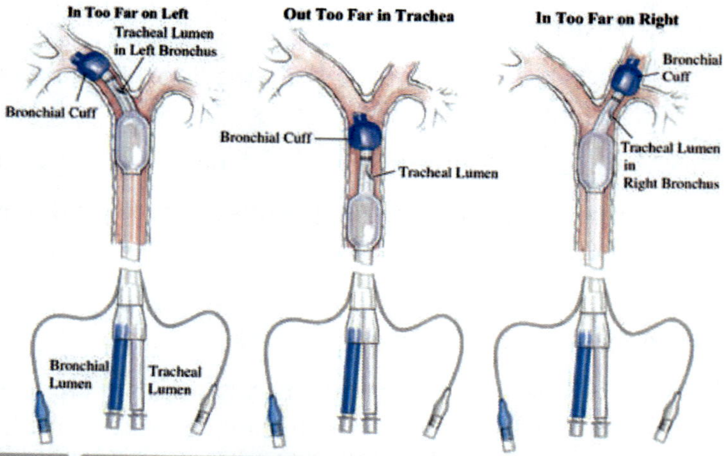

Procedure	Breath sounds		
Clamp Tracheal lumen Both Cuffs Inflated	Left	Left and right	Right
Clamp Bronchial Lumen Both Cuffs Inflated	None or very diminished	None or very diminished	None or very diminished
Clamp Bronchial Lumen Deflate Bronchial Cuff	Left	Left and right	Right

Figure 9-2 – Auscultation results for common malpositions of a left-sided DLT.

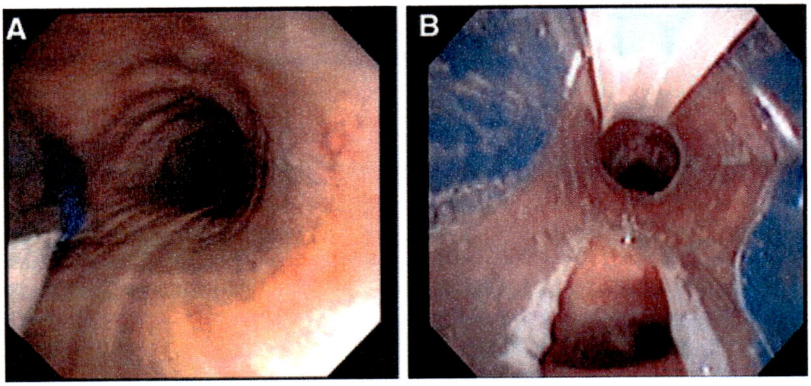

Figure 9-3 – (**A**, **B**) Bronchoscopic views of *left* and *right* double-lumen tubes (DLTs) positioned correctly. (**A**) *Left-sided DLT* (via tracheal lumen) with minimally visible *blue bronchial cuff* in the left mainstem. (**B**) *Right-sided DLT* (via bronchial lumen) with the ventilation side port aligned with the RUL orifice (06:00 h) and patent bronchus intermedius (*center*).

- Bronchial lumen (Fig 9-3B): A visible right upper lobe bronchus, aligned with the ventilation side port, as well as a clear view of the right middle and lower lobe bronchi distally from the bronchial lumen.

Any manipulation in patient position should be followed by reconfirmation of DLT position by bronchoscopy.

Troubleshooting Left-Sided DLTs

Generally speaking, there are three major types of malposition. These include in too deep, out too far, and in the wrong bronchus. This section discusses how to identify these malpositions, how to correct them, and what to do if you are uncertain of the position, as well as discusses options for difficult passage of the DLT through the airway.

Note: Prior to manipulating, the cuffs of the DLT should be deflated to aid in tube positioning and limit trauma.

In Too Deep

- Recognition.
  - Tracheal-lumen view (Fig 9-4):
    - Mucosal wall abuts tracheal outlet (medial wall of left mainstem bronchus).
    - Shadow of right mainstem may be visible through the tube above tracheal outlet on the right.
    - Bronchial-lumen view abuts secondary carina on left.
- Correction.
  - With scope positioned at tracheal outlet, withdraw DLT until primary carina comes into view.
  - Inflate bronchial cuff/fine-tune correct depth and cuff volume.

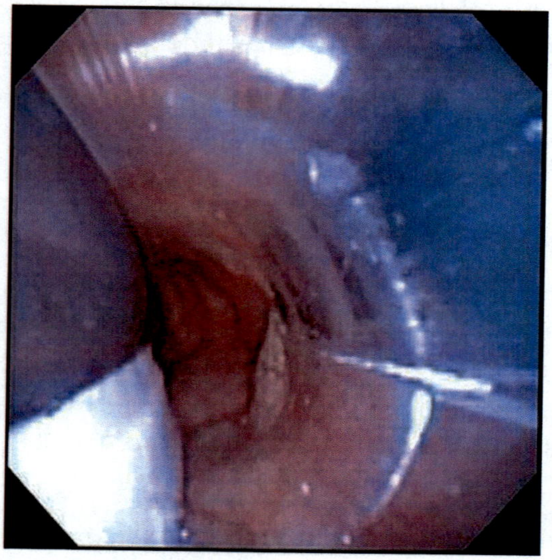

Figure 9-4 – Bronchoscopic view via the tracheal lumen of L-double-lumen tube that is in too deep. The tracheal orifice is abutting mucosa and a *shadow* is noted on the *right-hand side* of the tracheal lumen. The visible mucosa is from the left mainstem bronchus and the *shadow* is the opening to the right mainstem bronchus.

Out Too Far

- Recognition.
  - Tracheal-lumen view (Fig 9-5):
    - Mucosal wall abuts tracheal outlet (wall of trachea).
    - No shadow of right mainstem visible on the right side of tube.
    - Blue cuff may or may not be visible depending on how closely the tracheal wall abuts tracheal outlet of DLT.
    - If able to drive bronchoscope past the blue bronchial cuff, the carina should come into view.
  - Bronchial-lumen view reveals secondary carina of left mainstem distant from the bronchial lumen tip (or possibly primary carina, if DLT is out very far).

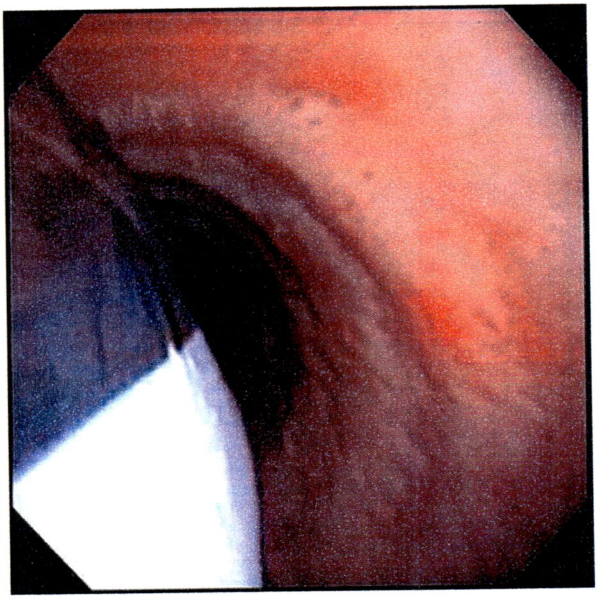

Figure 9-5 – Bronchoscopic view via tracheal lumen of L-double-lumen tube (DLT) that is out too far. Mucosa is abutting the tracheal orifice of the DLT. The *blue cuff* is visible in this example, with no view of the carina. The mucosa is that of the tracheal wall. If the bronchoscope is advanced past the *blue cuff*, one would likely encounter a view of the primary carina. Simply advancing the tube and bronchoscope together would also likely bring the carina into view and correct the position.

- Correction.
  - With scope positioned at tracheal outlet, advance DLT until primary carina comes into view. Rotation of the DLT may be required to maneuver the bronchial lumen into the left mainstem bronchus.
  - Inflate bronchial cuff/fine-tune correct depth and cuff volume.
  - (If advancement of DLT results in right endobronchial intubation, see below).

Incorrect Bronchus (Left-Sided DLT in the Right Mainstem)

- Recognition.
  - Tracheal-lumen view:
    - Mucosal wall abuts tracheal outlet (right mainstem lateral wall).

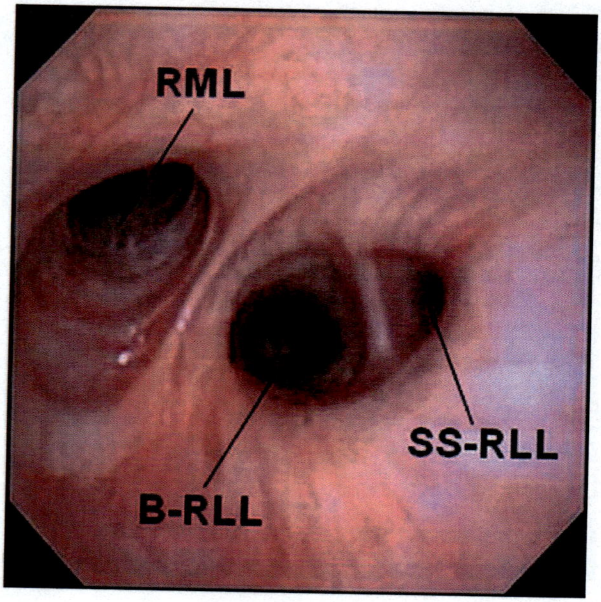

Figure 9-6 – Bronchoscopic view via the bronchial lumen of a L-double-lumen tube (DLT) that has passed into the right mainstem bronchus. The ability to recognize this view of the bronchus intermedius allows early recognition that the tube is in the *right (incorrect) bronchus*. There are typically three openings arranged more or less in a line: right middle lobe (RML), basilar segments of the right lower lobe (B-RLL), and superior segment of the RLL (SS-RLL).

- No shadow of right mainstem visible on the right side of tube.
- Bronchial-lumen view reveals anatomy of the bronchus intermedius (Fig 9-6) (Chapter 8).

Correction (two techniques):

- Technique 1:
  - With scope at tracheal-lumen outlet, withdraw DLT about 5 cm.
  - Rotate DLT toward the left mainstem bronchus.
  - Advance DLT. Carina should come into view with bronchial lumen in the left mainstem.
  - Inflate bronchial cuff/fine-tune depth and cuff volume.
- Technique 2:
  - With scope at bronchial-lumen outlet, withdraw DLT until primary carina comes into view.
  - Advance scope into left mainstem.
  - Advance DLT over scope into left mainstem.
  - Place scope in tracheal lumen. Obtain view of primary carina with the bronchial lumen in the left mainstem.
  - Inflate bronchial cuff/fine-tune depth and cuff volume.

Note that the initial view via the tracheal lumen is of mucosal wall in all the above malpositions. Most commonly, the DLT is in too far. In any case, with the scope at the tracheal outlet, withdrawal or advancement of the DLT generally brings the carina into view. If still unable to identify DLT position, see below for "Unsure of DLT position."

Unsure of DLT Position

- Position scope in bronchial-lumen at outlet.
- Withdraw scope and DLT together until primary carina comes into view.
- Confirm that the carina is the primary carina by examining the right mainstem.

- Advance scope down left mainstem.
- Advance DLT over scope.
- Place scope in tracheal lumen to confirm position.
- Inflate bronchial cuff/fine-tune depth and cuff volume.

Difficulty Passing DLT Through Glottis (Difficult Airway)

- Secure airway with SLT by difficult airway tool of your choice.
- Exchange to DLT (err on smaller size) using tube exchange catheter (Chapter 10) or use bronchial blocker (see below).

Difficulty Advancing DLT Beyond Glottis

- Causes:
    - DLT is too large.
    - DLT hangs up on tracheal rings (most common).
    - Solutions.
        - Use a smaller tube.
        - Rotation of DLT by 90–180°. This aligns bronchial tip toward the posterior membranous trachea for smooth advancement.
            - Once advancement is possible, correct for the exaggerated rotation, so the DLT enters the left mainstem bronchus.
            - Take care to remove stylet before rotating and advancing.

Difficulty Advancing into Left Mainstem Bronchus

- Causes.
    - DLT hangs up on sharp or broad carina.
    - Acute left mainstem angle takeoff.
    - Left-shifted carina.
    - DLT is too large for mainstem bronchus.
    - Solutions.

      - Use a smaller sized DLT.
      - Turn head to right while advancing DLT.
      - Drive DLT into left mainstem over bronchoscope (via bronchial lumen).
      - Revert to right-sided DLT (depending on case) or an SLT with bronchial blocker.

Troubleshooting Right-Sided DLTs

Note:

- The right mainstem bronchus needs to be at roughly >10 mm in length to be able to obtain an adequate seal.
- Partial alignment of fenestration with right upper lobe is preferable to a bronchial cuff that is herniated over the carina. Cuff herniation may lead to an air leak and inadequate lung isolation.

Difficulty Aligning Fenestration with Right Upper Lobe

- Causes.
  - Rarely, DLT is in wrong side (see above).
  - Usually, DLT is too deep (Fig 9-7) and/or rotated.
  - Solution.
    - With scope in bronchial lumen and with view of ventilation side port, withdraw and/or rotate DLT.
    - Recheck the view of primary carina via tracheal lumen to confirm that bronchial cuff is still well-seated.

Difficulty Due to Short Right Mainstem Bronchus

If aligning fenestration with right upper lobe results in withdrawal of DLT to the point where the bronchial cuff herniates over the primary carina and fails to isolate the lung (i.e., air leaks past the bronchial cuff), there are two options.

- Convert to SLT and bronchial blocker.
- Position a bronchial blocker in the left mainstem bronchus such that the cuff completes the air seal.

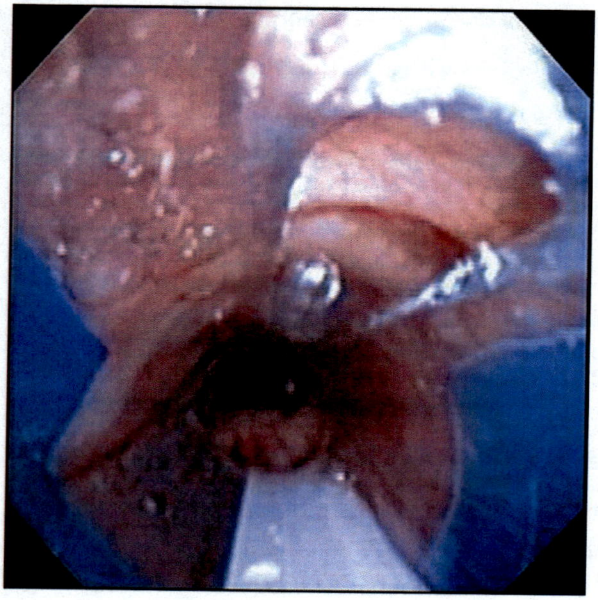

Figure 9-7 – Bronchoscopic view via bronchial lumen of a R-double-lumen tube (DLT) that is in too deep. The ventilation side port is abutting the mucosa of the *right-sided bronchus* and not aligned with the RUL bronchus. Correction requires withdrawal of the DLT until the RUL bronchus comes into view. Confirmation that the DLT is in the correct side is obtained by identifying the primary carina via the tracheal lumen.

Box 9-5 – Complications of DLTs

Hoarseness.

Vocal cord or upper airway injury.

Trauma or perforation of trachea or bronchus (usually, the membranous portion).

Hypoxemia.

Hypercarbia.

Air trapping, dynamic hyperinflation (leading to hemodyamic compromise).

Mucosal ischemia from cuff overinflation (strictures).

Bronchial Blockers and Blocker Systems

Knowledge of bronchial blockers may allow one to circumvent the disadvantages associated with DLTs (Box 9-2B). Blockers are advantageous for patients with difficult airway anatomy, who require lung isolation. See Box 9-6 for advantages/disadvantages for bronchial blockers.

Box 9-6A, B – Advantages and Disadvantages of Bronchial Blockers

A: Advantages

Can be placed through an existing SLT or through tracheostomy.

Easier than DLT for difficult intubations.

No need for ETT exchange at end of procedure if postoperative ventilation is required.

May be used for selective lobar blockade.

Useful in the pediatric population.

Can rescue an ill-fitting DLT.

Most have central lumens to allow air egress, insufflation, CPAP, or jet ventilation.

SLT single-lumen tube, *ETT* endotracheal tube, *CPAP* continuous positive airway pressure.

B: Disadvantages

Longer time for lung collapse (often clinically insignificant).

Longer time to position (operator dependent).

Potential for dislodgement leading to tracheal occlusion during patient positioning and surgical manipulation.

Not ideal for right-sided procedures (right mainstem anatomy precludes positioning of BB deeply into the right, predisposing to dislodgement).

Inclusion of the BB into the staple line.

Small lumen for suctioning/CPAP.

BB bronchial blocker, *CPAP* continuous positive airway pressure.

Design

All bronchial blockers have the same general features, but each differs in its mechanism for blocker placement. See Table 9-3 for specific design characteristics of the individual blockers/blocker systems.

General Features

- 50–78-cm hollow bore catheter (internal diameter 1.4–2.0 mm).
- Bronchial cuff on the distal end with a corresponding pilot balloon.

Once placed into the bronchus and cuff is inflated, the blocker prevents ventilation to that bronchus. The hollow catheter allows for deflation of the lung, application of CPAP, and for suctioning (although each is limited due to the small internal lumen of the catheter).

Of the available blockers on the market, all require an independent SLT, with the exception of the Torque Control Blocker (TCB) Univent Tube® (Vitaid, Lewiston, NY). The TCB Univent is a specialized tube that has a bronchial blocker incorporated into an endotracheal tube (see below).

Arndt Bronchial Blocker® (Cook Inc., Bloomington, IN) (Fig 9-8A, B)

This bronchial blocker system is designed to pass through a SLT using a multiport adapter. IT is steered by a nylon wire looped around the bronchoscope. When in place, the wire is removed, leaving a patent central lumen for air egress, CPAP, air insufflation, jet ventilation, or suction.

Table 9-3 – Types and characteristics of various bronchial blockers

CHARACTERISTIC	ARNDT WEB BLOCKER	COHEN BLOCKER	UNIBLOCKER WITH TCB	TCB UNIVENT TUBE
Size	5F, 7F, and 9F	9F	9F	Adult: 6.0–9.0mm Pediatric: 3.5 and 4.5mm
Balloon shape	Spherical	Pear shaped	Spherical	Spherical
Cuff inflation volume	5F (0.5–2cc) 7F (2.0–6.0 cc) 9F spherical (4.0–8.0 cc) 9F elliptical (6.0–12.0 cc) (recently discontinued)	5–8cc	5–8cc	Adult: 4–8cc
Cuff type	High volume/low pressure	High volume/ low pressure	High volume/low pressure	High volume/low pressure
Guidance mechanism	Nylon wire loop (replaceable in 9F only)	Wheel device to deflect the tip	None, preshaped tip	None, preshaped tip

(continued)

Table 9-3 – (continued)

CHARACTERISTIC	ARNDT WEB BLOCKER	COHEN BLOCKER	UNIBLOCKER WITH TCB	TCB UNIVENT TUBE
Smallest recommended ETT for coaxial use	5F (4.5 ETT)* 7F (7.5 ETT)* 9F (8.0 ETT)*	9F (8.0 ETT)*	9F (8.0 ETT)	N/A
Murphy eye	Present in 9F	Present	Not present	Present
Center channel internal diameter	1.4 mm (7–9F) 0.7 mm (5F)	1.6 mm	2.0 mm	2.0 mm

F=French, *WEB*= wire-guided endobronchial blocker, *TCB*=torque control blocker, *FOB*=fiberoptic bronchoscope, *ETT*=endotracheal tube.

*Using a small pediatric FOB (3.4 mm) can decrease ETT by 0.5mm (Per www.cookmedical.com).

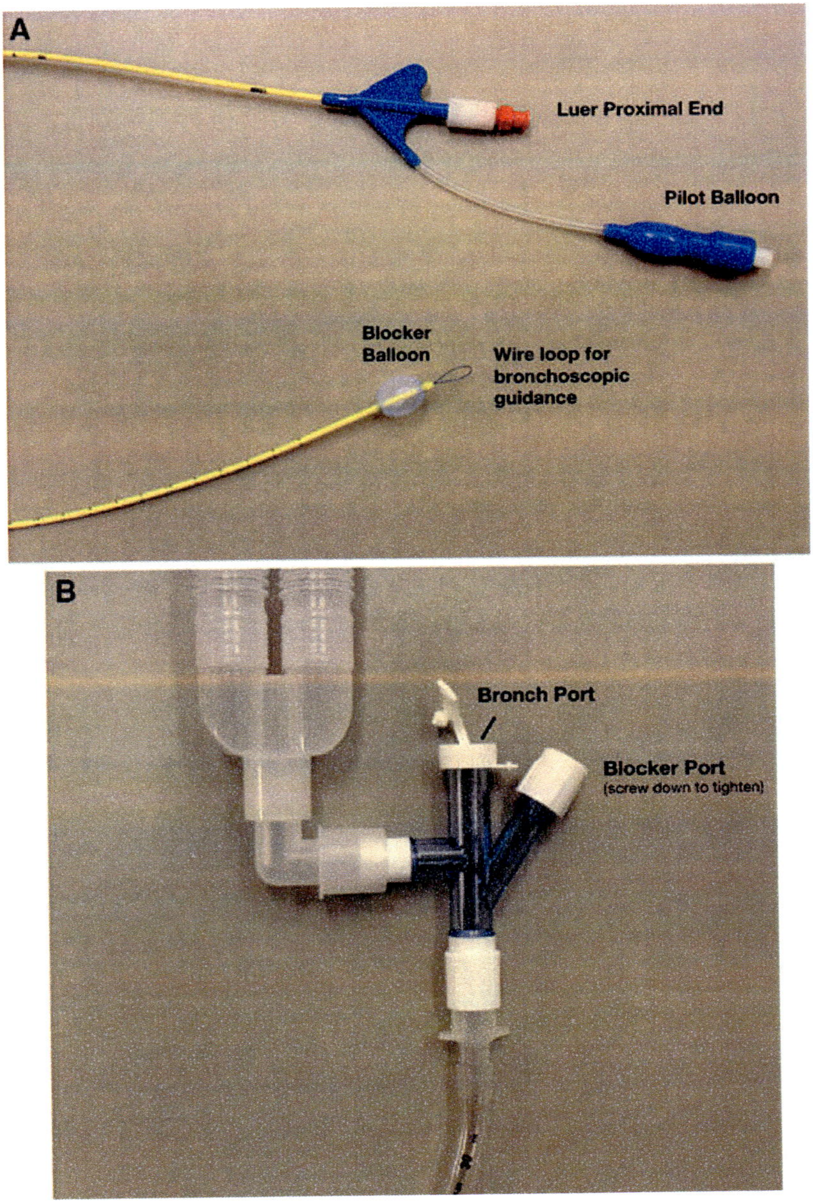

Figure 9-8 – (**A**, **B**) The Arndt bronchial blocker system and multiport adapter.

The multiport adapter has three ports:

1. A port with a luer-lock mechanism for the blocker to eliminate an air leak, when tightened
2. A port with a diaphragm for the bronchoscope
3. A port with a 15-mm connector for the anesthesia circuit

Insertion Technique (Box 9-7)

Box 9-7 – Insertion of Arndt Bronchial Blocker

Recommended Steps for Placement of an Arndt Bronchial Blocker

- Preassemble blocker and scope through the multiport adapter. Couple the blocker and bronchoscope by passing scope through wire loop (Fig 9-9).
- Attach assembly to the ETT.
- Attach the anesthesia circuit onto the circuit connector of the adapter.

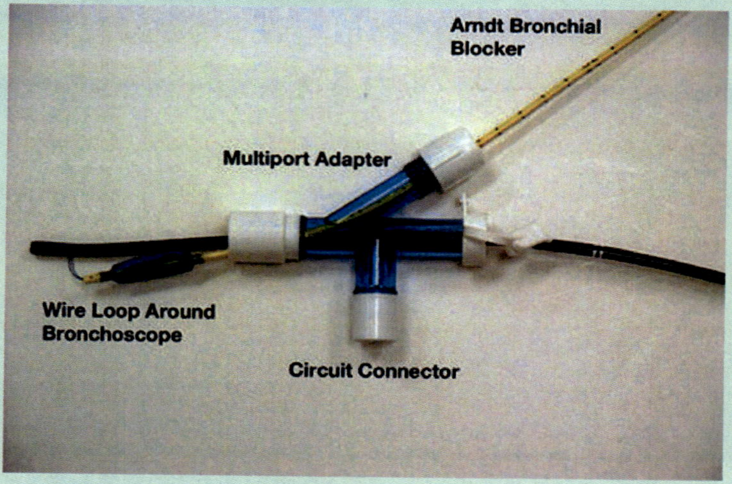

Figure 9-9 – Bronchoscope and blocker loaded through multiport adapter and coupled.

(continued)

Box 9-7 – (continued)

- Placement[1,2]: Two Methods
  - 1: Advance the bronchoscope into the desired bronchus, and then advance the coupled blocker along the bronchoscope into the bronchus[3].
  - 2: Tightly couple the blocker to the bronchoscope by pulling on the proximal end of the nylon wire and advance the assembly together into the desired bronchus.
- Screw tighten the variable orifice mechanism to fix the blocker and prevent air leak.
- Inflate balloon under direct vision with 6–10-cc air (lung isolation begun).
- Cuff should be approximately 2 mm below the carina for left-sided lung isolation and just below the carina for right-sided lung isolation.
- Remove nylon wire to assist lung deflation[4].
- Bronchoscopically reconfirm blocker position with any position change of the patient.

[1-4]**Notes**

1. Right-sided blockers are easier to place, but isolation may be variable depending on the location of the RUL takeoff.
2. Attempts at left mainstem placements may occasionally fail because the BB becomes "hung up" on the carina (see below).
3. Ventilation can be continuous during placement of a bronchial blocker, but an air leak is present until the diaphragm is closed around the blocker.
4. The nylon wire is replaceable in the 9 Fr size only.

General Troubleshooting of Blocker Placement

The principal technical problem with the Arndt BB system is that it can get "hung up" on the carina when attempting to advance it into the left mainstem bronchus. A solution is to turn the patient's head to the right side, and then advance the tightly coupled scope/blocker into the left mainstem with the bronchoscope flexed toward lateral aspect of left mainstem. This technique can assist in positioning any of the blocker or blocker systems described in this text.

Cohen Tip Deflecting Endobronchial Blocker® (Cook Critical Care, Bloomington, IN) (Fig 9-10)

Specific Design Considerations

- See above (Table 9-3).
- Like the Arndt Bronchial Blocker, it is packaged with a multiport adapter to allow for coaxial use with a SLT.
- 3-cm nylon tip that is deflected up to 90° by rotation of a proximal wheel.
- 2-cm external plastic sleeve (gripper) to aid in blocker maneuvering/rotation.

Insertion Technique

Placement of the Cohen Bronchial Blocker has the same general considerations as placing the Arndt Bronchial blocker (Box 9-7). Once the blocker is placed through the SLT via the multiport adapter, the proximal wheel is rotated counterclockwise to create tip deflection. The blocker itself is turned toward, and inserted into the desired

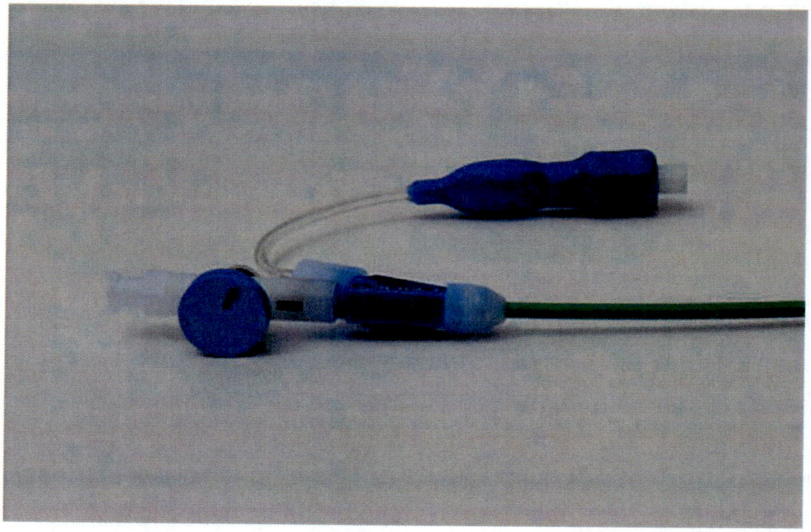

Figure 9-10 – Cohen tip deflecting endobronchial blocker counterclockwise rotation of the wheel deflects the tip. To return the blocker tip to neutral, rotate the wheel clockwise, until the two black lines align.

bronchus, under fiber-optic visualization. Once positioned, the balloon is inflated (desired position 1–2 mm below the carina), initiating lung isolation. The multiport adapter is tightened around the blocker to eliminate leaks, and the bronchoscope is removed.

The TCB Univent® Tube with (Vitaid, Lewiston, NY) (Fig 9-11)

The TCB Univent Tube is essentially a SLT with an incorporated bronchial blocker. The tip of the blocker has a preformed bend which allows some directional control by exerting torque at the proximal end. The larger external-to-internal diameter imposed by the encorporated blocker may increase airway resistance or risk of airway

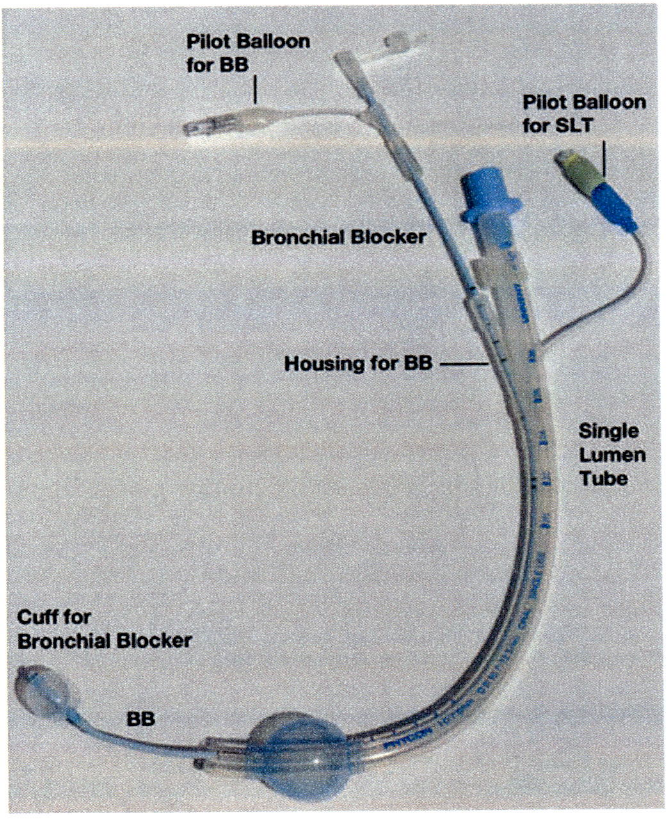

Figure 9-11 – Torque Control Blocker Univent tube.

injury. Advocates tout its ease of use. A variation called the Uniblocker® (Vitaid) is an attachment for traditional SLTs that houses a blocker system similar to the Univent.

Specific Design Considerations

- See above (Table 9-3) and Fig. 9-11.
- SLT that has a separate attached lumen on the concave surface that houses a bronchial blocker.
- External shape is oval. A 7.0 TCB Univent® tube has external diameters of 10.7/12.5 mm. The larger diameter reflects the anterior-posterior dimension. In contrast, a 7.0 SLT has an external diameter of 9.6 mm.
- Malleable blocker with preformed distal bend to aid positioning.
- A blocker cap connector, on the proximal end of the blocker, prevents air leakage during two-lung ventilation.
- Constructed of medical-grade polymeric silicone.
- Available in a variety of sizes, from pediatric to adult.

Insertion Technique

The TCB Univent Tube is placed under direct laryngoscopy. Once intratracheal placement has been confirmed, the blocker is directed toward the desired bronchus by rotating the blocker under bronchoscopic visualization. If blocker placement proves challenging:

- Intubate the desired bronchus with the bronchoscope (through the Univent tube).
- Advance the tube over the bronchoscope into the bronchus.
- Place the blocker into the bronchus.
- Retract the tube to the trachea.
- Evaluate blocker position bronchoscopically.

Fogarty Arterial Embolectomy Catheter® (Edward Lifesciences, Irvine, CA) (Fig 9-12)

Although not designed as a bronchial blocker, an 8/14 or 8/22 Fr Fogarty® embolectomy catheter can be used to achieve lung isolation.

Specific Design Considerations

- Does not have a central lumen (precludes suctioning/CPAP and impairs air egress).
- Malleable wire stylet may be bent 45° at the distal end to provide a directionality for placement.

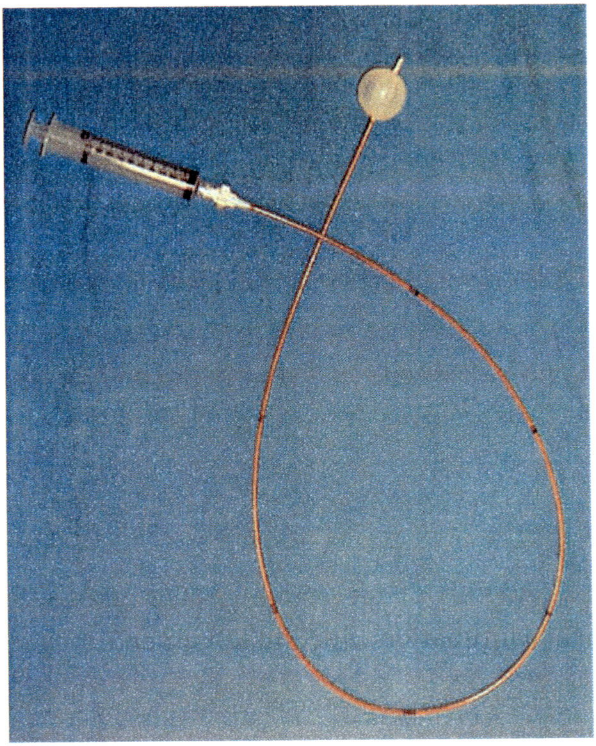

Figure 9-12 – Fogarty embolectomy catheter.

Insertion Technique: See Box 9-8

Box 9-8 – Insertion of a Fogarty Catheter

Preparation of the Fogarty:

- Test cuff.
- Lubricate the Fogarty with water-based lubricant.
- Make a 45° bend at the distal end, 3 cm from the tip.

Insertion of a Fogarty catheter:

- Perform direct laryngoscopy.
- Intubate the trachea first with the Fogarty catheter.
- Place a single-lumen 8.0 ETT *alongside* the catheter.
- Pass a pediatric fiber-optic bronchoscope through the lumen of the ETT to guide the blocker into the mainstem bronchus of choice.

Alternative method:

- Utilize the multiport adapter from the Arndt blocker set (Cook) to allow for the Fogarty to be placed through the SLT.

ETT endotracheal tube, *SLT* single-lumen tube.

Complications of Bronchial Blockers: Box 9-9

Box 9-9 – Complications of Bronchial Blockers

Malposition/dislodgement of the blocker.

Inclusion into the staple line.

Hypoxia/hypercarbia.

Mucosal ischemia from excessive cuff pressure.

Endobronchial Intubation with Single-Lumen Tubes

It is often forgotten that lung isolation can be achieved by advancing an SLT into a mainstem bronchus. Endobronchial intubation for lung isolation has advantages and disadvantages (Box 9-10).

This technique is principally employed in emergent situations (e.g., massive hemoptysis). Blind advancement of a SLT intubates the right mainstem, but the right upper lobe is typically occluded by the cuff. To intubate the left mainstem, two techniques are employed:

1. Advancing the SLT over a bronchoscope that is positioned in the left mainstem to serve as a stylet.
2. With the head turned to the right and the SLT rotated 180° (bevel pointing to the left), blind advancement of the SLT often enters the left mainstem.

If tube length is a limiting factor, extended tubes may be fashioned (Chapter 30) or nasal rae tubes may be used orally. Specifically designed endobronchial tubes are available in Europe, but not FDA approved for the USA at the time of this writing.

Box 9-10 – Advantages and Disadvantages of Endobronchial Intubation

A: Advantages of Endobronchial Intubation

Can be easily and rapidly performed in emergencies (especially, right endobronchial intubation).

Useful in small children.

May be useful in tracheal resection surgery (Chapter 30).

Obviates the need for tube exchanges.

Large, low-resistance conduit for ventilation or unilateral suction.

B: Disadvantages of Endobronchial Intubation

Left mainstem intubation can be challenging (esp. with copious blood/pus).

Unable to administer CPAP.

Unable to suction or pass bronchoscope into the contralateral lung without losing lung isolation.

Difficult to know the depth of insertion relative to carina.

Relies on passive deflation of the nonventilated lung.

ETT too short for naso-tracheobronchial intubation.

Right endobronchial intubation usually occludes right upper lobe.

Selected Special Lung Isolation Situations

RUL Anomolies

Congenital aberrancies of the tracheobronchial tree occur in roughly 10% of the general population. The most common of these aberrancies include an abnormal location and/or configuration of the RUL bronchus.

- Short, right mainstem bronchus:

  Normally, the right mainstem bronchus is 18 mm in length. In some patients, the right upper lobe bronchus may emerge from the right mainstem bronchus <10 mm from the primary carina.

- Tracheal bronchus (TB):

  A tracheal bronchus (TB) is any airway that emerges from the lateral tracheal wall. Tracheal bronchi are present in 1–3% of the general population. The airway may consist of one or more of the segmental bronchi of the right upper lobe or the right upper lobe in its entirety.

  Tracheal bronchi are classified according to the distance the airway emerges from the carina and the presence or absence of tracheal narrowing distal to the airway. Type I is >2 cm from the carina with a narrowed trachea distally. Type II is >2 cm from the carina with a normal tracheal diameter distally. A type III TB emerges at or near the carina (also called carinal bronchus) (Fig 9-13).

  Tracheal bronchi can be displaced or supernumerary. Displaced indicates that one or more of the segmental bronchi are located on the lateral tracheal wall instead of the right upper lobe. Displacement of the entire right upper lobe bronchus is referred to as a "pig bronchus," as this is the normal morphology in swine. Supernumerary refers to the presence of one or more of the segmental bronchi on the lateral tracheal wall in addition to the presence of a normal right upper lobe bronchus off of the right mainstem bronchus.

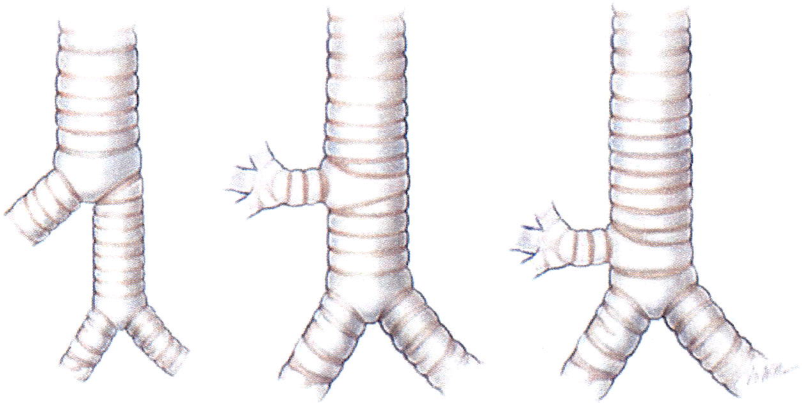

Figure 9-13 – Types of tracheal bronchi categories of tracheal bronchi. See text for explanation. From Wiser and Hartigan (4) (original artwork by Marcia Williams; reproduced with permission).

Anesthetic Implications

Right-sided DLTs fit poorly in patients with a short, right mainstem bronchus or TB. The right upper lobe fenestration of the right-sided DLT is unlikely to be aligned with the RUL bronchus in a patient with a short, right mainstem bronchus while maintaining an adequate air seal. Likewise, it is not possible to ventilate a TB with a right-sided DLT. Since there is insufficient alignment of the fenestration with the RUL, poor ventilation and atelectasis ensue with significant risk of hypoxemia.

Most procedures can be safely performed with a left-sided DLT. For left mainstem procedures (e.g., sleeve resection, left-sided pneumonectomy, or left-sided lung transplant), one could use a left-sided DLT or bronchial blocker, provided the device is withdrawn as needed, i.e., for surgical resection of the bronchus. A right-sided DLT may be required if an exophytic tumor of the left mainstem is present. In this circumstance, the RUL would not be ventilated, and the ability to provide CPAP to the nondependent lung may be required to mitigate hypoxemia.

Tracheostomy

Options for lung isolation, when there is a tracheostomy, include placement of a BB through (using a multiport adapter), alongside the tracheostomy tube, or past the tracheostomy cuff via the oral or nasal route while ventilating through the tracheostomy. One can also remove the tracheostomy tube and replace it with a DLT via the glottis or the stoma. Securing a DLT placed through a stoma can be awkward. The size and maturity of the stoma may also influence these decisions.

Tracheal Deviation

Tracheal deviation may occasionally make lung isolation more challenging if the curvature directs the DLT toward the unintended bronchus. Bronchoscopic guidance may be needed to direct the DLT into the proper location.

Tracheal Stenosis

Tracheal stenosis can be fixed or dynamic (see Chapters 20 and 30). The length of narrowing may be short or encompasses the majority of the trachea. A saber sheath trachea typically has a narrowing of the width of the distal 2/3 of the trachea. In general, tracheal stenosis may hinder the placement of large endotracheal tubes, including DLTs. Often, a bronchial blocker is more convenient.

Left-Shifted Carina

Patients with a left-shifted carina may make placement of a left-sided DLT challenging. If a left DLT cannot be placed, one could consider a bronchial blocker or right-sided DLT, depending on the clinical circumstances.

Selected References

1. Hannallah MS et al. The resting volume and compliance characteristics of the bronchial cuff of left polyvinyl chloride double-lumen endobronchial tubes. Anesth Analg. 1993;77:1222–6.

2. Slinger PD, Lesiuk L. Flow resistances of disposable double-lumen, single lumen, and Univent tubes. J Cardiothorac Vas Anesth. 1998;12:142.

3. Alliaume B, Coddens J, Deloof T. reliability of ausculatation in positioning of double-lumen endobronchial tubes. Can J Anesth. 1992;39(7):687–90.

4. Wiser SH, Hartigan PM. Challenging lung isolation secondary to aberrant tracheo-bronchial anatomy. Anesth Analg. 2011;112:688–92.

Further Suggested Reading

Campos. Current techniques for perioperative lung isolation in adults. Anesthesiology. 2002;97:1295–301.

Campos. An update on bronchial blockers during lung separation techniques in adults. Anesth Analg. 2003; 97:1266–74.

Neustein SM. The use of bronchial blockers for providing one-lung venitlation. J Cardiothorac Vas Anesth. 2009;23(6):860–8.

Slinger PD. Lung isolation in thoracic anesthesia, state of the art. Can J Anesth. 2001;48:R110.

Chapter 10
Special Airway Devices for Thoracic Anesthesia: CPAP, PEEP, and Airway Exchange Catheters

Sarah H. Wiser

Keywords CPAP • PEEP • Airway Exchange Catheters • Positive End-Expiratory Pressure Tube Exchange Catheters • Continuous Positive Airway Pressure

Introduction

Treatment of hypoxemia during OLV and tube exchanges between single and double lumen tubes are situations unique to thoracic anesthesia which require special airway devices. This chapter focuses on technical aspects of the following devices:

- Positive End-Expiratory Pressure (PEEP) valve for OLV
- Continuous Positive Airway Pressure (CPAP) device for OLV
- Tube Exchange Catheters (TEC) for double lumen tubes

PEEP and CPAP Devices for OLV

Common causes of hypoxemia during OLV include V/Q mismatch and shunt in both the dependent and nondependent lungs (Chapter 5). PEEP and CPAP are commonly employed techniques to mitigate hypoxemia. The technical application of each is described below. Selected physiologic aspects of PEEP and CPAP are briefly

P.M. Hartigan (ed.), *Practical Handbook of Thoracic Anesthesia*,
DOI 10.1007/978-0-387-88493-6_10, © Springer Science+Business Media, LLC 2012

presented for context, but the reader is referred to Chapter 5 for clinical application essentials.

PEEP Valve Devices

A *PEEP valve* is a device which maintains airway pressure at end-exhalation.

Physiology and Rationale for PEEP

During two-lung mechanical ventilation, PEEP is well known as a means to potentially enhance oxygenation by preventing small airway closure. Optimal PEEP may also improve compliance and potentially decrease cyclic alveolar collapse-related lung injury (atelectotrauma) (1). Excessive PEEP may cause barotrauma or impair venous return and cardiac output by increasing intrathoracic pressure.

During OLV, the dependent lung is prone to atelectasis due to anesthesia (reduced FRC), the lateral position, gravity, and surgical pressure on the mediastinum. In some patients, PEEP selectively applied to the *dependent lung* may diminish atelectasis and improve oxygenation. Excessive dependent-lung PEEP during OLV may over-distend dependent-lung units, increase dependent-lung vascular resistance, and redirect perfusion to the nondependent lung. In addition to exacerbating hypoxemia, excessive PEEP may cause barotrauma and impair cardiac output, as can occur in two-lung ventilation. The quantity of PEEP must therefore be titrated during OLV based on the patient's respiratory compliance and response (Chapter 5).

How Does a PEEP Valve Work?

The simplest PEEP valve consists of a spring exerting tension on a diaphragm (Fig 10-1). The diaphragm allows flow as long as the airway pressure exceeds the counterforce of the spring against the

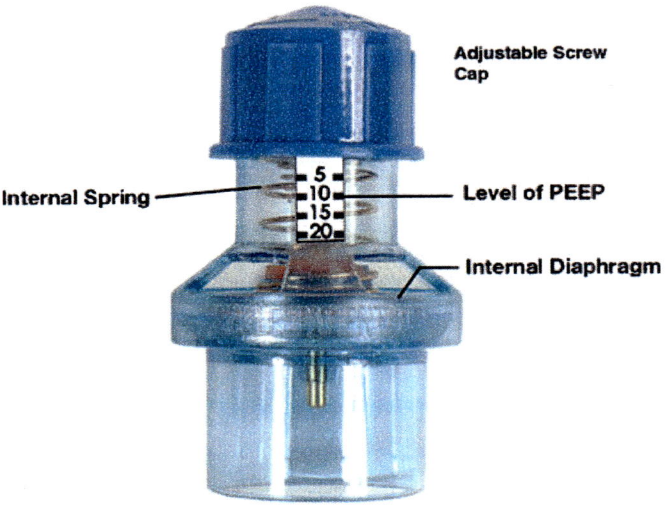

Figure 10-1 – The pictured simple, disposable spring PEEP valve allows for variable levels of PEEP. Clockwise rotation of the adjustable screw increases the level of PEEP applied. The approximate amount is indicated by the numbers on the side. The rotation increases the force by which the spring exerts pressure onto the diaphragm, impeding airflow during exhalation, thereby providing end-expiratory pressure.

diaphragm. During exhalation, as the airway pressure declines to below the set PEEP value, the diaphragm closes, preventing further decline of end-expiratory pressure.

An ideal PEEP valve (which does not exist) would be independent of gas flow. All PEEP valves are, to some extent, governed by flow through the device, according to Ohm's Law, where expiratory pressure established is proportional to resistance times flow. For a given resistance, the pressure exerted is proportional to the flow of the device. Therefore, at higher flows, the PEEP applied will be higher than the set value and prolong exhalation. Some mechanisms of generating PEEP are more efficient than others (see below).

Spring systems, as described above, electronic, pneumatic, magnetic, and ball valve systems are the various mechanisms used to generate PEEP. PEEP devices may be integrated into the ventilator or may be separate devices that are attached directly into the anesthesia circuit, CPAP device, or manual resuscitator bag.

Attachable PEEP Valves

If one is using an older anesthesia machine, one must obtain a PEEP valve that attaches to the *expiratory limb* of the anesthetic circuit. PEEP valves are either uni- or bidirectional. They may have an adjustable amount of PEEP or may come in fixed increments of PEEP (usually 2.5, 5, 7.5, 10 cm H_2O, etc.). Attachable PEEP valves are less efficient than integrated systems. They are set at a specific amount of PEEP, thus are highly subject to the effects of Ohm's law. The amount of PEEP delivered by attachable PEEP valves may be inaccurate at low or high airflows, and prolong the expiratory phase of the ventilatory cycle.

In order to deliver PEEP, one must orient the PEEP valve properly in the circuit. Proper orientation requires the arrows on the PEEP valve to follow the direction of airflow in the *expiratory limb* of the anesthesia circuit (Fig 10-2). Improper placement of PEEP valves will lead to the lack of application of PEEP or ZEEP (Zero End-Expiratory Pressure).

This is an improvement over the original unidirectional mechanical PEEP valves, which obstructed airflow if placed backwards in the circuit. Severe airway obstruction, and death, has been reported following such misapplication of unidirectional PEEP valves (2). Misapplication of current bidirectional PEEP valves does not obstruct airflow, but fails to deliver PEEP.

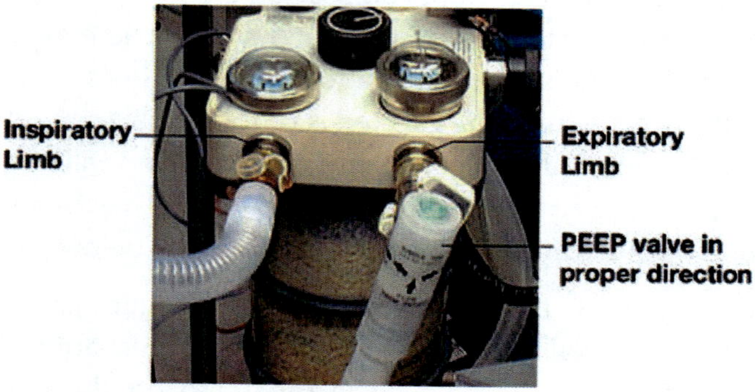

Figure 10-2 – Attachable fixed PEEP valve located on expiratory limb of circuit. *Note*: *Arrows* on the PEEP valve indicating the direction of air flow. Photo by James H. Philip, MD, jim@lifename.com.

Advantages of attachable PEEP valves include: simplicity, low expense, applicability to any standard anesthesia breathing circuit, and ability to attach to manual resuscitator bags for transport or to separate devices for the application of CPAP during OLV (see below).

Integrated PEEP Valves

In modern anesthesia machines, PEEP can be applied by push-button or dial, using the machine's electronic menu. In integrated systems, the PEEP is generated through the expiratory valve by either an electronic (proportional linear solenoid) or pneumatic mechanism that alters the force exerted on the diaphragm. These mechanisms are actively controlled during the expiratory phase of the ventilatory cycle. Due to the active control of PEEP, these devices are more accurate at high and low airflows, and the efficiency of exhalation is better maintained, minimizing the prolongation between peak inspiratory pressure to baseline airway pressure.

Depending on the machine, the application of PEEP may have varying effects on ventilation during pressure control ventilation. Two examples (Fig 10-3A and B):

1. Aisys® (General Electric Healthcare, Madison, WI)
   - The PEEP selected will be additive to the selected driving pressure, thus increasing the peak inspiratory pressure ceiling. Delta pressure would be unchanged and tidal volume would be preserved (assuming no change in compliance).
2. Fabius GS® (Drager Medical AG & Co. KG, Lübeck, Germany)
   - The PEEP selected will be incorporated into the selected driving pressure. Thus, the peak inspiratory pressure ceiling remains unchanged, but the tidal volume will diminish due to a decrease in the delta pressure.

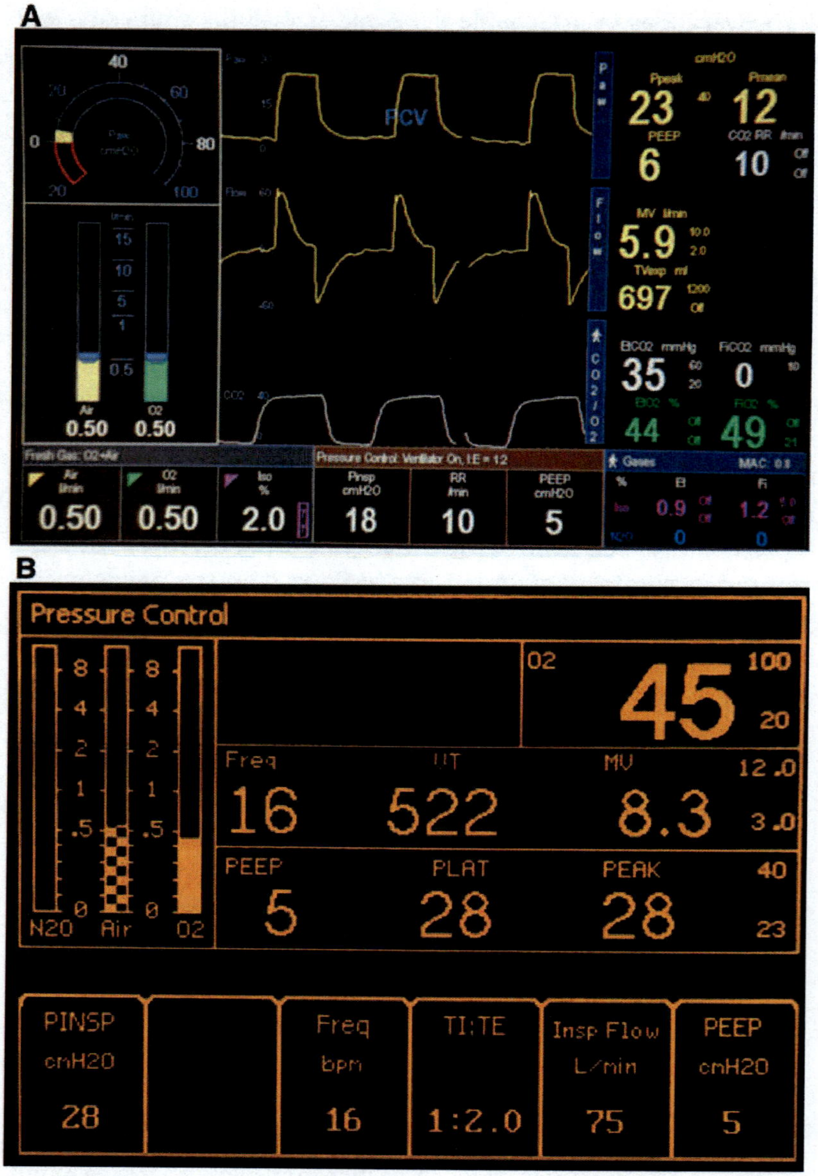

Figure 10-3 – Effect of PEEP on ventilation in: (**A**) Aisys and (**B**) Fabius during pressure control mode. (**A**) Aisys: Note set inspiratory pressure = 18 cm H_2O, set PEEP = 5 cm H_2O, and measured peak pressure = 23 cm H_2O. The PEEP is additive to the set driving pressure, but delta pressure remains 18 cm H_2O. Barring compliance change, tidal volume would be unaffected by PEEP. (**B**) Fabius: Note set inspiratory pressure = 28 cm H_2O, set PEEP = 5 cm H_2O, and measured peak pressure = 28 cm H_2O. The PEEP is incorporated into the driving pressure. Adding PEEP to this system results in reduced delta pressure and reduced tidal volumes unless the inspiratory pressure limit is similarly increased.

The above effect on ventilation is avoided if one utilizes volume control. However, peak and mean airway pressures will be affected by the addition of PEEP.

The advantages of integrated PEEP valves, besides convenience of use, include improved accuracy and elimination of misapplication errors.

PEEP applied by integrated or attachable PEEP valves is sometimes referred to as *Extrinsic PEEP*, to be distinguished from *Intrinsic PEEP*, or *Auto PEEP* which results from air trapping due to expiratory airflow resistance from the patient's own airways. Intrinsic PEEP results from obstructive lung disease and/or inadequate expiratory time for the tidal volumes delivered. Intrinsic PEEP is common during OLV and there are important potential interactions between intrinsic and extrinsic PEEP to be aware of (Chapter 5).

CPAP Device

A CPAP Device in OLV is a device that provides continuous oxygen to the nondependent lung in a nonventilatory fashion. There are various commercial CPAP devices on the market. Generally speaking, the device should have a (Fig 10-4):

1. Fresh gas inlet
2. Mechanism that retards egress of flow from the lung (e.g., PEEP valve)
3. Manometer
4. Inline reservoir bag for intermittent ventilation/inflation (optional)

CPAP to the nondependent lung improves oxygenation by reducing nondependent lung shunt without fully reinflating or ventilating that operative lung. The application of CPAP to the *nondependent* (nonventilated) lung can be very effective in treating hypoxemia (3). However, CPAP can hinder surgical exposure, especially in thoracoscopic procedures, therefore may not be the first

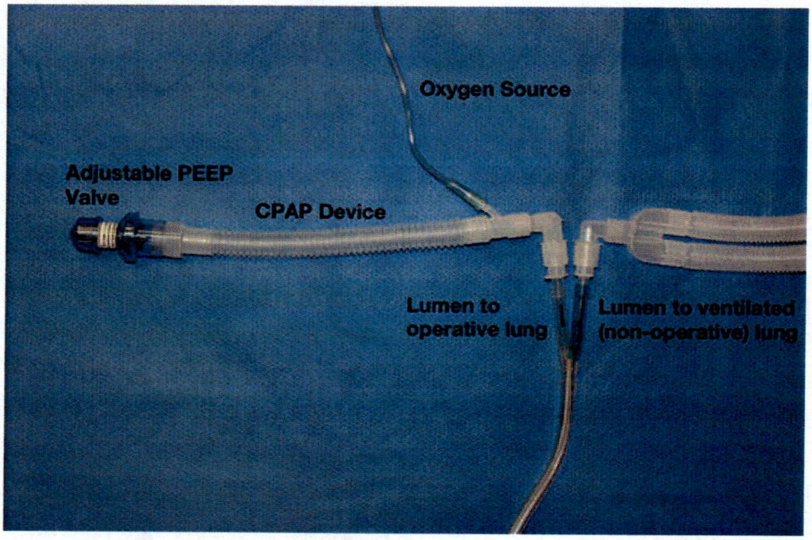

Figure 10-4 – Anatomy of a basic CPAP device. Figure shows how to connect the device to a DLT. Here the CPAP device is attached to the nondependent lumen (operative lung) of the DLT, and the anesthesia circuit is attached to the dependent lumen (non operative lung) of the DLT.

Box 10-1 – How to initiate CPAP during OLV

Initiating CPAP during OLV:

- Set the PEEP valve to the desired amount of CPAP (5–10 cm H_2O)
- Connect the fresh gas inlet to an auxiliary oxygen source
- Set auxiliary oxygen source to a flow of 5 L/min
- Connect the CPAP device to the 15 mm connector of the nondependent side of the DLT (or to the 15 mm connector for the bronchial blocker)

choice of therapy for minimally invasive thoracic procedures (Chapter 5).

Box 10-1 provides the steps to initiate CPAP during OLV. *Note: To obtain the best results, CPAP should be applied prior to lung deflation or following a partial recruitment maneuver.*

Disadvantages of Intraoperative CPAP Include:

- Hindrance of lung deflation, obscuring surgical exposure
- Risk of airway fire with the use of electrocaudery

Double Lumen Tube Exchange Catheters

During the course of an anesthetic for thoracic surgery, one generally needs to change the endotracheal tube for pre- and/or postoperative bronchoscopy and/or postoperative ventilation. Each of these encounters bears the risk of losing the airway due to edema or difficult anatomy. In addition, conditions for laryngoscopy (anesthetic depth and paralysis) may be suboptimal if one is planning emergence immediately following terminal bronchoscopy. If postoperative ventilation is planned, one must always consider the risks of leaving a DLT in place vs. changing the DLT to a SLT (Table 10-1).

Whether the plan is for postoperative ventilation, or extubation following terminal bronchoscopy, it is the practice at the authors' institution to change the DLT to a SLT. The following precautions are emphasized for safety:

- Clear communication with the surgeon and OR staff regarding the level of concern over the airway
- Surgeon in the room during tube change
- Readily available fiberoptic bronchoscope, LMA, and/or other rescue device(s)
- Optimal patient conditions:
    - Paralysis (goal 1 twitch on train of four monitor at the time of tube change, if plan to extubate following postoperative bronchoscopy)
    - Optimal positioning

The use of a tube exchange catheter can aid in the transition from a DLT to a SLT, but does not guarantee protection against the loss of airway. Experience and attention to details of the technique are essential to ensure success and safety.

Table 10-1 – Risks vs. benefits of tube exchange.

Risks of Postoperative DLT	Risks of Tube Exchange
▪ ICU personnel unfamiliar with DLT ▪ Higher airflow resistance (Mallinckrodt DLT) can impede weaning (see Chapter 9) ▪ Dislodgement causing hypoxemia ▪ Risk of mucus plugging in the lumen ▪ Difficulty in suctioning (requires a smaller and longer suction catheter) ▪ Airway trauma and edema ▪ Need to readdress airway at a later date ▪ Vocal cord injury	▪ Loss of airway ▪ Damage to airway by exchange catheter
Benefits of Postoperative DLT	**Benefits of Tube Exchange**
▪ No loss of airway by avoiding tube exchange	Changing to SLT: ▪ Improved suctioning ▪ Ability to perform bronchoscopy ▪ Improved mechanics for weaning ▪ Less risk of airway trauma/edema ▪ Obviates confusion from ICU personnel who may be unfamiliar with DLT management

DLT Double lumen tube, *SLT* single lumen tube, *ICU* intensive care unit.

Advantageous Design Features of DLT Airway Exchange Catheters (Fig 10-5)

- Length at least 90 cm
- Blunt-tipped (to minimize airway trauma)
- Flexible enough (particularly at tip) to minimize airway trauma, yet sufficiently rigid to be a reliable stylet
- Centimeter marks clearly denoted along the length of the catheter

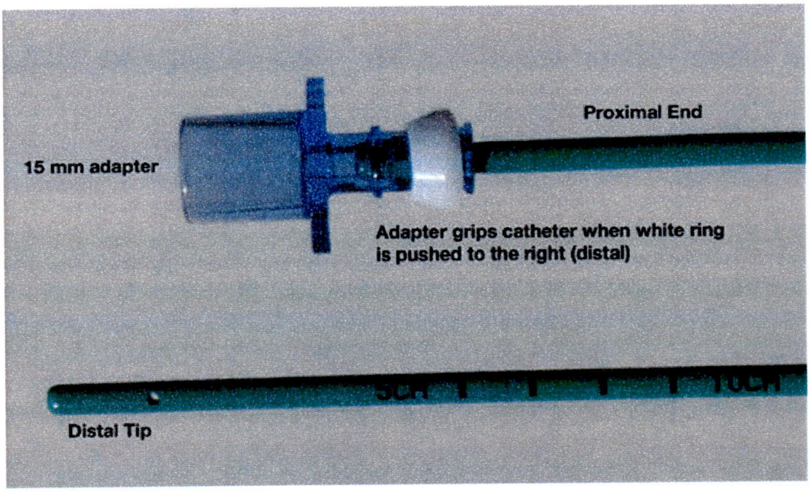

Figure 10-5 – Example of a double lumen tube exchange catheter® (Cook Airway Exchange Catheter with 15 mm Rapi-Fit adapter) (Cook Critical Care, Bloomington, IN). Proximal and distal tips are pictured. Also available in different sizes and stiffness, and with flexible tips. Proximal luer connectors for jet ventilation also available.

- Diameter and material to allow smooth passage through DLT lumen
- Hollow bore with adapters to allow rescue delivery of oxygen
  - Adapters for 15 mm anesthesia circuit
  - Adapters for jet ventilator

Technique: Tube Exchange of DLT to SLT

Recommended steps for a tube exchange from DLT to SLT are listed in Box 10-2.

The *most common cause of failure* is inability to get the tube to pass through the glottis. The difference in diameter between the exchange catheter and the tube produces a "shelf" which hangs up on the airway structures. This is exacerbated by incomplete paralysis and imperfect positioning. The steep bevel at the tip of the SLT

Box 10-2 – Recommended steps for a tube exchange from a DLT to a SLT

- Lubricate catheter with water-based lubricant
- Place patient on 100% FiO_2
- Suction mouth/pharynx
- Disconnect DLT from circuit
- Insert exchange catheter down the either lumen of the DLT to a depth of 22 cm (at the teeth)[1,2]
- Deflate balloon(s) of DLT
- Stabilize catheter while removing ETT (an assistant is required)
- Place new SLT over the catheter[3]
- Perform direct laryngoscopy to displace tissues[4]
- Insert SLT into the trachea, gentle rotation of the SLT 90° may be required[5]
- Remove catheter
- Confirm tracheal placement with $ETCO_2$ and breath sounds, or immediate bronchoscopy

[1–5]Clinical pearls:

1. Depth of insertion is especially important if one is transferring a DLT for a SLT after a pneumonectomy due to the risk of disrupting the new bronchial stump (22 cm at the teeth is roughly appropriate depth for most adults, but must be adjusted for tall or short stature)
2. The markings on the DLT exchange catheter are difficult to visualize through the ETT. The authors recommend marking the range on the catheter from 21 to 25 cm with a permanent marker to help identify the desired depth
3. If exchanging from a SLT to a DLT, place catheter through the *bronchial lumen* to allow entry through the glottis
4. Attention to prevent rupture of tube cuff on teeth during insertion of new tube
5. Avoid back and forth movements with the ETT while attempting advancement through the glottis over an exchange catheter. Back and forth movements can dislodge the catheter from the trachea or advance it potentially causing airway trauma. Perform rotational movements of the ETT instead

allows one to overcome this obstacle through a sequence of simple maneuvers:

- Slightly withdraw the SLT by 1–2 cm
- Rotate the tube at least 90° (angles the bevel of the SLT toward the glottis)
- Advance the tube forward through the glottis

Advancing a DLT over an exchange catheter requires more technical experience due to its stiffness and less advantageous bevel. The same maneuvers (90°–180° rotation and gentle forward pressure) are recommended until one feels the "give" as it passes through the cords.

Complications/Risks

The use of an airway exchange catheter does carry a risk, including:

- Loss of airway
- Injury to bronchial stump/airway

One must be mindful of the risks involved and be prepared with a backup plan, should loss of airway occur.

Selected References

1. The Acute Respiratory Distress Syndrome Network. Ventilation with lower tidal volumes as compared with traditional tidal volumes for acute lung injury and the acute respiratory distress syndrome. N Engl J Med. 2000;342(18):1301–8.

2. Kacmarek RM, Chipman D. Basic principles of ventilator machinery (Chapter 3). In: Tobin MJ, editor. Principles and practice of mechanical ventilation. 2nd ed. New York: McGraw-Hill; 2006.

3. ECRI Institute. PEEP valves in anesthesia circuits hazard. Health Devices. 1983;13(1):24.

Further Suggested Reading

Hogue CW. Effectiveness of low levels of non-ventilated lung CPAP in improving arterial oxygenation during one-lung ventilation. Anesth Analg. 1994;79:364–7.

Chapter 11
Alternative Ventilatory Techniques

Gyorgy Frendl

Keywords Ventilatory management • Alternative ventilatory techniques • Jet ventilation • Bernoulli's Principle • Venturi Effect • High frequency ventilation • High frequency positive pressure ventilation • High frequency jet ventilation • High frequency oscillatory ventilation • High frequency flow interruption • Apneic insufflation • Differential ventilation • Noninvasive positive pressure ventilation

Introduction

Most patients undergoing thoracic surgical procedures suffer from some degree of pulmonary disease which impacts their ventilatory management. Traditional modes of positive pressure mechanical ventilation are familiar to the general practitioner (Box 11-1) (Fig 11-1) and have been well reviewed (1). Variations on these common modes, dictated by pathophysiology (e.g., longer expiratory time for obstructive pulmonary disease, etc.) should also be familiar (2). The focus of this chapter will be alternative ventilatory techniques that may be necessary during specific thoracic surgical procedures or situations, when traditional ventilatory techniques are inadequate. Such alternative techniques (e.g., jet ventilation, high frequency ventilation (HFV), etc.) may be used as the primary mode of ventilation, or as an adjunct in various thoracic surgical situations.

P.M. Hartigan (ed.), *Practical Handbook of Thoracic Anesthesia*,
DOI 10.1007/978-0-387-88493-6_11, © Springer Science+Business Media, LLC 2012

Box 11-1 – Traditional Modes Positive Pressure Ventilation During Surgery

Volume-Control

- AKA "volume-cycled," "volume-limited," and "volume-targeted"
- Constant inspiratory flow rate
- Inspiration terminated when set volume is achieved
- Passive expiration
- Potential for high peak and plateau pressures when compliance is low, or resistance is high
- Requires closed or semi-closed system
- Designed to deliver guaranteed minute ventilation and avoid excessive tidal volumes
- Excessive lung volumes may nonetheless occur due to air trapping
- Convenient for situations of variable compliance

Pressure-Control

- AKA "pressure-cycled," "pressure-limited," and "peak pressure-targeted"
- High initial flow rate, as needed to achieve set peak inspiratory pressure
- Decelerating flow pattern during inspiration, as needed to maintain set pressure
- Inspiration is terminated by duration, as set by respiratory rate and I:E ratio
- Potential for high and low volumes delivered, depending on resistance and compliance
- Peak and plateau pressures are essentially equal
- Requires closed or semi-closed system
- Designed to prevent excessive inspiratory pressures
- May deliver variable volumes in situations of varying compliance
- Minute volume of ventilation must be carefully monitored
- Soft correlation between airway pressures and lung injury (transmural pressure and volume are more reflective)
- High initial inspiratory flows are advantageous in the presence of large air leak

(continued)

Box 11-1 – (continued)

- Higher flows early in inspiratory phase may provide improved recruitment of lung units with long time constants
- Convenient when switching back and forth between one and two lung ventilation

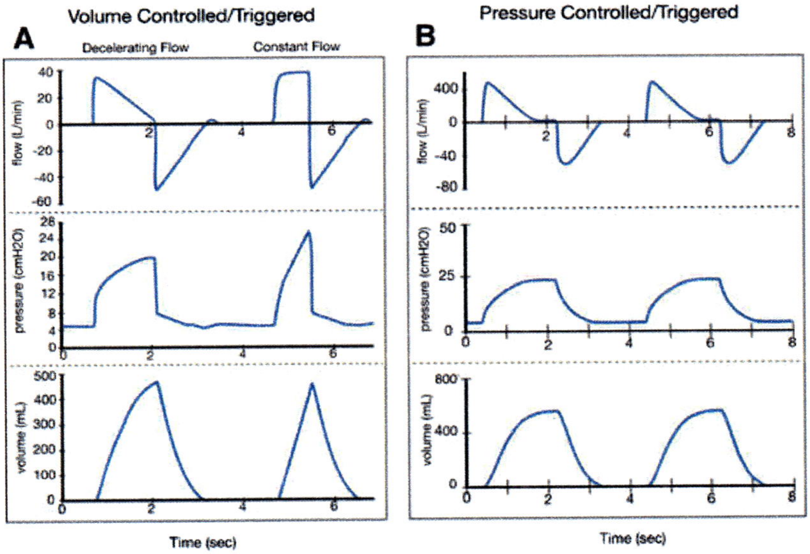

Figure 11-1 – Pressure-time, flow-time, and volume-time diagrams characterizing volume limited (Panel **A**) and pressure limited (Panel **B**) modes of ventilation.

Alternative Ventilatory Techniques

In general, alternative techniques are employed to help achieve the goals of ventilation (Box 11-2) when there is a large air leak, an open airway, an excessive concern of lung injury, as an adjunct to single-lung ventilation, or when there is need to avoid an endotracheal tube (e.g., laser surgery of airway). Common alternative techniques discussed here include:

- Jet ventilation
- High frequency jet ventilation

Box 11-2 – Management Goals of Ventilation

- Satisfactory Gas Exchange
  - Oxygenation
  - CO_2 elimination
- Avoidance of Lung Injury (3)
  - Volutrauma
  - Barotrauma
  - Atelectotrauma

- High frequency positive pressure ventilation
- High frequency oscillatory ventilation
- High frequency flow interruption
- Air insufflation (apneic oxygenation)
- Differential independent ventilation

Common situations when such techniques may be advantageous include:

1. Surgery of the major airways (tracheal resection or reconstruction, carinal resection)
2. When motionless field is required for the surgical procedure of the thorax or the airway
3. Procedures when the airway has to be shared by surgeons and anesthesiologists (i.e., rigid bronchoscopy)
4. Airway injury or when a large bronchopleural fistula is present

When using alternate ventilatory strategies, anesthesia is most often delivered via the intravenous route. Anesthetic consideration for rigid bronchoscopy is discussed in Chapter 26.

Jet Ventilation

Jet ventilation is a broad term for positive pressure ventilation delivered through a small orifice catheter (or device) with high orifice velocity, which relies on entrainment of ambient air to supplement the delivered tidal volume. Jet ventilation must be employed in open systems (e.g., rigid bronchoscopy, open tracheal resection, etc.) to allow air entrainment, and to allow passive exhalation (prevent air trapping). Oxygen concentrations of 30–100% and gas delivery pressures of 10–50 psi are used commonly.

In its simplest form, the Sanders jet system (Fig 11-2) employs a narrow orifice nozzle attached to a rigid bronchoscope or operative laryngoscope, with a hand-held trigger to deliver intermittent inspiratory bursts at high pressure. This system was developed in the 1960s to allow uninterrupted access by the surgeon. Modern systems allow for regulation of delivery pressure, frequency, duration, FiO_2, and other variables. Traditionally, jet ventilation at a frequency greater than 1 Hz is referred to as high frequency jet ventilation (HFJV) (see below).

Jet ventilation can be delivered through modern rigid bronchoscopes via a built-in channel (Fig 11-3), attachment, or via narrow tubing placed into the airway with or without the placement of an endotracheal tube. When used alone, these catheters can be placed through the vocal cords (translaryngeal-infraglottic access), through the neck (transtracheal-infraglottic access) or through a gas delivery nozzle placed just above the vocal cords (supraglottic access). Jet ventilation catheters may also be placed "over-the-field" into an open trachea or bronchus during tracheal or carinal resection (Chapter 30). Using jet ventilation, sufficient oxygenation can be maintained to allow the completion of procedures. One typical setup for low frequency jet ventilation is shown in Fig 11-4. Jet ventilation allows access to the airway with enough space for surgeons to perform endobronchial or laryngeal procedures. While jet ventilation may be the primary mode of ventilation, more often it is used as a rescue maneuver or a means of supplementing oxygen delivery to delay or prevent desaturation in order to allow surgery to be completed during a period when conventional positive pressure ventilation is impractical.

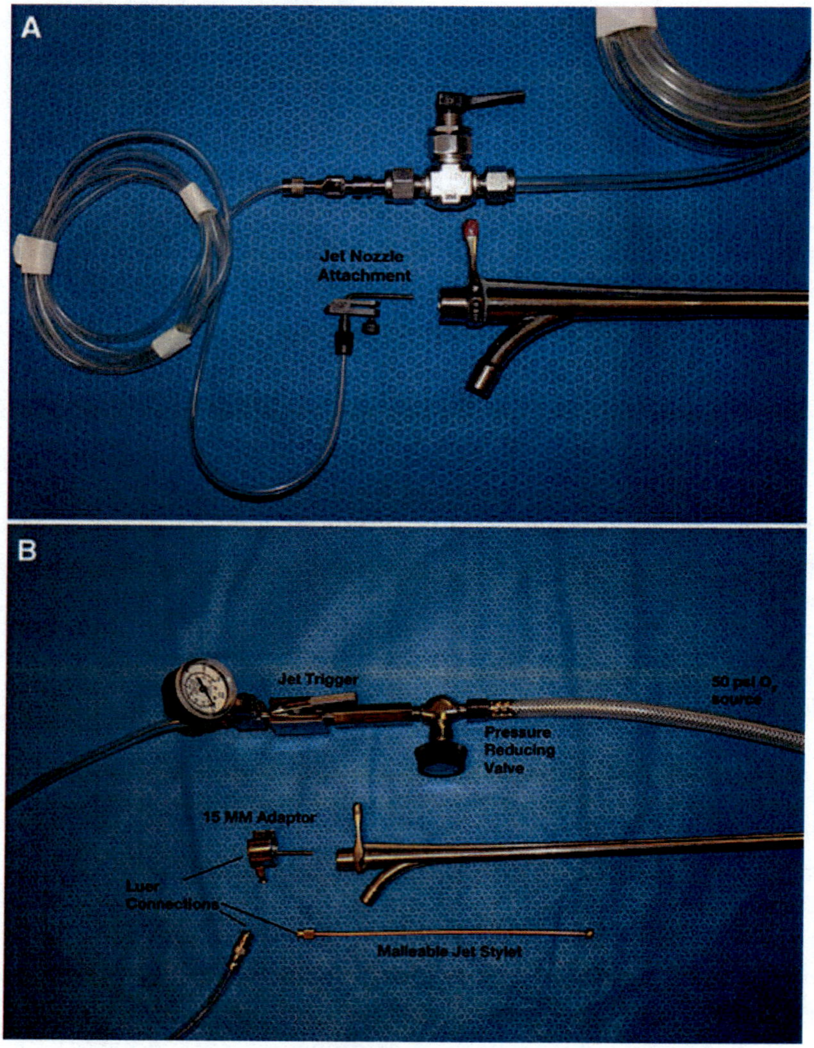

Figure 11-2 – Some examples of Sanders jet injection systems. Jet nozzle may be directly mounted on rigid bronchoscope (**A**), or attached by luer connector to circular attachments compatable with the proximal end of a rigid bronchoscope or 15 mm ETT connector (**B**). Also depicted is a malleable cannula with proximal luer connector for jet ventilation. Some rigidity of jet cannulae is desirable.

Commonly sited advantages and disadvantages of jet ventilation are listed in Table 11.1. When used for brief periods, or as an adjunct (e.g., intermittent jet ventilation of the operative lung during one-lung ventilation of the opposite lung), or as a rescue

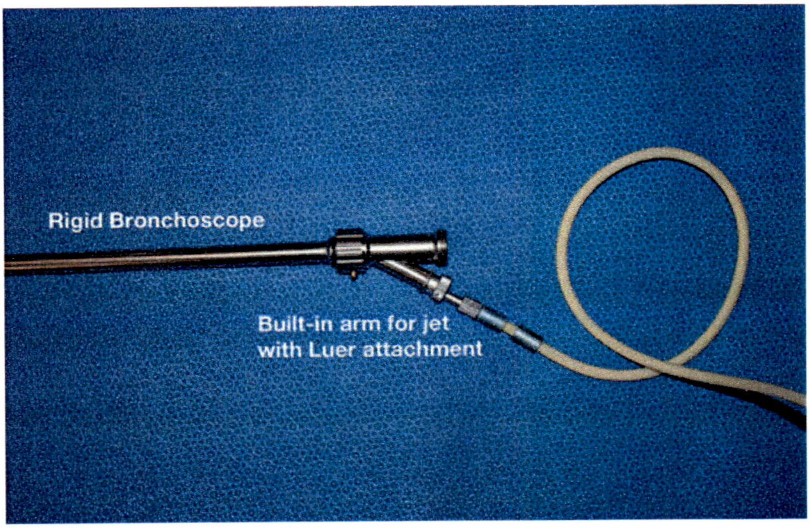

Figure 11-3 – Rigid bronchoscope with built-in jet ventillation channel (luer connection).

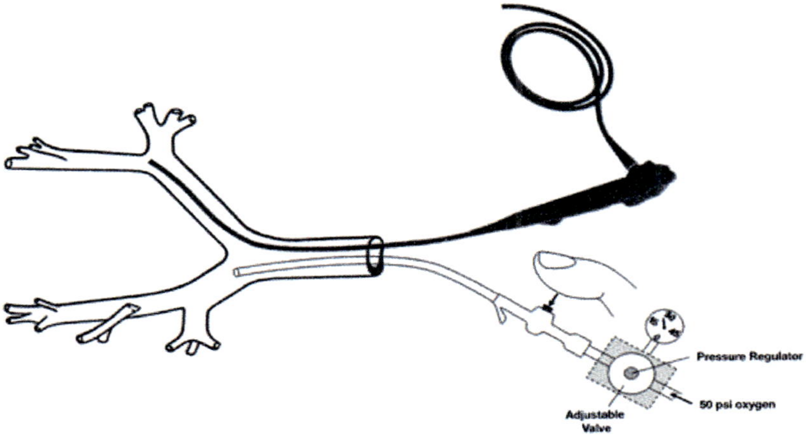

Figure 11-4 – Example of setup for low frequency jet ventilation demonstrating one type of placement of oxygen delivery catheter.

maneuver, the advantages tend to outweigh the disadvantages. It is essential that the operator be familiar with the equipment, and that adequacy of ventilation is monitored by observation of chest rise (or lung inflation) and arterial blood gas analysis (or transcutaneous CO_2 monitoring if available). When using jet ventilation the operator

Table 11.1 – Advantages and disadvantages of jet ventilation

Advantages of jet ventilation

- Can be delivered to an open system (high air leak)
- Avoids combustible plastic endotracheal tubes in the proximity of ignition sources (laser, electrocautery, etc.)
- Less interruption of surgery

Disadvantages of jet ventilation

- Potential for hypercapnia and hypoxemia
- Risk of barotrauma (subcutaneous emphysema, pneumothorax, disruption of stump or fistula)
- Unknown FiO_2 (depends on air entrainment)
- Unknown end-tidal CO_2
- Unknown tidal volume (entrainment dependent)
- Risk of blowing blood and debris distally within airway
- Limited lung expansion when restrictive (open system unable to generate large positive pressure)
- Unable or difficult to deliver agents by inhalational route (anesthetic agents, bronchodilators, inhaled nitric oxide, etc.)

must confirm that there is sufficient escape of ventilating gases from the airway to avoid barotrauma and over inflation of the lungs.

The mechanism of air entrainment by jet ventilation is governed by *Bernoulli's Principle*, which forms the basis of the *Venturi Effect*. A simplified explanation is provided in Fig 11-5. In short, the high velocity of air exiting the narrow jet orifice generates low pressure in that proximity, which serves to draw in (entrain) surrounding gas which increases the volume delivered by bulk flow. The precise ratio of jet-to-entrained air depends on the local physics; thus the final oxygen concentration and tidal volume are not easily controlled. Bernoulli's Principle has multiple applications within medicine (Venturi mask) and outside medicine (airplane lift, sailing, carbureters of cars, etc.).

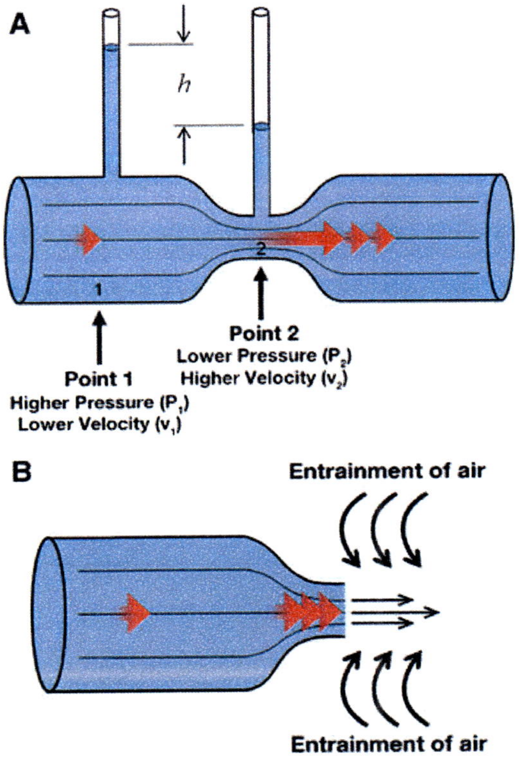

Figure 11-5 – (**A**) The Venturi Effect is the drop in pressure that occurs when a fluid flows through a region of constriction or stenosis at high velocity. The continuity equation requires that the sum of potential and kinetic energy be equivalent at any point along a pipe of continuous flow (law of conservation of energy). Since velocity must be greater within the region of stenosis, pressure must be reduced. The degree of pressure drop is derived from Bernoulli's Equation. (**B**) By the same principle, the low pressure around a jet of fluid (gas) exiting a narrow orifice at high velocity leads to entrainment of surrounding gas during jet ventilation.

High Frequency Ventilation

HFV is a loosely defined, umbrella term to describe alternative ventilatory techniques which have in common high frequencies and low tidal volumes (often less than anatomic dead space). The earliest and simplest form is *high frequency positive pressure ventilation* (HFPPV). This technique was initially developed to reduce respiration-related hemodynamic changes for research purposes, but was found to be surprisingly effective for gas exchange. HFPPV typically employs conventional ventilators (time cycled with flow rates of 175–250 L/min), with respiratory rates of 60–100 breaths per minute delivering tidal volumes from 3 to 4 mL/kg. This results in oscillatory gas movements around a set (optimal) mean airway pressure. The result is enhanced mixing of fresh gas with alveolar gas at lower mean airway pressures. Uncuffed, large bore catheters are usually used rather than cuffed ETTs, and exhalation is passive. A theoretical advantage of this and other forms of HFV is that lung volumes can be maintained within the "safe zone" between overdistension and derecruitment, potentially protecting against volutrauma and atelectrauma. HFPPV is rarely used clinically today, but serves as useful conceptual prototype for other forms of HFV.

High Frequency Jet Ventilation

HFJV is essentially jet ventilation delivered at higher frequency. A solenoid valve converts source oxygen of a constant drive pressure into bursts, or jets of oxygen at a set frequency, pressure, and I:E (on-off) ratio (Fig 11-6). As with low frequency jet ventilation, small orifice catheters are utilized enabling surgical access and ventilation through stenotic regions. Characteristics of HFJV include:

- Frequencies of 100–400/min (1.7–6.7 Hz) via a high pressure "jet" (70–350 kPa), resulting in entrainment and tidal volumes of 1 mL/kg or less.
- Passive exhalation with I:E ratios as high as 1:12.
- Relatively low airway pressures (compared to low frequency jet or conventional positive pressure ventilation).

HFJV has all the advantages and disadvantages of jet ventilation (Table 11.1). In addition, there is less motion of the operative field (though there can be a shimmering effect). Decreased mean airway pressures may potentially reduce adverse hemodynamic effects and the risk of barotrauma. Modern devices have a means of monitoring airway pressures downstream from the jet pressure.

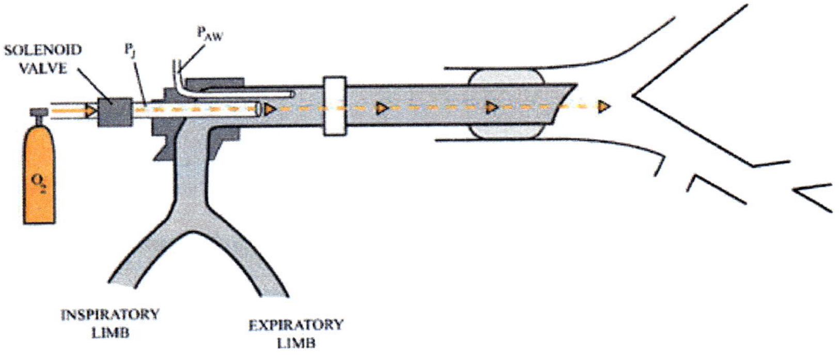

Figure 11-6 – Schematic depiction of HFJV system applied to an intubated patient. The solenoid valve modulates the high pressure oxygen-air supply into intermittent bursts of set frequency and duration. Low pressure fresh inspired gas is typically provided by the anesthesia circuit. Jet pressure (P_J) is monitored to detect malfunction of the solenoid or jet. A surrogate of airway pressure (P_{AW}) is measured downstream of the jet to detect excessive airway pressure. Low P_{AW} may indicate circuit disconnect or other source of air leak. *Modified with permission from Miller RD (Editor). Miller's Anesthesia, 6th Edition. Elsevier, Churchill Livingstone, Philadelphia, 2005.*

HFJV has been associated with less ventilator induced lung injury in certain specific situations in the ICU in some studies. The claim that HFJV for patients with a large bronchopleural fistula results in improved ventilation at reduced mean airway pressures and airflow through the fistula, has not been consistently demonstrated. HFJV may be combined with conventional mechanical breaths to recruit areas of atelectatic lung. When HFJV is used as an adjunct, and is combined with conventional mechanical ventilation, PEEP can be employed to increase "end-expiratory lung volume" (reducing atelectasis).

Examples of situations in which HFJV might be used include:

- Rigid bronchoscopy
- Open airway situations (tracheal resection, etc.)
- Stenotic airways
- Laryngeal and tracheobronchial laser airway surgeries
- Patients with bronchopleural fistulae (in both the operating room and in the ICU).

The mechanisms by which HFJV results in gas delivery to alveoli likely involves some combination of mass movement, enhanced molecular diffusion (Taylor Dispersion), high velocity gas flow, coaxial gas flow, gas trapping, and pendelluft movement (asynchronous movement of gas from one lung region to another). Airway pressures are in part determined by the frequency. As with pressure control ventilation, decreases in compliance result in decreased lung expansion and ventilation.

High Frequency Oscillatory Ventilation

The unique feature of high frequency oscillatory ventilation (HFOV) is the fact that both expiration and inspiration are active (gas is pushed in and pulled out). This oscillation is produced by a piston or diaphragm which pulsates like a loudspeaker (Fig 11-7). This active expiration theoretically improves efficiency of CO_2 elimination and reduces gas trapping. Other characteristics of HFOV include:

- Frequency range is typically 400–2,400 breaths per minute (6.7–40 Hz).
- Set power determines the distance that the piston or diaphragm moves, thus affecting tidal volume.
- "Tidal Volumes" are determined by set power, frequency, and compliance/resistance characteristics determined by lung and ETT size. Tidal volumes are less than anatomic dead space.
- Ventilating pressure oscillates around a constant distending pressure (P_{AW}), which is typically 25–35 cm H_2O.
- Lungs visibly wiggle, or shimmer during HFOV, potentially interfering with lung surgery.
- "Bias Flow" of fresh gas is typically set at 20–40 L/min.
- Oxygenation is primarily determined by FiO_2, P_{AW}, and lung volume.
- CO_2 elimination is improved by increasing set power or reducing frequency to increase tidal volumes.

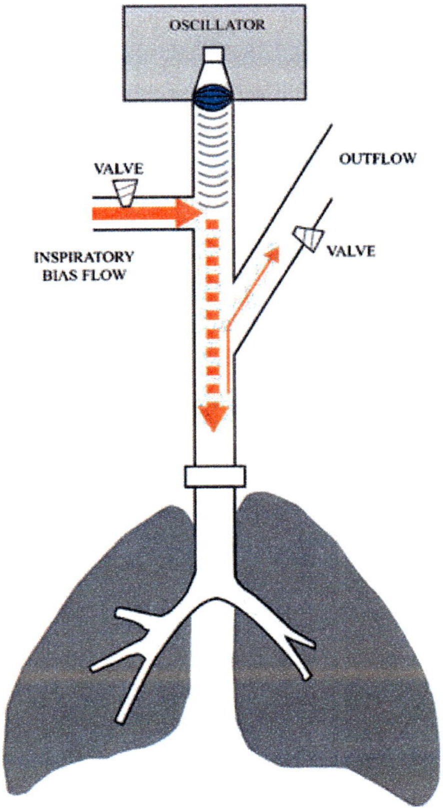

Figure 11-7 – Simple schematic of high frequency oscillatory ventilation system. Oscillations generated by a piston or diaphragm agitate air within the ETT and conductive airways. A bias flow of fresh gas mixes with alveolar gas, facilitated by the oscillations, and "flushes" out the more CO_2-rich gas exiting the lungs. Mean airway pressure may be regulated by adjustments to bias flow rate or the outflow valve. *Modified with permission from Tobin MJ (Editor). Principles & Practice of Mechanical Ventilation, 2nd Edition. McGraw Hill, New York, 2006.*

Expertise and familiarity with the equipment are essential for safe use of HFOV. Counterintuitively, reductions in frequency enhance CO_2 elimination. This occurs because the resultant increased tidal volume effect offsets the reduction in number of tidal "breaths" per minute. Deflating the ETT cuff may also enhance CO_2 elimination, but at the cost of reduced P_{AW}, and possibly reduced oxygenation.

Currently, HFOV is principally used as a lung protective strategy for preterm and neonatal infants at risk for acute lung injury. The use of HFOV was proven beneficial in randomized studies for preterm infants (of sizes both less than or equal to 1 kg and more than 1 kg) when used early with a lung recruitment strategy, after surfactant replacement. HFOV treatment resulted in clinical outcomes consistent with a reduction in both acute and chronic lung injury. HFOV is also used for pediatric patients with severe hypoxemia (ARDS) unresponsive to conventional mechanical ventilation (3).

For adult patients, HFOV is most commonly used when conventional mechanical ventilation is insufficient to support ventilation and oxygenation in cases of severe hypoxemia due to ARDS or acute lung rejection following lung transplant. Currently, there is no clear evidence that the use of HFOV provides a survival benefit for these adult patients. HFOV may be useful for ventilating patients with bronchopleural fistula. Any theoretical lung protective advantages of HFOV may be compromised if oxygenation requirements necessitate increasing airway pressures approaching those of conventional mechanical ventilation. HFOV is more commonly used in the ICU; its utility during surgical procedures is limited by the fact that the oscillatory movements create a moving surgical field.

Other commonly cited disadvantages of HFOV include:

- Complex, unfamiliar machine to many clinicians
- Difficult to use in transport
- Patients often require deeper sedation
- Secretions can reduce the efficacy of HFOV
- Hyperinflation of lungs can occur if significant COPD is present (relative contraindication)
- Necrotizing tracheobronchitis has been seen with HFOV
- Auto-PEEP may develop especially if patients develop unrecognized airway obstruction

High Frequency Flow Interruption

High frequency flow interruption (HFFI) is similar to HFJV in that rapid, brief pulses of fresh gas are delivered and expiration is passive. The mechanism for creating the pulses is different. HFFI uses a rotating bar or ball with a channel which aligns permitting a pulse of flow with each rotation. The velocity and frequency of gas pulses are typically less than HFJV (up to 15 Hz). There is limited data comparing efficacy of HFFI with other alternative forms of HFV. Usage is currently limited to premature and neonatal patients in centers where there are clinicians familiar with the technique.

Apneic Insufflation (Low- and High-Flow Apneic Ventilation)

Air and oxygen maybe delivered to nonventilated lungs in a continuous (low or high velocity) flow via small catheters placed into the airways. In the context of thoracic surgery, it is sometimes employed in an attempt to augment one-lung oxygenation (via a catheter to the operative lung) or as the sole source of oxygenation/ventilation during a period of apnea when the airway is surgically divided, or the surgeon needs a motionless field.

As a means of oxygenating patients, apneic insufflation by itself is only an adjunct which may augment oxygenation or delay desaturation. The mechanism is thought to be enhanced mass movement. As oxygen is consumed and removed from alveoli, the concentrated oxygen insufflated into conducting airways is drawn distally. The rise in CO_2 (6 mmHg during the first minute of apnea, followed by 3–4 mmHg/min thereafter) tends to be the limiting factor in tolerated duration of apnea. With low flow insufflation, the effectiveness of oxygenation is limited in the presence of a large shunt (>25%). Thus, when employed during OLV, oxygen insufflation through a small catheter to the nondependent, collapsed lung is unlikely to be effective unless higher flows are employed resulting effectively in CPAP to that lung with recruitment of atelectatic lung. In situations of more limited shunt, or imperative apnea for a motionless surgical field, oxygen insufflation may significantly delay desaturation for a number of minutes, enabling critical surgical steps to be completed.

Differential (Independent) Ventilation of the Two Lungs

Differential ventilation of the two lungs is performed by the use of two separate ventilators, and it requires the isolation of the lungs with a double lumen endotracheal tube. This technique is often a last resort and calls for expert ventilator management. Timing and coordination of two ventilators, both delivering PPV, can be challenging. Situations in which this option might be considered include:

- When the compliance of the two lungs is significantly different.
- When there is an air leak in from one lung (e.g., mainstem bronchopleural fistula).
- When lung isolation is required (e.g., to prevent cross-contamination), but gas exchange is unsatisfactory with one-lung ventilation despite CPAP and other traditional maneuvers.

Noninvasive Positive Pressure Ventilation

This modality is more and more frequently used for short-term (few hours to days) ventilation in the PACU or ICU and is delivered via a tight fitting face mask. It is most beneficial for patients with reversible atelectasis, or COPD flare and heart failure as a means of avoiding reintubation. It is akin to the mask ventilation used in the operating rooms, but the breaths are programmed to be delivered by a ventilator. CPAP, BiPAP, PSV, or controlled modes of ventilation can be delivered this way. The most common problem leading to failures of this mode is uncooperative patients who do not tolerate the facemask long term.

Selected References

1. Tobin MJ, editor. Principles and practice of mechanical ventilation. New York: McGraw-Hill; 2006.

2. Lumb AB, editor. Nunn's: applied respiratory physiology. Philadelphia: Butterworth & Heinemannn; 2000.

3. The Acute Respiratory Distress Syndrome Network. Ventilation with lower tidal volumes as compared with traditional tidal volumes for acute lung injury and the acute respiratory distress syndrome. N Engl J Med. 2000;342:1301–8.

4. Benumof JL, editor. Anesthesia for thoracic surgery. Philadelphia: WB Saunders; 1995.

Further Suggested Reading

Kaplan JA, Slinger PD, editors. Thoracic anesthesia. Churchill-Livingston: Elsevier Science; 2003.

Ritacca FV, Stewart TE. Clinical review: high-frequency oscillatory ventilation in adults – a review of the literature and practical applications. Crit Care. 2003;7: 385–90.

Hess D, Mason S, Branson R. High frequency ventilation. Respir Care Clin North Am. 2001;7:577–98.

MacIntyre NR. High frequency jet ventilation. Respir Care Clin North Am. 2001;7:599–610.

Chapter 12
Respiratory Therapy Devices

David A. Silver

Keywords Nasal cannula • Venturi mask • Simple face mask • Nonrebreather • High-flow O_2 mask • ETT • Noninvasive positive pressure ventilation • Thoracic walker • INOmax DS • Flolan

Specialized respiratory therapy devices are crucial to the perioperative care of the thoracic surgery patient. Some, such as continuous positive airway pressure (CPAP) attachments for double-lumen endotracheal tubes, described elsewhere, are used primarily in the operating room (OR). Others, such as the INOmax DS™ nitric oxide delivery system, described below, may be initiated in the OR but continued in the intensive care unit (ICU) for hours to days postoperatively. Many specialized pieces of equipment, such as the "thoracic walker," are used exclusively in the postoperative period and are critical to the successful postoperative recovery of the thoracic surgery patient.

Oxygen delivery devices and approximate maximum FiO_2 delivered:

▪ Nasal cannula	0.4
▪ Venturi mask	0.5 (maximum)
▪ Simple face mask	0.5
▪ Nonrebreather	0.8–0.9
▪ High-flow O_2 mask	0.8–0.9
▪ ETT	1.0

P.M. Hartigan (ed.), *Practical Handbook of Thoracic Anesthesia*,
DOI 10.1007/978-0-387-88493-6_12, © Springer Science+Business Media, LLC 2012

Nasal Cannula

- *Order flow in liters per minute (L/min)*, usually from 2 to 6 L/min.
- In theory: 2 L/min gives $FiO_2=0.24$, and each 1 L/min adds approximately 0.04 up to 6 L/min (i.e., 0.28, 0.32, 0.36, 0.40).
- Higher liter flows are often uncomfortable, so switching to a face mask is recommended if 6 L/min is inadequate for the patient's needs (though high-flow nasal cannulae are also available).
- *Humidification* is important for comfort and to prevent drying of mucus membranes, which can lead to epistaxis, as well as inspissation of secretions.
- Successful use of this device (Fig 12-1) is NOT dependent on "Nasal breathing," though it is *dependent on patent nasal passages*. Oxygen is drawn down a pressure gradient into the posterior nasopharynx during inspiration, even in a patient who is a "mouth breather," enriching the oxygen content of inspired air.

Venturi Mask

- Provides "Plug In" FiO_2 via various inserts for the mask, using the Venturi Effect (see Chapter 11) to entrain room air, which

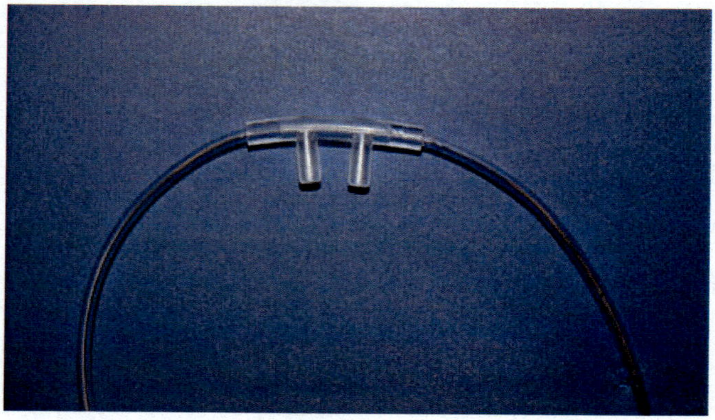

Figure 12-1 – Nasal cannula.

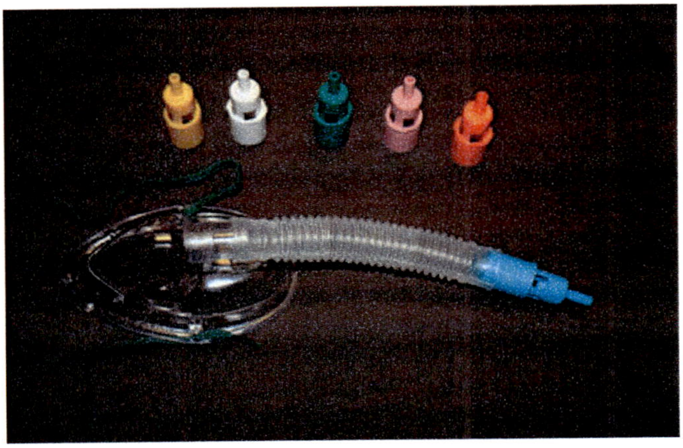

Figure 12-2 – Venturi mask.

mixes with the oxygen liter flow recommended by the manufacturer.

- Available FiO_2: 0.24, 0.28, 0.31, 0.35, 0.40, 0.50
- Color coding is not universal! Check the FiO_2 stamped on the insert.
- Some devices (Fig 12-2) deliver various FiO_2 levels with a single insert, based on different liter flows set by the user.
- Do not humidify at 0.24, 0.28, as this will reduce the FiO_2 delivered.

Simple Face Mask

- *FiO_2 delivered depends on the patient's inspiratory effort* (a larger tidal volume will entrain more room air, and dilute the oxygen delivered from the mask); the maximum FiO_2 that can be delivered is approximately 0.5.
- *The liter flow selected should be at least 5 L/min*. Lower flows may result in rebreathing of exhaled CO_2; higher flows will increase the FiO_2 delivered.

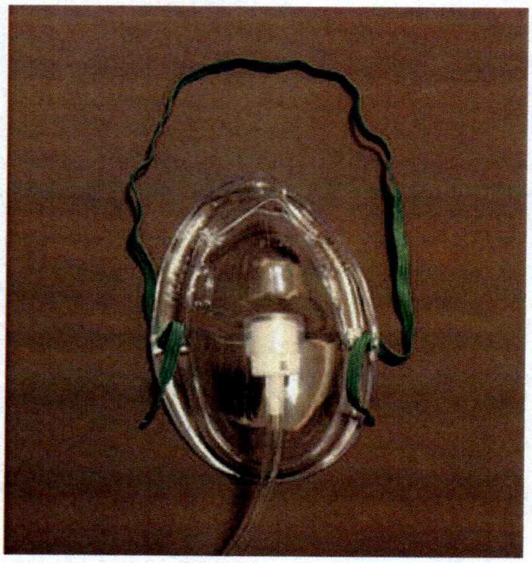

Figure 12-3 – Simple face mask.

- The maximum delivered FiO_2 is based on the fact that the patient's inspiration is intermittent, while the liter flow is constant so that even if the liter flow exceeds the patient's minute ventilation, higher FiO_2 is not delivered. Excess oxygen delivered during exhalation is spilled from the mask into the room. On inspiration, the patient will first inspire the oxygen accumulated in the oro- and naso-pharynx as well as the volume of the mask; this may total approximately 200–250 mL. Further inspiratory effort up to a full tidal volume entrains room air, thus diluting the effective FiO_2 delivered.
- This device (Fig 12-3) is comfortable and well-tolerated by most patients.

Nonrebreather Mask

- This device (Fig 12-4) adds a reservoir to the mask so that a greater percentage of the patient's tidal breathing is supplied with oxygen, up to an FiO_2 of 0.8–0.9.
- Oxygen flow should be adequate to prevent emptying of the reservoir bag during inspiration, usually 12–15 L/min.

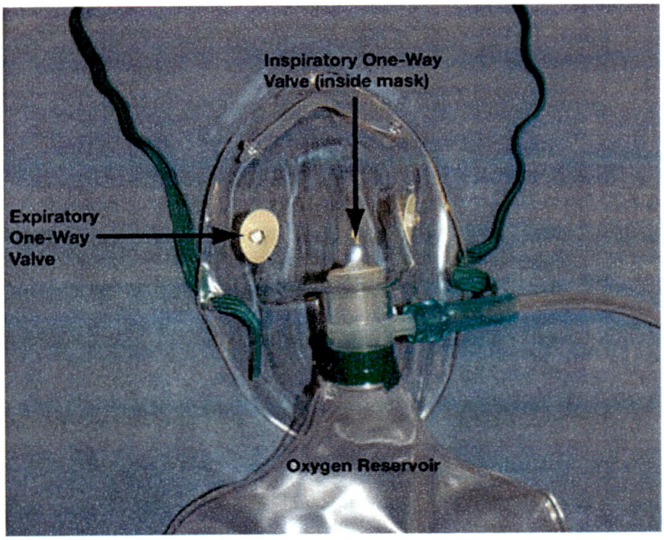

Figure 12-4 – Nonrebreather mask.

- Humidification is not an option with this device.
- A one-way valve from the reservoir prevents exhalation into the bag.
- One-way valves on the mask prevent entraining room air during inspiration, and allow exhalation to the atmosphere.
- The high liter flows associated with this device somewhat limit its utility with portable oxygen tanks.

High-Flow Oxygen Mask

- Designed primarily for use with wall-source oxygen, as it will rapidly exhaust a portable tank
- FiO_2 up to 1.0 "dialed in" at the wall source.
- Humidification very important given the high flows of dry gas delivered.

Noninvasive Positive Pressure Ventilation

- Positive pressure ventilation via a mask (which requires good fit and low air leak)
- Can deliver close to $FiO_2 = 1.0$
- Can add PEEP, pressure support, and a respiratory rate
- *Risk of pulmonary aspiration*, particularly in the immediate postoperative setting in patients who may have iatrogenic vocal cord dysfunction, or may be partially obtunded due to hypercarbia or medications.
    - Demonstrated utility in management of acute exacerbations of COPD
    - Favored by some to avoid reintubation in patients requiring temporary mechanical ventilatory support.
    - May result in gastric distension, further increasing aspiration risk
    - Endotracheal intubation provides a more secure airway, providing desired FiO_2, positive pressure and PEEP while reducing aspiration risk.

The "Thoracic Walker"

- Early and frequent ambulation in the postoperative period can greatly improve "pulmonary toilet" and mechanics, reducing atelectasis, improving ventilation, and increasing clearance of pulmonary secretions.
- This is a physical therapy device which enables the patient to ambulate while largely supporting his weight on his arms.
- The walker (Fig 12-5) is designed to hold two oxygen cylinders, and may also be rigged with a portable ventilator. Alternatively, for the intubated patient or one with a tracheostomy, a respiratory therapist may accompany the patient and provide bag-valve respiratory support.

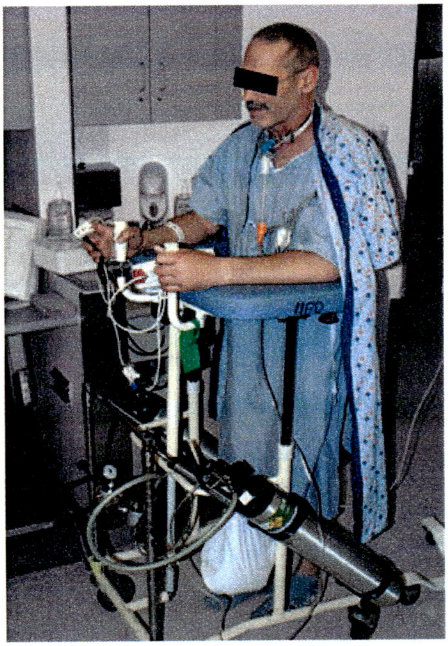

Figure 12-5 – The "Thoracic walker".

Inhaled Nitric Oxide: The INOmax DS™ Delivery System (INO Therapeutics, Inc., and Ikaria)

- Inhaled nitric oxide (iNO) is a potent inhaled vasodilator with a half-life in vivo of seconds, due to its potent affinity for and inactivation by hemoglobin. As such, inhaled NO is a selective pulmonary vasodilator.
- *iNO is FDA-approved for the treatment of term and near-term (>34 weeks) neonates with hypoxic respiratory failure associated with clinical or echocardiographic evidence of pulmonary hypertension*, where it improves oxygenation and reduces the need for extracorporeal membrane oxygenation.
- *iNO has been used off-label* to attempt to optimize ventilation-perfusion (V/Q) matching, and in the treatment of pulmonary hypertension following pneumonectomy, pulmonary resection, and pulmonary transplant.

- Levels of iNO may be adjusted from 2 to 80 parts per million (ppm), with most vascular reactivity occurring at 20 ppm or less, and many experts recommending 10 ppm as the appropriate starting level of therapy. The medication should be tapered with careful monitoring of clinical status as the patient's condition improves. Rebound pulmonary hypertension may occur with rapid weaning.
- iNO is expensive, and is billed based on duration of use. Thus, administration should be discontinued in patients who do not demonstrate a rapid clinical response to initiation of therapy. Liter flows and levels of iNO delivered do not affect the cost of care under the current system.
- The INOmax DS measures and displays levels of NO, nitrogen dioxide (NO_2) and O_2 in the circuit.
- Serum methemoglobin levels should also be periodically checked, as this byproduct will accumulate during iNO therapy in a dose-dependent fashion.
- *When connected to an anesthesia machine, flows should be set to at least 5 L/min to ensure delivery of set NO and to minimize the formation of NO_2 in the circuit.*
- The machine is easily connected to a wall source of oxygen when not being used for transport so that the limited life of the mounted oxygen cylinder is not an issue.

Use of iNO with a Circle Anesthesia System

The INOmax DS (Fig 12-6) allows the user to adjust the concentration of iNO delivered via a ventilator or (for transport) an attached Ambu™ bag.

The delivery system is connected to the anesthesia machine by adding the injector module to the inspiratory limb of the anesthesia circuit. A standardized 330 mm length of 22 mm hose is interposed between the injector and the patient gas sample line.

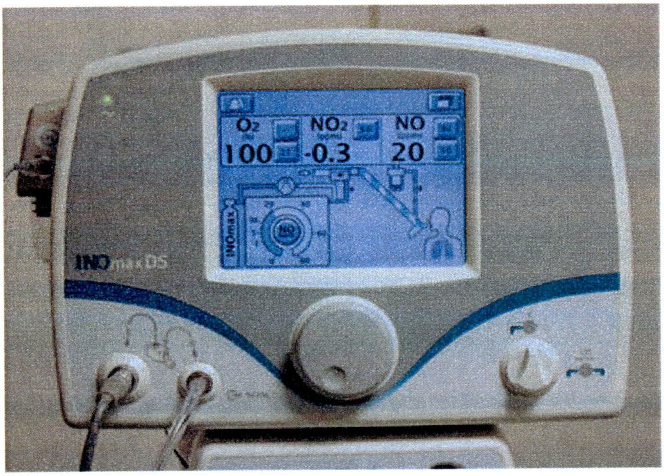

Figure 12-6 – INOmax DS.

The reader is cautioned to refer to the latest user's manual provided by the manufacturer (Ikaria holdings, Clinton, NJ) for updated guidance on the operation of the INOmax DS. The schematic in Fig 12-7 is provided for general reference.

Flolan™ (Epoprostenol Sodium), Inhaled

- Epoprostenol (PGI_2, prostacyclin) is a metabolite of arachidonic acid, with potent pulmonary and systemic arterial vasodilatory effects, as well as inhibitory effects on platelet aggregation.
- Epoprostenol is rapidly hydrolyzed at neutral pH in blood and is subject to enzymatic degradation, with metabolites which are excreted in the urine. Its half-life in vivo is on the order of minutes.
- The drug is FDA approved for long-term intravenous treatment of primary pulmonary hypertension and pulmonary hypertension associated with the scleroderma spectrum of disease, in NYHA Class III and IV patients who do not respond adequately to conventional therapy.

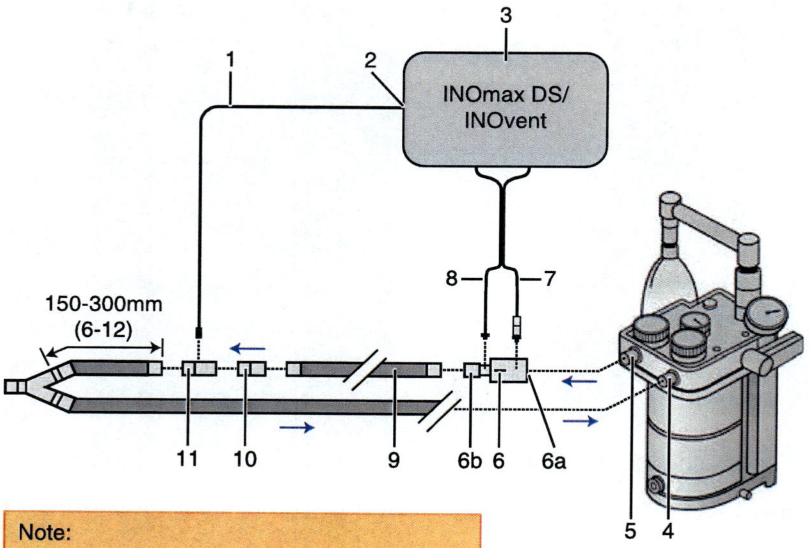

Note:

1. With a circle anesthesia breathing circuit, the INOmax DS / INOvent delivery system will perform as specified in the technical specifications with ***fresh gas flow rates equal to or greater than the patient minute volume.***

2. The breathing circuit between the sample tee and the patient Y should be between 6 and 12 inches (150-300mm) long: greater than 6 inches to minimize the sampling of mixed inspired/expired concentrations and less than 12 inches to help ensure correct NO_2 measurement.

3. For OR ventilation systems with the inspiratory flow measurements at the inspiratory port of the absorber, place the Injector Module upstream of the inspiratory flow sensor.

1. Gas sample line
2. Sample line inlet
3. INOmax DS/INOvent delivery system
4. Absorber expiratory port
5. Absorber inspiratory port
6. Injector module
   a. Input
   b. Output
7. Injector module cable
8. Injector module tubing
9. Inspiratory limb of anesthesia circuit
10. 22M / 15F x 22M /15F Adapter
11. Sample Tee

Figure 12-7 – Schematic for connection of INOvent or INOmax DS to a standard anesthesia circuit. (*After* http://inomax.com/assets/pdf/IKARIA_Anesthesia_Cards_Rev2_final.pdf. *Used with permission*).

- *Inhaled use of epoprostenol is an off-label use of the drug*. When administered by intermittent auto-injection into the ventilator circuit, it is a fairly selective pulmonary vasodilator, similar to iNO. It is less expensive than iNO, but also less selective for the pulmonary circulation, with a significant incidence of systemic hypotension.
- *Indications*: Inhaled epoprostenol may be helpful in the management of perioperative acute right ventricular failure, as in the settings of heart and lung transplant, ARDS, and acute pulmonary hypertension.
- *Contraindications*: Some patients with pulmonary hypertension develop pulmonary edema during intravenous dose initiation. Patients receiving the drug via inhalation should be carefully monitored for the development of pulmonary edema.
- *Common side effects* of intravenous administration include flushing (58%), headache (49%), nausea/vomiting (32%), and hypotension (16%).
- *Dosage*: A typical starting dose is 0.05 mg/kg/min (ideal body weight), reducing by 0.01 mg/kg/min if systemic hypotension results.
- Patients should be assessed for clinical response 30 min after initiation of therapy. If no improvement is evident, it may be discontinued.
- Rebound pulmonary hypertension has been described with abrupt discontinuation of epoprostenol, so in patients who do respond to treatment, it is usually weaned by 0.01 mg/kg/min every 2 h as tolerated.

Chapter 13
Technical Aspects of Common Pain Procedures for Thoracic Surgery

Nelson L. Thaemert

Keywords Thoracic epidural catheters • Midline approach • Paramedian approach • Paramedian thoracic epidural • Midline thoracic epidural • Intercostal nerve blocks • Thoracic paravertebral nerve blocks

Introduction

For patients undergoing thoracic surgery, postoperative analgesia with local anesthetics can be provided in a variety of forms, including epidural catheters, intercostal blocks, paravertebral blocks, and infusions of local anesthetic within the incisions. When compared to systemic analgesia alone, these techniques can provide many advantages, including reduced opioid use, less respiratory and central nervous system depression, and potentially improved pulmonary mechanics. While analgesia from thoracic epidural catheters is the gold standard for pain relief following thoracic surgery, each of these routes should be considered as potential elements of a comprehensive anesthetic plan.

Thoracic Epidural Catheters

Thoracic epidural analgesia has a central role in pain management after major thoracic surgery. Insertion of thoracic epidural catheters has generally been regarded as more difficult than that of

P.M. Hartigan (ed.), *Practical Handbook of Thoracic Anesthesia*,
DOI 10.1007/978-0-387-88493-6_13,

lumbar placement, but should be a familiar and reliable component in the skill set of a thoracic anesthesiologist. The physiology, complications, and contraindications are discussed in Chapter 37; technical aspects are discussed below.

Anatomy

Developing an understanding of the anatomy of the mid-thoracic vertebrae is essential for successful placement of a thoracic epidural catheter. The anatomy of the thoracic vertebral bodies and ligaments is depicted in Figs 13-1 and 13-2.

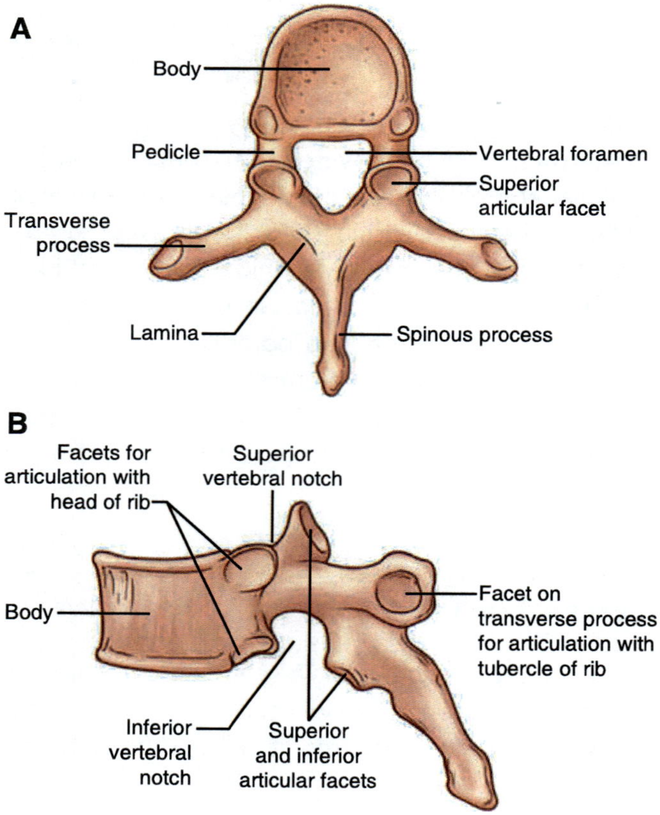

Figure 13-1 – Thoracic vertebral bodies.

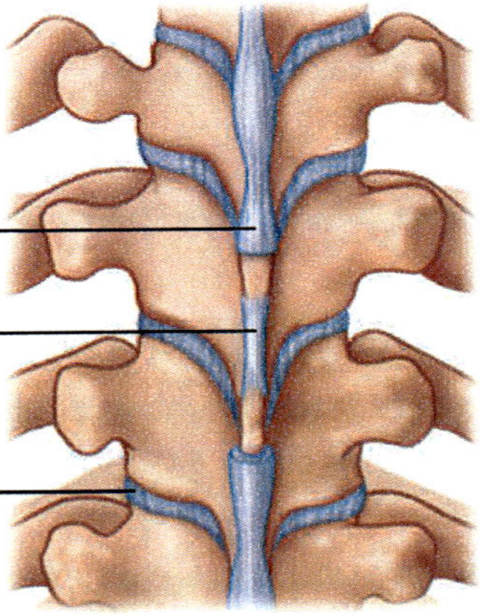

Figure 13-2 – Posterior thoracic spine ligaments.

The most pertinent differences between thoracic and lumbar vertebral anatomy are summarized below:

- 45° caudad angulation of spinous processes with narrow interspace between processes
- Narrower thoracic interlaminar foraminae
- Less robust ligamentum flavum
- Narrower and less well-defined thoracic interspinous ligament
- Narrower thoracic epidural space
- Narrower thoracic nerve root foraminae
- Larger thoracic laminae

Patient Preparation

Thoracic epidural catheters should be placed in patients that are conscious and mildly sedated when possible, and are commonly placed preoperatively. If unexpected surgical events prompt postoperative placement, attempts should be made to provide adequate analgesia with other techniques before emergence from anesthesia. Placement under general anesthesia is discouraged.

Monitors for blood pressure and pulse should be in place before placement. Supplemental oxygen and resuscitative drugs should be available.

Positioning

Patients can be positioned in a sitting or lateral decubitus position for catheter placement. Placement in the sitting position aids identification of the midline, especially in obese patients. Positioning in the lateral decubitus position allows comfortable sedation without patient movement and, if indicated, simultaneous placement of a radial arterial line by a second practitioner.

Landmarks and Choice of Insertion Site

Choice of interspace depends on the type and location of surgery. Generally, epidural local anesthetic will spread for several dermatomes above and below the location of the catheter tip. For most thoracic surgery, an entry point between T5 and T7 is recommended. Unlike lumbar epidurals, thoracic epidural catheters fairly reliably thread in the cephalad direction due to the angle of entry.

When the patient's shoulders are relaxed, the tip of scapula rests at the level of T7. Interspaces can be counted down from C7 or up from iliac crest and other lumbar landmarks (Fig 13-3).

Midline vs. Paramedian Approach

The midline approach is more familiar to clinicians from lumbar experience. However, arguments in favor of the paramedian approach for thoracic epidurals include the following:

- Caudad angulation of spinous processes and narrow interlaminar foraminae allow only for a narrow window to pass a needle with the midline technique
- Interspinous ligament is narrow, and difficult to keep engaged within (with midline approach). Slipping off can give false loss of resistance

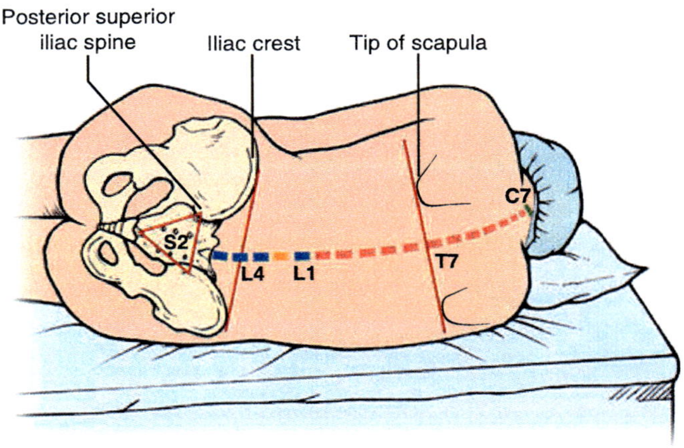

Figure 13-3 – Thoracic epidural positioning and landmarks.

- Interspinous ligament may be calcified obstructing needle advancement
- Interspinous ligament may be cystic or discontinuous, with areas of false loss of resistance
- Paramedian technique allows ligamentum flavum to be approached at more acute angle, and interspinous ligament avoided

Procedural Steps: Paramedian Thoracic Epidural

1. Entry point should be 1–1.5 cm lateral and 1 cm caudad to the midpoint of the chosen interspace. Place a generous skin wheal of local anesthetic at the entry point.
2. Infiltrate local anesthetic into the paraspinous muscle, fascia, and periostium of lamina by inserting the needle perpendicular to the skin.
3. Insert an epidural needle perpendicular to the plane of the skin and advance until lamina is encountered.
4. Withdraw the epidural needle slightly and redirect in a medial and rostral direction until you feel the needle "walk

off" the lamina and engage the ligamentum flavum (often subtle). One or two further readjustments of needle direction are commonly needed. The final angle of the needle after insertion is usually 15–20° ± 5° off mid-sagital, and 45° ± 10° off the plane of the back (see Fig 13-4). If unable to locate window, methodically search vicinity of the ideal angle with minor needle angle adjustments. If only lamina is encountered, reevaluate insertion site or consider different interspace.

5. The ligamentum flavum should be encountered immediately after walking off the lamina. The feel and compliance of the ligamentum flavum can be variable. Engaging compliant l. flavum may require advancing the needle an additional 1–1.5 cm beyond the "ledge" of lamina.

6. Once the ligamentum flavum is engaged, the epidural space is identified by standard loss of resistance to air or saline techniques. The loss of resistance at the thoracic level tends to be more subtle than the lumbar level. The distance from skin to thoracic epidural space is 6 ± 2 cm in most adults with the paramedian approach.

7. Catheter insertion is typically silky smooth due to the steep angle of entry. Any resistance should raise the suspicion of incorrect site. Depth of catheter insertion beyond needle should be approximately 5 cm.

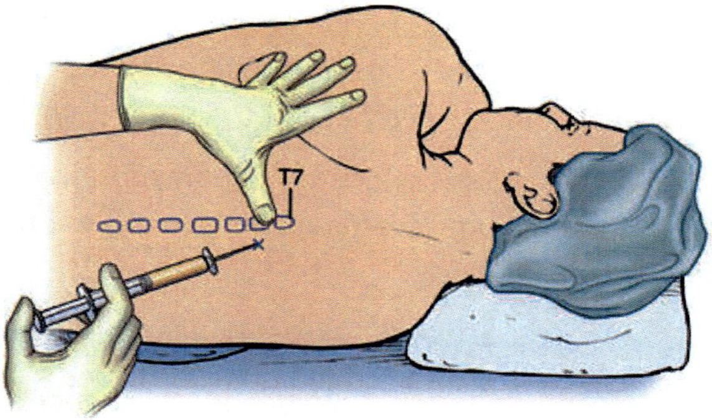

Figure 13-4 – Paramedian thoracic epidural placement.

Procedural Steps: Midline Thoracic Epidural

1. Entry point should be directly over or slightly cephalad to the lower spinous process of the desired interspace. An entry point that is too high (midinterspace) is a common cause of failure, unless kyphosis is extreme. Infiltrate local over entry site (wheal) and down to the spinous process, then redirect, walking off the north side of the spinous process within the mid-sagital plane.
2. Insert an epidural needle along the same path, walking off the spinous process to engage the interspinous ligament at an angle of roughly 45° from the plane of the back (mid-sagital).
3. Identify the epidural space by typical loss of resistance to air or saline techniques. Distance from skin to epidural space is typically deeper by midline approach than paramedian (6–8 cm). Early loss of resistance may be due to slipping off of the thin thoracic interspinous ligament. Should this occur, one can try to re-engage the ligament (redirect) or just continue parallel to the interspinous ligament until ligamentum flavum is engaged. If bone is encountered, redirecting in a more rostral fashion may be fruitful.
4. As with paramedian approach, the catheter should thread without resistance to a depth of 5 cm beyond the needle.

Intercostal Nerve Blocks

Intercostal nerve blocks can provide excellent analgesia after chest surgery, and are generally placed postoperatively by the anesthesiologist (percutaneously), or intraoperatively by the surgeon (either from inside the chest prior to chest closure, or from outside the chest). Because of their limited duration, preoperative placement is strategic only for short duration cases.

Anatomy

The intercostal nerves provide somatic sensation to the lateral and anterior thoracic muscles and skin, ribs, sternum, parietal pleura, and motor innervation to intercostal muscles and portions of the rectus sheath. The anatomy is depicted in Fig 13-5.

Technique

Intercostal nerve blocks can be performed either in the awake, sedated patient, or while under general anesthesia.

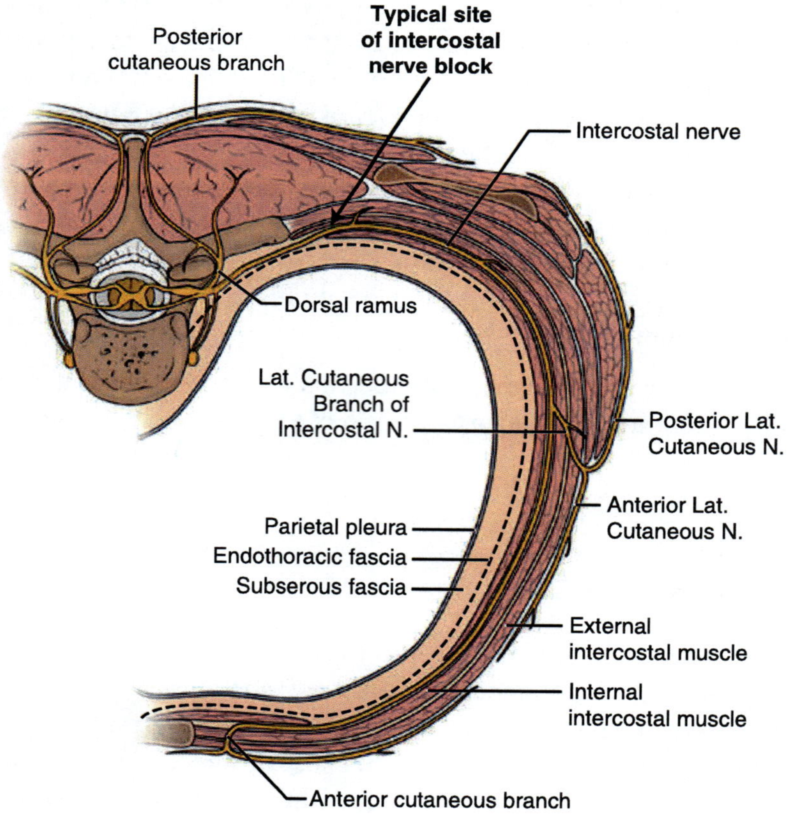

Figure 13-5 – Intercostal anatomy.

Location and Positioning

Intercostal nerve block should be performed proximal to (closer to spine) the midaxillary line, where the lateral cutaneous branch originates (Fig 13-5). In adults, the most common site for blockade is 6–8 cm from the spinous process.

Procedural Steps: Percutaneous Intercostal Nerve Blocks (Fig 13-6)

1. Under aseptic conditions, identify the ribs targeted for blockade.
2. Insert a 22-guage short bevel needle at a 20° cephalad angle, walking off the inferior border of the rib.
3. Advance the needle 3 mm. A subtle "pop" of the fascia of the internal intercostal muscle may be felt.
4. Aspirate for blood, and if negative, inject 3–5 mL of local anesthetic.
5. Blockade of adjacent intercostal nerves (cephalad and caudad) is recommended, as overlapping cutaneous innervation is common.

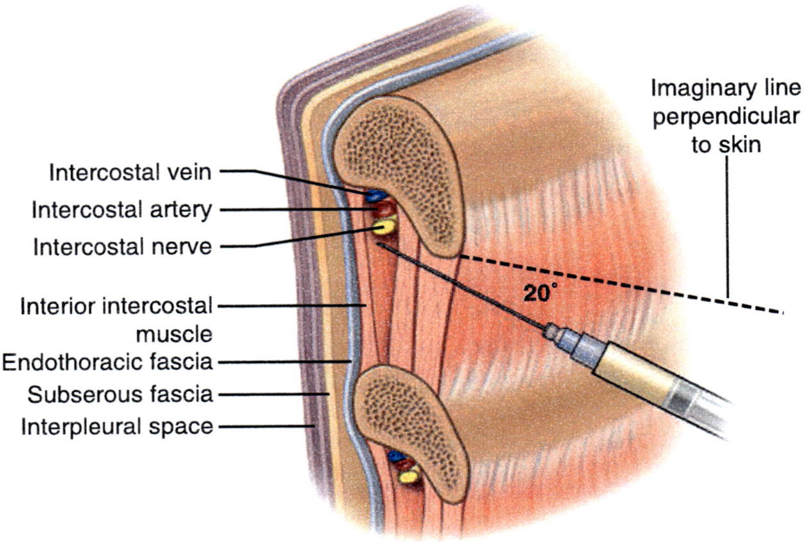

Figure 13-6 – Intercostal nerve blockade.

After the block, the patient should be monitored for potential complications, including pneumothorax, local anesthetic toxicity, hematoma, nerve damage, and rarely, subarachnoid block.

Thoracic Paravertebral Nerve Blocks

Paravertebral nerve blockade is the technique of injecting local anesthetic in the paravertebral space where the spinal nerves exit the intervertebral foraminae. It results in the blockade of both somatic and sympathetic nerves over multiple contiguous thoracic dermatomes. It is useful in the treatment of acute postoperative pain following thoracic surgery.

Anatomy

The thoracic paravertebral space is a wedge-shaped space that lies on either side of the vertebral column (Fig 13-7).

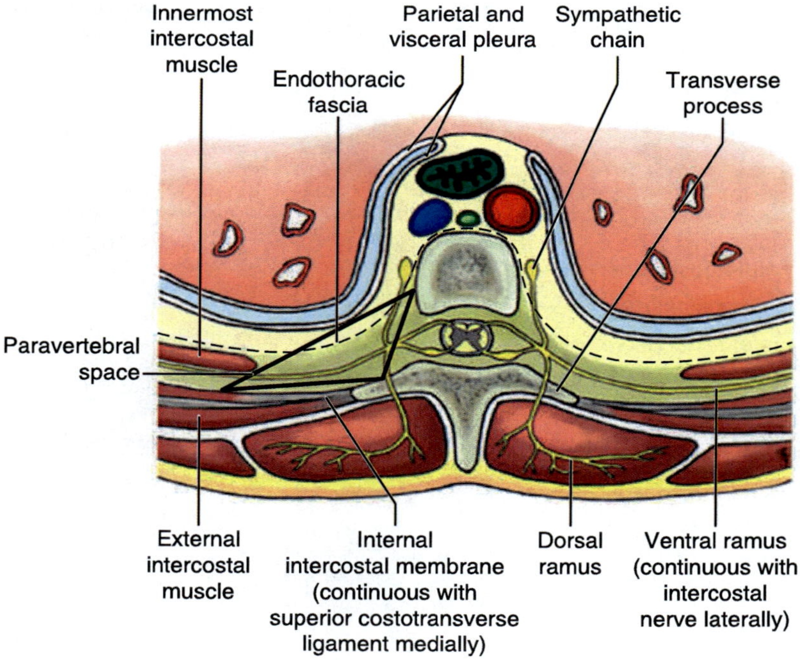

Figure 13-7 – Paravertebral anatomy.

The thoracic paravertebral space communicates with a number of other adjacent spaces, including:

- Intercostal space, laterally
- Epidural space, medially, via the intervertebral foramen
- Contralateral paravertebral space, via the epidural space and prevertebral space
- Cranial extension ends in the cervical spine
- Caudal extension is bound by the origin of the psoas muscle

Patient Preparation

Thoracic paravertebral blocks are best placed in patients that are awake or mildly sedated. Potential exists for nerve root trauma, intravascular injection, pleural puncture, and intrathecal injection, symptoms of which can be reported by an awake patient. Patients are positioned sitting, with BP and HR monitors, and rescue drugs and supplemental oxygen available.

Procedural Steps: Thoracic Paravertebral Blocks

1. Identify vertebral levels that block(s) are desired. Injections may spread for several dermatomal levels, or remain localized to the injected level.
2. With a skin marker and ruler, mark patient's spinous processes (Fig 13-8), then measure, identify, and mark locations of transverse processes 2.5 cm laterally. Due to the inferiorly angled geometry of the thoracic spinous processes, the marked transverse process belongs to the vertebral body below (Fig 13-1).
3. After sterile cleansing, insert either a 22-guage spinal needle (or an epidural needle if a catheter is desired), with tubing or syringe attached perpendicular to the skin where the transverse process is marked. Advance until contact is made with the transverse process, usually 2–4 cm depth. Locating the transverse process before advancing the needle further

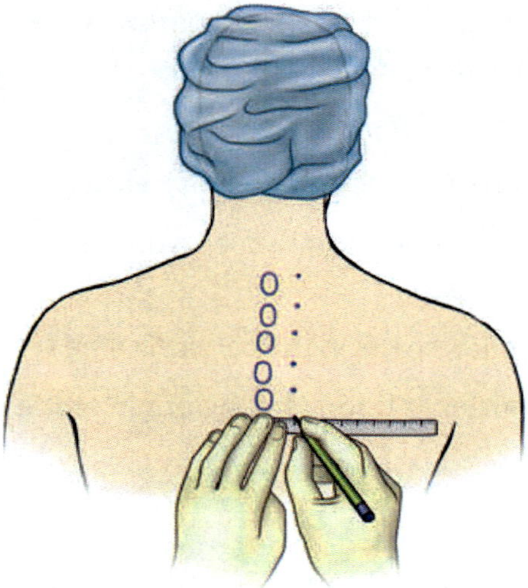

Figure 13-8 – Paravertebral marking and landmarks.

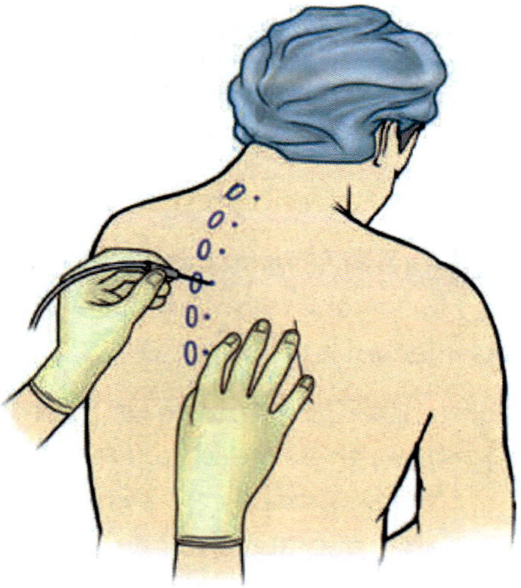

Figure 13-9 – Paravertebral nerve block.

is important to prevent inadvertent pleural puncture. Repositioning of the needle may be necessary (Fig 13-9).

4. Walk off the superior or inferior aspect of the transverse process until loss of resistance to air or saline is encountered, or subtle "pop" is felt as needle tip traverses the thin

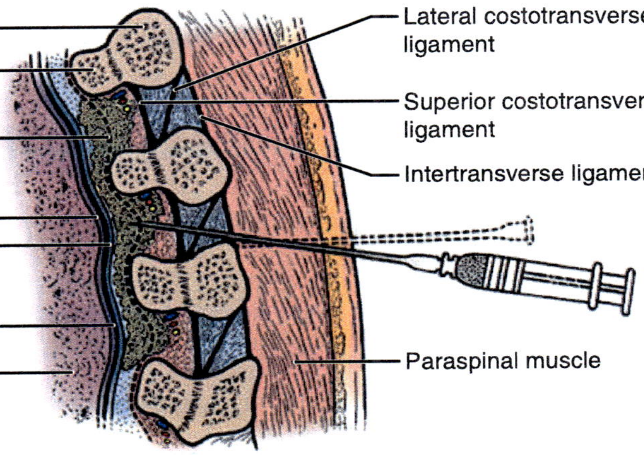

Figure 13-10 – Needle placement during paravertebral nerve blockade.

superior costotransverse ligament. The usual depth is 1–1.5 cm beyond the edge of the transverse process. Any loss of resistance may be subjective and indefinite.

5. If no pop is felt, limit insertion to less than 2 cm past the depth of the transverse process (Fig 13-10).
6. If injecting at a single level, deliver 15–20 mL (divided doses with intermittent aspiration) of local anesthetic after negative aspiration. If performing a multiple level block, inject 3–4 mL, then repeat the procedure at the adjacent levels. If inserting a catheter, manipulation of the needle or injection of saline to create a cavity may be necessary. Very easy catheter passage may be an indication of intrapleural placement.

Mechanism and Spread of Anesthesia

Local anesthetic injected into the paravertebral space typically spreads for several dermatomal levels. However, potential patterns of spread include:

- Remaining localized
- Contiguous levels above and below

- Intercostal space, laterally
- Epidural space, medially

Note that a single injection of 15–20 mL may be as effective as multiple injections of 3–4 mL/site. However, if a wide block (>5 dermatomes) is desired, it is preferable to perform two injections several dermatomes apart or multiple injections at several levels. Missing the paravertebral space at any given level can likely be compensated for via contiguous spread from adjacent levels.

Contraindications

Similar to other regional anesthetic techniques, contraindications to paravertebral blockade include:

- Infection at the site of insertion
- Empyema
- True allergy to amide local anesthetics
- Tumor occupying the thoracic paravertebral space
- Coagulopathy, bleeding disorder, or therapeutic anticoagulation

Pain Pumps

Local anesthetic can also be continuously delivered by proprietary delivery devices and catheters designed to be placed by the surgeon. Such "pain pumps" include the On-Q Pain Buster (*I-Flow Corp., Lake Forest, California*), Stryker Pain Pump *(Stryker Corp., Kalamazoo, Mich.)*, and DonJoy Pain Control Device *(DonJoy, Inc., Vista, California*). The nature and efficacy depend largely on the position of the catheters, which may be placed within muscle layers of the incision, in intercostal spaces, or through a rent in the parietal pleura to an approximation of the paravertebral space. Parasternally placed catheters are increasingly used for sternotomy incisions, and may be superior to thoracic epidurals in coverage of manubrial pain.

Pain pumps are a useful alternative where thoracic epidurals are either contraindicated, technically unfeasible, or unavailable. Pain pumps are an excellent, long-lasting rescue maneuver for the patient whose incision was unexpectedly extended to thoracotomy (without pre-operative epidural). More than one catheter can be attached to a single pump, in which case the delivery of local anesthetic may be affected by differential resistances. Catheters are positioned in sterile fashion under direct vision by the surgeon either prior to or after chest wall closure.

Generally, pumps are designed to provide local anesthetic such as bupivicaine 0.25% or ropivicaine 0.5% at a programmable or set rate, typically 4 cc/h. Thus, local anesthetic toxicity is unlikely in normal sized adults, unless additional local anesthetic is infused by another source.

Suggested References

Gottschalk A, Cohen SP, et al. Preventing and treating pain after thoracic surgery. Anesthesiology. 2006;104(3):594–600.

Karmakar M. Thoracic paravertebral block. Anesthesiology. 2001;95(3): 771–800.

III

Essential Principles of Clinical Management

Chapter 14
Preoperative Evaluation of the Thoracic Surgical Patient

Nicholas Sadovnikoff

Keywords Preoperative assessment • Respiratory mechanics • Gas exchange • Cardiopulmonary interaction • Split-lung function tests

Introduction

The anesthetic preoperative evaluation of a patient prior to thoracic surgery can be challenging, but is frequently fruitful. Advances in anesthetic management, noninvasive surgical techniques, and intensive care have gradually but progressively lowered the threshold for declaring patients to be surgical candidates. When it is felt that a patient's disease is amenable to complete surgical excision, the term "*resectable*" is employed; when it is felt that the patient can tolerate the proposed procedure, the term "*operable*" is utilized. The fact that surgical techniques have improved has increased the number of resectable patients, while the improvements in anesthetic and perioperative care have lowered the barriers to operability. Of the only roughly 13% of patients diagnosed with lung cancer who will be cured, virtually all be as a result of surgical resection. Thus, the incentive on the part of the patient to accept a risky operative intervention is greatly increased. The net result is that of a decreasingly robust population appearing in the preoperative evaluation clinic.

P.M. Hartigan (ed.), *Practical Handbook of Thoracic Anesthesia*,
DOI 10.1007/978-0-387-88493-6_14, © Springer Science+Business Media, LLC 2012

The patient presenting for evaluation has already had an extensive discussion with the thoracic surgeon regarding the risk–benefit ratio for the planned surgery. The decision to proceed is based on an algorithm that takes into account the maximal loss of functional lung that is compatible with satisfactory functional status (see below). It is not the role of the anesthesiologist to make the decision whether or not to go forward. Rather, the anesthesiologist is in a position to identify issues that may have been overlooked, that might preclude the planned surgical intervention (this is rare), or that might favor postponement (less rare). In addition, the preoperative visit is an opportunity to identify the patients at highest risk for perioperative complications and to optimize their management to the fullest. It is essential that on the day of surgery, the operative anesthesiologist, who may be meeting the patient for the first time, will have confidence that the patient has been fully evaluated and that all possible measures have been taken to optimize the patient's outcome.

General Approach

The cornerstones of preoperative assessment involve consideration of two realms of risk: *procedure-specific* and *patient-specific*. The latter constitutes the major concern of this chapter, but the former deserves attention as the patient-specific issues modify the degree of risk inherent in the procedure.

Procedure-Specific Issues

The spectrum of thoracic surgical procedures is quite broad, and the attendant risks and need for anesthetic preparation is likewise variable. The surgeries are summarized in Table 14-1. For procedures categorized as low-risk and intermediate-risk, the incidence of postoperative pulmonary complications (PPCs) is so low that little preoperative preparation is necessary. Surgeries classified as high-risk have a higher incidence of PPCs, and more careful preoperative assessment and preparation is warranted. For individual procedure-related concerns, refer to the chapters in this volume addressing the

Table 14-1 – Thoracic surgical risk categories; procedure-based

Low risk	Esophageal dilatation
	Cervical mediastinoscopy
	Laparoscopic reflux procedures
	Pleuroscopy/pleural drainage
Intermediate risk	VATS pulmonary resection
	Sympathectomy
	Open reflux procedures
	Nonemergent airway procedures (Dilation, core-out, laser, etc.)
	Tracheostomy
	Limited thoracotomy/lobectomy
High risk	Open thoracotomy for major pulmonary resection, bilobectomy, pneumonectomy, extrapleural pneumonectomy, pleurectomy, etc.
	Esophagectomy
	Sleeve resection
	Tracheal resection/reconstruction
	Emergency cases:
	Lung transplantation
	Esophageal perforation
	Tracheal/bronchial resection/repair
	Penetrating chest trauma
	Massive hemoptysis
	Rigid bronchoscopy for relief of acute obstruction (foreign body, mass, etc.)

specific surgeries (*Section IV*). Obviously, even procedures involving limited physiologic trespass may carry substantial risk if patient risk factors are severe.

Patient-Specific Issues

The health status of the patient scheduled for intermediate and high-risk thoracic surgery is the focus of the remainder of this chapter. First and foremost is the evaluation of a patient's respiratory function. There is no better assessment tool in this regard than a carefully obtained history, focusing upon exercise capacity. Patients in ASA classes I or II who have reasonable exercise capacity, that is who can climb three flights of stairs without stopping or perform ≥4 METS of physical activity, in many instances do not warrant further screening tests, as their likelihood of postoperative pulmonary complications is low; this should, however, be considered carefully for patients facing high-risk surgery. In reality, thoracic surgical patients commonly have respiratory impairment as well as other comorbidities. Further, unlike for other surgeries, *the most common complications are pulmonary in nature*, placing substantial emphasis on the lungs in the preoperative evaluation.

Three fundamental elements constitute what Slinger has called the "three-legged stool" of preoperative evaluation: respiratory mechanics, gas exchange, and cardiorespiratory interaction (1). This concept, presented here as a Venn diagram (Fig 14-1) emphasizes the fact that the three components can interact, overlap, and combine to increase the patient's risk profile.

Respiratory Mechanics – The assessment of respiratory mechanics is accomplished by spirometry. While these tests can be problematic in that they are dependent to some degree on the patient's ability to cooperate and are effort-dependent, they remain the mainstay of the surgeon's assessment of operability. The most important test in surgical planning is the Forced Expiratory Volume over one second (FEV_1), usually expressed as a percentage of what is predicted for the patient's size and gender (FEV_1%). This is then used to calculate the predicted postoperative FEV_1% as follows:

$$\text{ppoFEV}_1\% = \text{preoperative FEV}_1\% \times \left(1 - (\%\text{ of resected lung})/100\right)$$

The % of resected lung is calculated by the maximum number of lung segments that may need to be excised. A ppoFEV_1% of >40% is considered acceptable, whereas values <30% are associated with

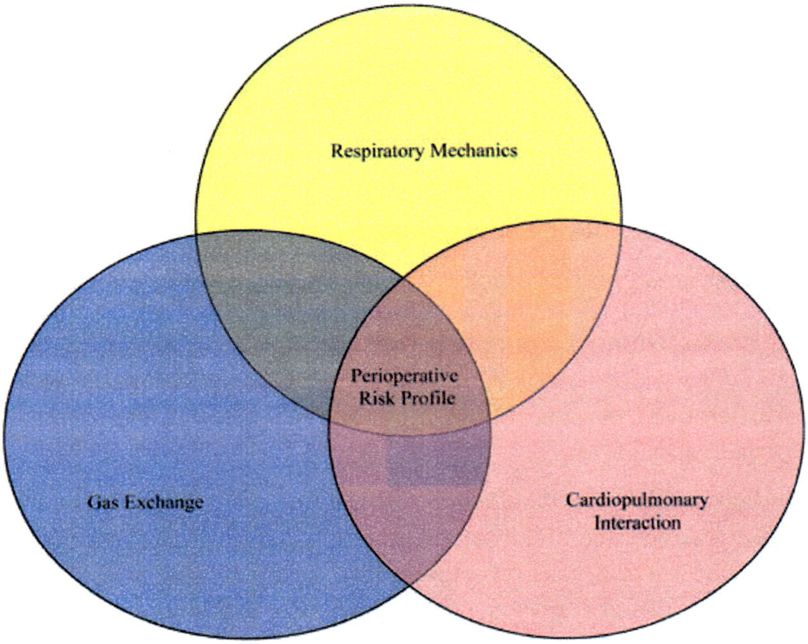

Figure 14-1 – Three-ringed circus of perioperative evaluation for thoracic surgery.

a high frequency of pulmonary complications and may deter the surgeon from operating. This threshold is not inviolable, for several reasons. First, the formula assumes homogeneity of lung function. Often, the lung tissue to be resected is less functional than the lung that will remain, leading to an underestimate of postoperative function. In these instances, radionuclide split-lung function testing may be helpful in indentifying differential function. Second, as noted above, the measurements are dependent upon effort and cooperation, and the results may be misleadingly low in patients who have pain or other impediments to optimal performance of the tests. Finally, as the outcome for patients who have nonsurgical management of lung cancer is poor, both patients and surgeons may to be willing to accept an unfavorable surgical risk profile in the face of a devastating nonsurgical prognosis.

Gas Exchange – With progression of pulmonary disease, the ability of the alveolar surface of the lungs to exchange oxygen and carbon dioxide may become impaired. This process is separate from the mechanical impairment just discussed. Arterial blood gases were traditionally used to assess this aspect of lung function, but time and experience have shown that even patients with an arterial PaO_2 of <60 mmHg or a $PaCO_2$ > 45, once thresholds for inoperability, can do well with careful attention to pain control, early mobilization, and pulmonary toilet postoperatively. A better assessment of the amount of functional alveolar surface is the *diffusing capacity for carbon monoxide* (*DLCO*). A predicted postoperative DLCO (ppoDLCO) can be calculated by the same percentage method as for the $ppoFEV_1$%, and a ppoDLCO of <40% of predicted correlates with postoperative complications independently from mechanical function ($ppoFEV_1$%).

Cardiopulmonary Interaction – This is arguably the most meaningful means of assessment of the patient, as it integrates the degree of mechanical and gas exchange impairment with cardiac function and overall physical fitness. Many methods of assessing this have been devised. The most quantitative of these is a measurement of maximal oxygen consumption (VO_2max). Patients able achieve a VO_2max of >15 ml/kg/min have been shown to have very low morbidity and those who can raise their VO_2max to >20 ml/kg/min have a low (10%) incidence of pulmonary complications. Patients with VO_2max of <10 ml/kg/min should probably not have pulmonary resection, as a very high mortality has been reported in this population (2). Because measurement of VO_2max requires substantial technology and is labor-intensive, it is not widely used. Stair climbing is another test of overall cardiopulmonary capacity, though it is somewhat harder to standardize. The simple 6-min walk with oximetry has been adopted by many as the simplest and most reproducible test. The patient walks as far as possible over 6 min while continuous pulse oximetry is monitored. A distance covered of <2,000 ft. correlates well with a VO_2max of <15 ml/kg/min as well as with a fall in oxygen saturation (SaO_2) (3).[1] A decrease in SaO_2 of >4% during exercise also has been shown to predict higher morbidity and

[1] Cahalin L, Pappagianapoulos P, Prevost S et al. The relationship of the 6-min walk test to maximal oxygen consumption in transplant candidates with end-stage lung disease. Chest 1995; 108:452–57.

mortality (4), but not all studies have demonstrated a link between exercise testing and outcomes (5).

Split-Lung Function Tests – When a major pulmonary resection or a pneumonectomy is being considered, differential evaluation of the operative and nonoperative lungs is valuable. Not only does such quantitation help more accurately predict the "worst case" functional result of resection, but it also provides guidance as to the challenges the anesthesiologist is likely to encounter intraoperatively. It was for a time popular to subject patients to simulated pneumonectomy by occluding the mainstem bronchus of the operative lung with a bronchial blocker and transiently occluding the ipsilateral pulmonary artery with an intravascular balloon. The lack of sufficient predictive power of this highly invasive test has kept it from being widely adopted. More commonly, radionuclide ventilation and perfusion scanning are performed to exclude the possibility that the nonoperative lung is differentially physiologically impaired.

Flow-Volume Loops – This spirometric test may be of value in the preoperative assessment of airway obstruction, in particular, severity of obstruction, fixed versus variable obstruction, and postural effects. Such information may guide the anesthetic induction technique employed (see Chapter 30); in particular, an approach that maintains spontaneous breathing may be preferred. In practice, however, most patients with significant airway compression/obstruction are identified by a history of positional dyspnea, and flow-volume loops are not mandatory for all patients with intrathoracic airway compromise (6).

Comorbid Conditions – Comorbidities add additional degrees of risk to thoracic surgical procedures. Some, such as age, simply cannot be modified, whereas others, such as coronary artery disease, may be possible to optimize prior to the surgical procedure. In the case of modifiable conditions, the time needed to fully optimize a patient's comorbidity must be weighed against the urgency of surgery.

Age – Chronological age does affect outcomes in the aggregate, but as a single factor is a poor predictor of outcome, especially when compared to measures of functional status described above. Studies have reported operative mortality rates of as low as 3% in patients aged 80–92 years, though their pulmonary and cardiovascular complication rates are two- to threefold higher than in younger patients (7). Thus, age alone is seldom used to define the threshold of operability (8).

Coronary Artery Disease (*CAD*) – The preoperative evaluation of the patient with coronary artery disease for noncardiac surgery has been extensively reviewed culminating in published guidelines by a joint task force of the American College of Cardiology and the American Heart Association, most recently in 2007 (9). Intrathoracic procedures fall into to the "intermediate risk" category (1–5%) for cardiac complications (defined as the combined incidence of cardiac death and nonfatal myocardial infarction). The recommendations do not favor extensive cardiac investigations in patients whose CAD is clinically stable. Only patients who have unstable or severe angina are recommended to undergo invasive testing, which they would undergo for such symptoms even in the absence of a planned surgery. If a patient's anginal history reflects a stable or improved pattern, no further cardiac investigation is warranted. If the history is unclear, or the patient's functional status is poor, then noninvasive testing (exercise or pharmacologic) may be warranted. Rarely, concurrent lung resection and coronary revascularization may be considered.

Timing of thoracic surgery for patients who have suffered a recent myocardial infarction (MI) is controversial. Older data suggested that surgery in the first 4 weeks after a MI is associated with a high degree of risk, but recent revascularization and medical optimization strategies may attenuate this elevated risk. The risk of delaying surgery should be compared with the cardiac risk of proceeding, in close collaboration with the patient's cardiologist.

Patients receiving statins and/or β-blockers should continue them through the perioperative period, if possible. An increasing body of evidence suggests that aspirin should be continued as well. The perioperative management of patients who have undergone angioplasty with or without stent placement is an evolving field, and the decisions regarding timing of surgery and discontinuation of antiplatelet therapy need to be made in concert with the patient's cardiologist.

A resting electrocardiogram (EKG), while of little diagnostic or prognostic value, is inexpensive, noninvasive, and is useful as a baseline study. Common practice is to obtain one in all patients undergoing major thoracic procedures within 30 days prior to the planned procedure.

Valvular Heart Disease – Severe valvular disease can present very high risk for both anesthesia and surgery. Symptomatic aortic stenosis (syncope, angina, or CHF) mandates postponement of surgery to consider intervention, which may consist of valve replacement or, in patients deemed not suitable for surgical repair, percutaneous valvuloplasty, prior to undertaking the proposed thoracic surgery. Patients with known but asymptomatic aortic stenosis should have an echocardiographic reevaluation of their aortic valve gradient and left ventricular function if this has not been done within the last year.

Severe mitral stenosis, now fairly rare, should also be evaluated carefully before proceeding with thoracic surgery. The risks and benefits of valve replacement or valvuloplasty should be weighed prior to proceeding with the thoracic surgery. Severe mitral regurgitation should be similarly evaluated. In general, correction of mitral valve disease should be undertaken only if it would be indicated in the absence of the planned thoracic surgery.

Congestive Heart Failure – Patients with a history of CHF or symptoms consistent with the onset thereof should not proceed directly to nonemergent surgery as this condition is subject to preoperative modification. Close collaboration with the patient's cardiologist is essential to ensure that the patient's volume status, medication management, and electrolyte levels are optimized. Attention should be paid to ensure that the patient does not undergo excessive diuresis and then present for surgery in a state of volume depletion.

Rhythm Disturbances – Cardiac dysrhythmias are extremely common after thoracic surgical procedures. Preexisting dysrhythmias or a history thereof further predispose patients to complications of this nature. The most common and vexing of these is atrial fibrillation (AF), which occurs in 30–70% of thoracic surgery patients (see Chapter 17). The incidence increases with patient age, magnitude of pulmonary resection, intraoperative blood loss, and intrapericardial surgical resection. Postoperative AF prolongs ICU and hospital length of stay, and is frequently associated with hypotension requiring significant interventions. Patients who present for surgery with chronic AF are nearly all managed with chronic anticoagulation. In general, this is discontinued prior to thoracic surgical procedures, both to limit surgical bleeding as well as to permit safe placement of thoracic epidural catheters for postoperative analgesia. The incidence of perioperative AF has recently been shown to be substantially lowered by the use of prophylactic administration of amiodarone (10). This may well gain wider acceptance with the growing body of evidence supporting this strategy

Diabetes – Patients with known diabetes should be managed carefully. Type I diabetics must never have parenteral insulin discontinued entirely. Studies addressing the value of aggressive intra- and postoperative glucose control have resulted in controversial conclusions. In the case of midline sternotomy incisions, intensive intraoperative and postoperative glucose control has been shown fairly definitively to lower the rate of sternal wound infections (11, 12). Aggressive intravenous insulin regimens to manage perioperative glucose levels have also been shown to result in an increased incidence of hypoglycemia, with accordant morbidity (13). Heightened awareness of glycemic control in diabetics with moderate intraoperative glucose targets (150–200 mg/dl) seems most appropriate. There exist no data to support preoperative optimization for glycemic control as a means to improve outcomes; hence, the diagnosis of diabetes alone should not delay surgery.

Obesity – While morbid obesity clearly increases the rates of diabetes, hypertension and CAD, studies of obese patients undergoing thoracic surgery have failed to show worse outcomes for that population (14). While the obese patient's habitus may lead to challenges in airway management, placement of epidural catheters, intraoperative ventilation, anesthetic retention, and postoperative mobilization, these have surprisingly not translated into worse outcomes when studied. Thus, while obesity is potentially a modifiable element preoperatively, the evidence supporting weight loss as a preoperative strategy is lacking.

Renal Impairment – The development of acute renal failure postoperatively dramatically increases perioperative mortality. Patients with preexisting renal insufficiency must be managed very carefully to avoid exacerbation of their renal disease. Nonsteroidal anti-inflammatory agents should be used with great caution. Patients on diuretics in particular should be assessed for their volume status, as hypovolemia and hypotension are strong risk factors for further renal injury. A high ratio of blood urea nitrogen (BUN) to creatinine should raise concerns for preoperative volume depletion. This issue is countered, particularly in the setting of a pneumonectomy, by the desire to administer intraoperative fluids parsimoniously out of concern for postpneumonectomy pulmonary edema, a complication which carries an approximate mortality of 50% (Chapter 6). Careful perioperative planning and avoidance of medications with renal toxicity is warranted.

Asthma – Well controlled asthma has not been shown to be associated with PPCs. On the other hand, poorly controlled asthma is highly associated with wheezing on induction and tracheal intubation, as well as an elevated rate of PPCs. Bronchospasm on induction may occasionally be so severe as to preclude adequate ventilation and cause postponement of the procedure.

Asthma is regarded as well controlled when a patient has daytime symptoms no more than four times a week and rarely has nighttime symptoms. Patients with more frequent attacks, recent need for corticosteroid treatment, recent hospitalizations, or frequent emergency department visits should be managed cautiously. The findings of cough, dyspnea, or wheezing on physical exam should trigger a consideration of a short course of corticosteroids prior to surgery. Prednisone at a dose of 0.5–1.0 mg/kg may be administered for the 1–3 days before the patient undergoes the procedure; this intervention is not associated with impaired wound healing and is generally well tolerated. Patients actively wheezing on the day of surgery should have the procedure postponed unless it is emergent, to allow time to medically optimize the reactive airways disease.

Chronic Obstructive Pulmonary Disease (*COPD*) – PPCs are strongly associated with COPD, and the more severe the patient's

COPD, the higher the risk of PPCs. The assessment of function and degree of risk was described earlier in this chapter, but the other role of the anesthesiologist is to determine whether the management of the COPD is optimized. Again the history is of paramount importance; any recent fever, increase in the quantity or purulence of sputum, or worsening of cough or dyspnea suggest the possibility of a lower respiratory tract infection. While prophylactic antibiotics in COPD patients have not been shown to decrease PPCs, treatment of active respiratory tract infections is warranted, whenever possible, until symptom levels return to baseline. Patients experiencing exacerbations of COPD without evidence of infections should have their management with long-acting anticholinergics, long-acting β-agonists, and inhaled corticosteroids optimized. A short course of prednisone preoperatively, as with asthma, may prevent or attenuate PPCs. When time permits, exercise training programs that can improve exercise tolerance and reduce dyspnea and fatigue may be able to lower the incidence of PPCs, though this remains controversial.

Obstructive Sleep Apnea (*OSA*) – This condition, characterized by frequent nocturnal episodes of hypopnea and apnea with attendant arterial O_2 desaturation due to upper airway obstruction, results in daytime somnolence and fatigue, and is associated with pulmonary hypertension, systemic hypertension, and right heart dysfunction. It is well described that patients with OSA are at increased risk of PPCs even when undergoing nonthoracic surgery. While the literature is scant with respect to patients with OSA undergoing thoracic procedures, it is reasonable to assume that they constitute a high risk population. Patients who use a nocturnal continuous positive airway pressure (CPAP) device should be counseled to expect to use it during the postoperative recovery period in the hospital. Strong consideration should be given to keeping such patients in the hospital overnight after procedures that are commonly performed as day surgeries.

Unfortunately, the vast majority of patients with OSA are undiagnosed. Patients who are obese, and in particular those who have a large neck circumference should generate an increased index of suspicion of this disorder. A simple instrument, the *STOP* questionnaire, has been devised that effectively identifies most patients suffering from this disorder. The acronym refers to questions regarding *S*noring, *T*iredness, *O*bserved apnea, and high blood *P*ressure and can readily be employed in the evaluation of patients being prepared for thoracic surgery. Patients who are found by this screening device to meet criteria for OSA should be referred for evaluation by a pulmonologist for consideration of perioperative CPAP and/or oxygen therapy. Ideally, such patients will then have successfully used the CPAP device at home prior to coming for their surgical procedure.

Smoking – Cigarette smoking is independently associated with increased risk of PPCs, even in patients who have not developed COPD (15). Its adverse effects include impaired macrophage functioning, impaired vascular endothelial function, decreased coronary flow reserve, and tachycardia. Smokers are more likely to manifest laryngospasm, severe coughing and oxygen desaturation with anesthesia, and they have significantly higher rates of wound infection. It is controversial, however, whether to recommend cessation immediately prior to surgery. In the first several weeks after stopping smoking, patients paradoxically experience an increase in sputum production, and some studies have shown an elevated incidence of PPCs in recent quitters. For this reason, it is recommended that, whenever possible, the patient stop smoking for at least 8 weeks prior to undergoing surgery. Patients unable to stop smoking prior to surgery put themselves at markedly increased risk for postoperative complications when they smoke postoperatively. Nicotine replacement therapy should be considered postoperatively, as it is relatively safe compared to smoking, and it starts the patient on a course that will potentially result in the cessation of smoking altogether.

Poor Nutritional Status – Patients who are malnourished have an elevated incidence of PPCs. In surgical patients in general, low serum albumin levels preoperatively (less than 3.5 mg/dl), are associated with an increased risk of PPCs compared to patients whose serum albumin is above 3.5 mg/dl (16). It is reasonable to propose aggressive nutritional supplementation in the preoperative period, but typically this requires several months to be effective, and for many thoracic surgery patients facing a known or possible malignancy, this is an unacceptable delay. For hypoalbuminemic patients, plans should be in place for aggressive nutritional support in the postoperative period.

Hematologic Disorders – Anemia is a common abnormality in patients presenting for thoracic surgery. Chronic anemia is often well tolerated due to compensatory mechanisms, and while it is rarely necessary to transfuse red cells preoperatively, there is little consensus as to what constitutes an adequate preoperative hemoglobin or hematocrit level.

Abnormalities of platelet count or function, as well as coagulation disorders, are of particular concern in thoracic surgical patients, as they may contraindicate epidural analgesic techniques. No consensus exists on safe threshold values. The risks/benefits of corrective transfusions must be individually weighed. Guidelines for cessation of anticoagulant therapy prior to neuraxial blockade are available in a recent consensus statement from the American Society of Regional Anesthesia (ASRA) (17) (see also Chapter 37).

Mediastinal Masses – Mass effects on major airways, vessels (SVC, PA), heart, or pulmonary outflow tract by mediastinal masses may be exacerbated by position and induction of anesthesia (Chapter 20). Assessment of risk hinges primarily on symptomatology and imaging data. The threshold for safe induction is not cleanly established. Generally, the absence of symptoms in the supine position, even with forced exhalation, is highly reassuring that tracheal patency is not critically threatened. The size and position of the mass on CT scan provides a sense of the risk for a mass effect. Too often, the focus is centered on airway compression forgetting that pulmonary artery or outflow tract obstruction may just as effectively preclude oxygenation. Anterior mediastinal masses compressing the distal trachea/carina are a greater threat than proximal tracheal compression (e.g., thymoma). Distal tracheal compression of greater than 50% normal and presence of positional symptoms are generally regarded as predictive of increased risk (18). Ultimately, the anesthetic plan must be tailored to the perceived risk and the experience level of the anesthesiologist. For high risk patients, options include awake topical anesthesia for biopsy, spontaneous breathing inhalational induction, awake bronchoscopy with stenting of the airway by an endotracheal tube prior to induction, and preoperative radiation therapy for radiosensitive tumors (with exclusion of biopsy target to preserve histology). This topic is discussed in more depth in Chapter 20.

Paraneoplastic Syndromes – Lung cancers are associated with a variety of paraneoplastic syndromes, and while these are more common in small-cell lung cancer, they may be seen in non-small-cell lung cancer (NSCLC) as well. They may require management prior to surgery, so the anesthesiologist should be alert to the possibility of the presence of one or more of these.

Hypercalcemia – Hypercalcemia may occur in the setting of a variety of malignancies, and it is fairly common in NSCLC, affecting 20–30% of patients with that diagnosis. Symptoms of hypercalcemia are relatively nonspecific and include lethargy, constipation, anorexia, nausea, vomiting, and polyuria/polydipsia. Untreated, extreme hypercalcemia can progress to coma and death. Normal serum calcium levels fall between 9.0 and 10.5 mg/dl (though corrections should be made in the setting of hypoalbuminemia), but symptoms of hypercalcemia do not generally occur until levels exceed 12 mg/dl. Calcium levels of >14 mg/dl constitute hypercalcemic crisis and mandate hospitalization. Fortunately, hypercalcemia is generally relatively easy to manage medically, with hydration and forced diuresis being the mainstays of therapy. It is desirable to normalize serum calcium levels prior to proceeding to surgical intervention.

Lambert-Eaton Myasthenic Syndrome (*LEMS*) – This neurologic syndrome is characterized by neuromuscular weakness that improves slightly with repetitive exercise. It is believed to be caused by autoimmune-mediated interference with presynaptic calcium channel function. It is of particular interest to the anesthesiologist because it results in exquisite sensitivity to nondepolarizing neuromuscular blockers (NNMBs). Patients with a clinical presentation consistent with LEMS should be managed intraoperatively either without NNMBs altogether or with substantially reduced doses thereof.

Syndrome of Inappropriate Antidiuresis (*SIAD*) – This is a syndrome associated with many conditions including lung malignancies that is characterized by inappropriate free water retention in the setting of hyponatremia. It was formerly referred to as the syndrome of inappropriate antidiuretic hormone (SIADH) until it became apparent that in only a minority of cases is the actual level of antidiuretic hormone (ADH or vasopressin) elevated when assayed. It is most often asymptomatic, in spite of markedly low serum sodium levels, and when symptoms are present, they are nonspecific, including fatigue, lethargy, and irritability. This disorder is extremely important to identify preoperatively, as overly rapid correction of the serum sodium has the potential consequence of the neurologically devastating phenomenon of central pontine myelinolysis. The diagnosis of SIAD is made by the finding of an inappropriately normal or high urine osmolality in spite of hyponatremic serum. Ideally, patients with this abnormality should have their hyponatremia gradually corrected preoperatively. If the urgency of surgery does not allow for this, the perioperative management should include very close attention to serum sodium such that it is not corrected overly rapidly.

Myasthenia Gravis (*MG*) – This disease is characterized by neuromuscular weakness that is aggravated by repetitive exercise. It is an autoimmune disorder in which a majority of patients can be demonstrated to have autoantibodies which directly interfere with the acetylcholine receptor at the neuromuscular junction. Thymic tumors or thymomas are highly associated with MG, and while the pathophysiology is incompletely understood, a significant number of patients who have MG but without thymoma improve following thymectomy. Hence myasthenics frequently present for this procedure.

The cardinal considerations in caring for these patients relate to their preoperative medical regimen and, of course, their neuromuscular weakness. Patients with MG are typically managed as outpatients with an oral acetylcholinesterase inhibitor, usually pyridostigmine, commonly in conjunction with glucocorticoids and/or immunosuppressive agents. In general, surgery should not be undertaken in patients whose medical regimen has not been optimized. Some patients with persistent weakness in spite of a maximal pharmacologic regimen may undergo plasmapheresis or receive immune globulin therapy preoperatively. Anesthetic management should include ensuring that the patients receive their daily glucocorticoid dose equivalent, though there is no evidence that elevated "stress dose" administration is necessary. Patients with MG are resistant to the pharmacologic effects of succinylcholine, so if this agent is used, doses two to four times the standard dosing are recommended. By contrast, MG patients tend to be exceptionally sensitive to the effects of NNMBs, giving rise to the concern for postoperative neuromuscular respiratory compromise. This gives substance to the approach of avoiding this class of drugs altogether in favor of either inhalational or deep intravenous anesthetic techniques.

The response to thymectomy is not immediate, so continuation of cholinesterase inhibitors intravenously through the operative period until the patient can resume oral intake is recommended to avoid myasthenic crisis. Because of pyridostigmine's poor bioavailability by the enteral route, the intravenous dose is 1/30th of the oral dose.

Anticipation of Problems with Lung Isolation – Successful lung isolation is essential to achieving satisfactory surgical conditions. Preoperative identification of impediments to achieving and maintaining lung isolation allows for better anesthetic planning and execution. There are two general categories of problems with lung isolation: *anatomic* and *physiologic*. Physiologic predictors of problematic one-lung ventilation are discussed in Chapter 5. Anatomic abnormalities with implications for lung isolation are listed in Table 14-2, and technical strategies for these are discussed in Chapter 9. Data from history, physical exam, chest CT, and (if available) prior anesthetics and bronchoscopic exams are of value in assessment of such issues. Not infrequently, the initial bronchoscopy on the day of surgery determines the final surgical and lung isolation plan.

Postoperative Pain Management – The plan for postoperative pain management should be established prior to surgery, subject to modification as circumstances change. The plan should essentially be based upon three considerations: the magnitude of the surgical incision(s), the degree of expected postoperative pulmonary compromise of the patient, and the preoperative pain management regimen. At one extreme, otherwise healthy, fit, and relatively young patients may tolerate a full thoracotomy incision for a complete

Table 14-2 – Anatomic abnormalities with implications for lung isolation planning

- Difficult upper airway anatomy
- Tracheal bronchus or short left mainstem bronchus
- Retracted left mainstem bronchus
- Left-shifted carina or acute take-off of left mainstem bronchus
- Tracheostomy
- Tracheal stenosis (intrinsic vs. extrinsic compression) (fixed vs. variable)
- Tracheal endoluminal tumor
- Tracheal stent, carinal Y-stent, or high endobronchial stent
- Central airway fistula (tracheoesophageal, bronchopleural, etc.)

pneumonectomy with little more than intravenous opioids, converting to an oral regimen once oral intake is possible. At the other extreme, patients with severe COPD undergoing a small thoracoscopic wedge resection with only "porthole" incisions may indeed benefit from thoracic epidural analgesia (TEA). In addition to TEA, numerous other techniques of postoperative pain management may be employed, including intercostal/paravertebral blocks and catheters, "soaker" local anesthetic catheters, and others (see Chapter 37).

Postoperative Intensive Care – While the decision to place a patient in an intensive care unit (ICU) postoperatively is frequently automatic based on the planned surgery, there are patients whose underlying disease issues mandate intensive postoperative monitoring and care in spite of a relatively minor planned surgery. These include patients with major organ system impairment, most commonly those with significant pulmonary, cardiovascular, or renal impairment. The preoperative anesthetic evaluation may recognize overlooked issues which warrant a planned ICU admission postoperatively. There is value to the patient, the patient's family, and to the hospital bed management system, of preventing an unanticipated ICU admission.

Selected References

1. Slinger PS, Johnston MR. Preoperative assessment for pulmonary resection, 2005. http://www.thoracic-anesthesia.com/?p=23.

2. Colice GL, Shafazand S, Griffin JP, et al. Physiologic evaluation of the patient with lung cancer being considered for resectional surgery: ACCP evidenced-based clinical practice guidelines (2nd edition). Chest. 2007;132:161S–77.

3. Cahalin L, Pappagianapoulos P, Prevost S, et al. The relationship of the 6-min walk test to maximal oxygen consumption in transplant candidates with end-stage lung disease. Chest. 1995;108:452–7.

4. Ninan M, Sommers KE, Landranau RJ, et al. Standardized exercise oximetry predicts post-pneumonectomy outcome. Ann Thorac Surg. 1995;60:603–9.

5. Win T, Jackson A, Groves AM, et al. Relationship of shuttle walk test and lung cancer surgical outcome. Eur J Cardiothorac Surg. 2004;26:1216–9.

6. Slinger PD, Karsli C. Management of the patient with a large anterior mediastinal mass: recurring myths. Curr Opin Anaesthesiol. 2007;20(1):1–3.

7. Osaki T, Shirakusa T, Kodate M, et al. Surgical treatment of lung cancer in the octogenarian. Ann Thorac Surg. 1994;57:188–93.

8. Dexter EU, Jahangir N, Kohman LJ. Resection for lung cancer in the elderly patient. Thorac Surg Clin. 2004;14:163–71.

9. Fleisher LA, Beckman JA, Brown KA, et al. ACC/AHA 2007 Guidelines on perioperative cardiovascular evaluation and care for noncardiac surgery: executive summary: a report of the American College of Cardiology/American Heart Association Task Force on practice guidelines. Circulation. 2007;116(17): 1971–96.

10. Tisdale JE, Wroblewski HA, Wall DS, et al. A randomized trial evaluating amiodarone for prevention of atrial fibrillation after pulmonary resection. Ann Thorac Surg. 2009;88:886–93.

11. Kramer R, Groom R, Weldner D, et al. Glycemic control and reduction of deep sternal wound infection rates: a multidisciplinary approach. Arch Surg. 2008;143:451–6.

12. Furnary AP, Zerr KJ, Grunkemeier GL, et al. Continuous intravenous insulin infusion reduces the incidence of deep sternal wound infection in diabetic patients after cardiac surgical procedures. Ann Thorac Surg. 1999;67(2):352–60.

13. Finfer S, Chittock DR, Su SY, et al. Intensive versus conventional glucose control in critically ill patients. N Engl J Med. 2009;360:283–97.

14. Smith PW, Wang H, Gazoni LM, et al. Obesity does not increase complications after anatomic resection for non-small cell lung cancer. Ann Thorac Surg. 2007;84:1098–105.

15. Warner DO. Perioperative abstinence from cigarettes. Anesthesiology. 2006;104:356–67.

16. Sweitzer BJ, Smetana GW. Identification and evaluation of the patient with lung disease. Anesthesiol Clin. 2009;27:673–86.

17. ASRA website. http://www.asra.com/consensus-statements/.

18. Shamberger RC, Holzman RS, Griscom NT, Tarbell NJ, Weinstein HJ, Wohl ME. Prospective evaluation by computed tomography and pulmonary function tests of children with mediastinal masses. Surgery. 1995;118:468–71.

Chapter 15
Overview: Surgeon's Approach to the Patient with Lung Cancer

Steven J. Mentzer

Keywords Lung cancer • Lung cancer staging

Introduction

In most thoracic surgery centers, lung cancer is the most common indication for surgery. For patients with suspected lung cancer, thoracic surgical procedures can establish a definitive diagnosis. For patients with a known diagnosis of lung cancer, thoracic surgery may contribute to local control of the primary tumor. In a third group of patients, thoracic surgery is useful for characterizing the anatomic extent of the disease – a process referred to as cancer staging. Staging is useful because the simple histologic diagnosis of lung cancer is associated with a wide range of possible outcomes. Staging procedures are designed to provide information that can clarify an individual patient's expected outcome (Fig 15-1). Patients with more advanced disease are candidates for more aggressive treatments. In the past two decades, patients with advanced disease are being offered multimodality therapy – that is, treatments that involve the combined use of chemotherapy, radiation therapy, and surgery.

P.M. Hartigan (ed.), *Practical Handbook of Thoracic Anesthesia*,
DOI 10.1007/978-0-387-88493-6_15, © Springer Science+Business Media, LLC 2012

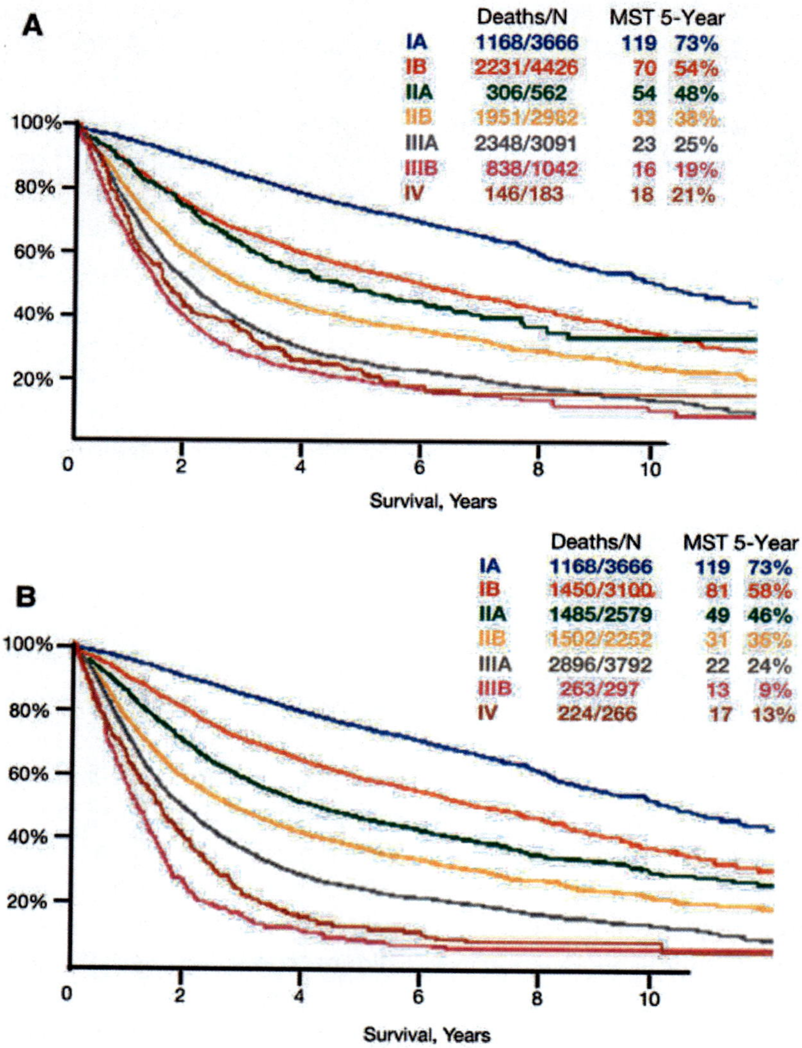

Figure 15-1 – Lung cancer survival curves by staging system – Overall survival expressed as median survival time (MST) and 5-year survival by pathologic stage using the sixth edition of TNM staging system (**A**) and the revised (proposed) International Association of the Study of Lung Cancer recommendations. Note the improved separation between survival curves for stage IIIA versus IIIB/IV (**B**) with the proposed new (7th Edition) staging system. *Reprinted with permission from Goldstraw P, Crowley J, Chansky K, et al, and the International Association for the Study of Lung Cancer (IASLC). The IASLC lung cancer staging project: Proposals for the revision of the TNM stage groupings in the forthcoming (seventh) edition of the TNM classification of malignant tumors. J Thorac Oncol 2007; 2(8): 706–14.*

Staging of Lung Cancer

Cancer staging is a descriptive shorthand that identifies distinct milestones in the natural history of the malignant disease. The natural history of each type of cancer is based on historical data; the underlying assumption is that each patient with a given type of cancer demonstrates a comparable pattern of disease progression.

For most cancers, the primary tumor progressively grows in size. As the tumor grows, genetic mutations and population dynamics within the tumor result in the development of a subpopulation of cells capable of tissue invasion and metastasis. The size at which the tumor develops a metastatic phenotype is a function of tumor biology; for example, small-cell lung carcinomas develop distant metastases at a much smaller tumor size than non-small-cell lung carcinomas. In most cancers, metastases develop by the embolic spread of metastatic cells to the lymphatic system and subsequently to the blood circulation.

The predictable sequence of tumor progression for each "type" of tumor has led to staging systems. The goal of the staging system is to provide consistent descriptions of the anatomic extent of cancers at specific times in their clinical progression. Denoix and colleagues first advocated the "TNM" classification in the 1940s (1). In 1986, the American Joint Committee on Cancer (AJCC) and the International Union Against Cancer (UICC) adopted a common TNM staging system (2). In 1997, this staging system was reconciled with the 1983 American Thoracic Society statement on clinical staging (3). The current staging system is based on the relative size and extent of the primary tumor (T), the absence, presence, and extent of regional lymph node involvement (N), and the absence or presence of distance metastases (M). The present TNM staging system has been universally adopted as the basis for therapeutic comparisons worldwide. The lung cancer TNM staging system was most recently revised in 2010 (Table 15-1).

In the evaluation of individual patients, a common approach is to systematically evaluate the anatomic extent of the cancer by first

Table 15-1 – Comparison of 6th- and 7th-edition lung cancer staging[a]

6TH EDITION T/M	7TH EDITION T/M	N0	N1	N2	N3
T1 (<2)	T1a	IA	IIA	IIIA	IIIB
T1 (>2–3)	T1b	IA	IIA	IIIA	IIIB
T2 (<5)	T2a	IB	**IIA**	IIIA	IIIB
T2 (>5–7)	T2b	**IIA**	IIB	IIIA	IIIB
T2 (>7)	T3	**IIB**	**IIIA**	IIIA	IIIB
T3 invasion	T3	IIB	IIIA	IIIA	IIIB
T4 [same lobe nodules]	T3	**IIB**	**IIIA**	**IIIA**	IIIB
T4 [extension]	T4	**IIIA**	**IIIA**	IIIB	IIIB
M1 [ipsilateral lung]	T4	**IIIA**	**IIIA**	**IIIB**	**IIIB**
T4 [pleural effusion]	M1a	**IV**	**IV**	**IV**	**IV**
M1 [contralateral lung] a	M1	IV	IV	IV	IV
M1 [distant]	M1b	IV	IV	IV	IV

[a]Changes in the staging system are highlighted in *bold*. Reprinted with permission from Goldstraw P, Crowley J, Chansky K, et al.: The IASLC Lung Cancer Staging Project: Proposals for the revision of the TNM stage groupings in the forthcoming (seventh) edition of the TNM classification of malignant tumors. J. Thorac Oncol 2: 706–14, 2007.

assessing the possibility of metastatic disease. In the case of lung cancer, the staging evaluation addresses three questions:

1. Is there metastatic disease outside the chest?
2. Is there metastatic disease within the chest, but outside the lung?
3. Is the disease confined to the lung?

Outside the Chest

A biological feature of lung cancer, and a practical explanation for the high mortality associated with the disease, is the tendency to give rise to blood-borne metastases. Non-small-cell lung cancers demonstrate a pattern of metastatic disease associated with brain, bone, adrenal gland, and liver metastases. Although there are slight variations in the pattern of disease associated with different histologic subtypes, the evaluation of any given patient with lung cancer must involve an assessment of these organs.

A systemic staging evaluation involves, at minimum, a head and chest computed tomography (CT) scan (with contrast dye) and a bone scan. The standard thoracic chest CT scan typically extends below the diaphragms to include the liver and adrenal glands. The limitation of nonmetabolic imaging is the relatively high incidence of false-positive findings; particularly, the presence of adrenal adenomas, liver hemangiomas, and benign bony abnormalities may falsely suggest metastatic disease. Metabolic imaging, such as positron emission tomography (PET) scanning, combines CT imaging with an assessment of metabolic activity (glucose uptake). PET/CT scans have largely replaced bone scans in major centers. Because of the intense metabolic activity of the brain, PET/CT scans are complemented with head MRI scans to complete the extrathoracic staging evaluation.

As a general rule, the PET/CT scan provides a map of potential metastatic disease; however, the presence of metastatic disease must be proven by a fine needle aspiration biopsy or a surgical tissue biopsy. Benign inflammatory diseases, such as sarcoidosis, are a common source of a falsely positive PET scan.

With few exceptions, patients with extrathoracic disease are stage IV and are not candidates for surgery. Notable exceptions are patients with solitary brain metastases. When carefully selected, a small subset of patients with a solitary brain metastasis may benefit from surgical resection. For most patients, however, the outlook is limited with life expectancy in the range of 8 months.

Inside the Chest/Outside the Lung

Lymph nodes. An interesting biologic feature of lung cancer is that extrathoracic disease is typically a result of hematogenous dissemation, whereas intrathoracic disease is the consequence of lymphatic metastases. Lung-to-lung blood-borne metastatic disease, except in advanced stages, is uncommon.

Another feature of intrathoracic spread, perhaps related to the defined hilar and mediastinal lymphatic anatomy, is the predictable sequence of metastatic lymph node progression. As a consequence, prognosis closely correlates with the anatomic extent of lymphatic disease. Disease limited to lymph nodes close to the tumor, the so-called hilar lymph nodes (N1), has a more favorable prognosis. Lymph nodes progressively further from the tumor – ipsilateral lymph nodes (N2) and contralateral/distant lymph nodes (N3) – have a progressively poorer prognosis.

In most cases, patients with N3 disease – including supraclavicular and contralateral nodal disease – are not surgical candidates. The presence of supraclavicular lymph node metastases can often be documented by outpatient fine needle biopsy. Contralateral lymph node involvement may require a cervical mediastinoscopy or, more rarely, a thoracoscopic biopsy. The documentation of N3 disease should not require a thoractotomy.

Patients with N3 disease are usually treated by a combination of chemotherapy and radiation therapy. Contemporary survival with chemoradiation therapy is in the range of 13 months.

Patients with ipsilateral (N2) mediastinal lymph node involvement (stage IIIA) are an important focus in lung cancer therapy. Because N2 lymph nodes represent disease presumed to be in the early phases of dissemination, these patients are the most likely to benefit from aggressive multidisciplinary treatment. Combined or multimodality therapy has been the focus of lung cancer therapeutic investigations for nearly 20 years. A common approach is to give the chemotherapy and radiation therapy prior to surgery – a so-called neoadjuvant chemoradiation treatment. Although there are biologic arguments supporting neoadjuvant therapy (preserved blood supply, etc.), the practical reality is that patients who fail to respond to chemoradiation therapy or develop interval systemic disease are spared surgery.

The development of neoadjuvant therapy has emphasized the importance of establishing N2 (stage IIIA) and excluding N3 (stage IIIB) prior to treatment. Preferably, this discrimination between stage IIIA and IIIB disease can be made with minimal surgical morbidity. The most commonly used modality of tissue diagnosis is cervical mediastinoscopy. Mediastinoscopy provides access to both ipsilateral and contralateral as well as upper and lower paratracheal lymph nodes. Endobronchial ultrasound and electromagnetic navigational bronchoscopy can be useful tools for obtaining nodal cytology, but provide a significantly more limited sample than mediastinoscopy.

Patients with N2 disease are optimally treated with both chemotherapy and radiation therapy. In patients demonstrating a response to therapy, surgery can be useful in consolidating the local control of the disease. The rationale for surgery, even in the setting of a significant radiographic response to therapy, is the common finding of viable residual cancer in the primary tumor. The survival of patients after combined therapy is in the range of 16 months.

Pleural effusions. The presence of a pleural effusion ipsilateral to a known lung cancer is worrisome for advanced malignant disease. Typically detected by chest radiograph, a unilateral opacity can represent either a pleural effusion and/or parenchymal lung collapse. Collapsed or atelectatic lung can be distinguished from pleural effusions by an assessment of the volume of the ipsilateral hemithorax. Collapsed lung is associated with tracheal deviation (mediastinal shift), an elevated hemidiaphragm, and decreased intercostal spaces. If there is evidence of a small hemithorax, chest CT scanning is useful to assess the relative contribution of the pleural effusion and atelectatic lung to the opacity observed on chest X-ray.

The most effective diagnostic approach involves thoracentesis and an examination of the cells in the pleural fluid. The diagnostic yield of cytologic examination of pleural fluid cells exceeds 50% in most types of malignant pleural effusion. The yield increases modestly with repeated thoracentesis. In some cases, thoracoscopy may play a role in establishing the etiology of the pleural effusion.

Patients with malignant cytology are candidates for surgery only in the context of multimodality clinical trials. The life expectancy of patients with malignant pleural effusions (stage IIIB) is in the range of 13 months.

Chestwall and mediastinal invasion. A subset of patients who have benefited from advances in surgical and anesthetic management are patients with mediastinal and chest wall invasion. A T3 tumor is a tumor of any size (T1 < 3 cm, T2 > 3 cm) that invades the chest wall or mediastinum. Common structures include the ribs, thoracic inlet (the so-called superior sulcus or Pancoast tumors), mediastinal pleura, pericardium, and mainstem bronchi without invasion of the carina. Because of advances in surgical and anesthetic management, T3 tumors are now classified in a more favorable prognostic category (stage II).

The diagnosis of chest wall invasion may be difficult to determine preoperatively. Tumor adhesion or simple contact with the parietal pleura may be indistinguishable from tumor invasion by preoperative imaging. Thoracoscopy can be useful to assess operability in a subset of patients. When a tumor has invaded the intrathoracic fascia, the surgical procedure typically involves an en bloc resection of the chest wall.

A small group of patients with local invasion of the heart, aorta, trachea, or esophagus may be judged to be unresectable at the time of surgery (T4); however, many patients with focal involvement of these structures can be successfully reconstructed.

Inside the Lung

Based on the staging assumptions of disease progression, the earliest evidence of metastatic disease should be reflected in peribronchial (N1) lymph nodes. An advantage of anatomic surgical resections, such as lobectomy and segmentectomy, is the opportunity to harvest N1 lymph nodes. In contrast, nonanatomic or "wedge" resections typically do not provide these lymph nodes for analysis.

Whereas most evidence indicates that regional lymphadenectomy has limited therapeutic benefit, regional lymph nodes do provide more complete staging information. The identification of N1 disease decreases the expected long-term survival by approximately 10%. Patients without lymph node involvement have approximately a 70% long-term disease-free survival; patients with N1 disease have a 60% long-term survival.

Because of the unacceptably high rate of recurrence, even in the most favorable stage (30%), there is a growing trend for adjuvant chemotherapy in almost all patients with lung cancer. Chemotherapy is the adjuvant treatment of choice because the pattern of recurrence in early-stage lung cancer (stage I and II) is typically distant disease (70–80%). Recent multicenter clinical trials indicate a 5% improvement in survival rates with adjuvant chemotherapy. Of note, the absolute statistical impact of adjuvant chemotherapy in lung cancer and breast cancer is similar; however, the overall survival in breast cancer is much better.

Because of the unlikelihood of lung-to-lung metastases, the presence of two or more tumors in the lung suggests either metastatic disease from an extrathoracic primary or synchronous lung cancers. PET/CT scans can be useful to exclude the presence of extrathoracic malignancy. The treatment of synchronous lung cancers is essentially based on the optimal treatment of each individual tumor. A notable consideration, however, is the patient's underlying lung function and the amount of functioning lung tissue at risk. For example, in staged surgical resections, it is often preferable to first perform the smaller parenchymal resection. Pulmonary resections removing a significant percentage of the patient's functional reserve often limit options for selective ventilation during subsequent procedures.

An increasingly recognized form of lung cancer, not suited for the TNM paradigm of disease progression, is "bronchioloalveolar carcinoma" (BAC) or "minimally invasive adenocarcinoma." BAC is notable for distinct patterns of disease progression. One form of BAC presents as indolent "ground glass opacities" on chest CT imaging. Another presentation is multifocal disease; that is, the presence of multiple independent nodules. A third presentation is diffuse airspace disease associated with copious mucinous bronchorrhea. There is significant interest in BAC because of a genetic fingerprint: mutations in the epidermal growth factor receptor (EGFR). The study of EGFR mutations has provided insights into carcinogenesis as well as a potential target for therapy.

Summary

Cancer staging provides a description of the anatomic extent of the cancer at specific times in their clinical progression. In lung cancer, these milestones or stages are practically divided into (1) extrathoracic hematogenous metastatic disease, (2) intrathoracic lymphatic metastatic disease, and (3) resectable intraparenchymal disease.

Selected References

1. Denoix PF. Sur l'organisation d'une statistique permanente du cancer. Bull Inst Nat Hyg. 1944;1:67–74.

2. Mountain CF. A new international staging system for lung cancer. Chest. 1986;89:225S–33.

3. Mountain CF. Revisions in the International System for Staging Lung Cancer. Chest. 1997;111:1710–7.

Chapter 16
Principles of Anesthetic Management for Pulmonary Resection

Philip M. Hartigan

Keywords Wedge resection • Lobectomy • Segmentectomy • Pulmonary resection • VATS • Limited thoracotomy • Open thoracoctomy • Video-assisted thoracic surgical approach

Note to Readers:

This chapter serves as a general model, and foundation for the individual thoracic surgical procedures which follow in Section IV of this text. Many of the management concepts and strategies discussed in this chapter are recurrent in thoracic surgery, and need not be repeated for each procedure. Such issues, discussed below, are prerequisite to Section IV, and are essential foundation concepts for thoracic anesthesia in general.

Introduction

Pulmonary resection, in one form or another, is the most commonly performed thoracic surgical procedure. This chapter discusses anesthetic considerations for lobectomy and lesser resections (segmentectomy, wedge resection) with attention to common anesthetic issues of thoracic anesthesia (Box 16-2).

P.M. Hartigan (ed.), *Practical Handbook of Thoracic Anesthesia*,
DOI 10.1007/978-0-387-88493-6_16,

Box 16-1 – Definitions; Lobectomy and Lesser Resections

- *Wedge Resection*: Nonanatomic resection of partial lobe (Fig 16-1)
- *Segmentectomy*: Anatomic resection of sublobar segment (Fig 16-2)
- *Lobectomy*: Anatomic resection of entire lobe (Fig 16-3)

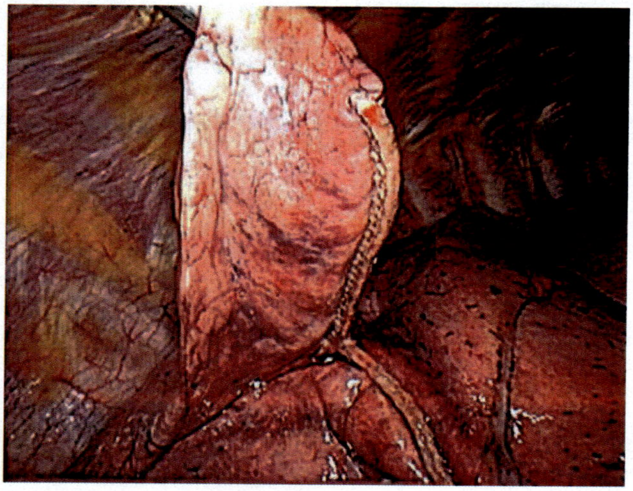

Figure 16-1 – Surgeon's view via thoracoscope (aimed toward the apex) of a right upper lobe wedge resection in progress.

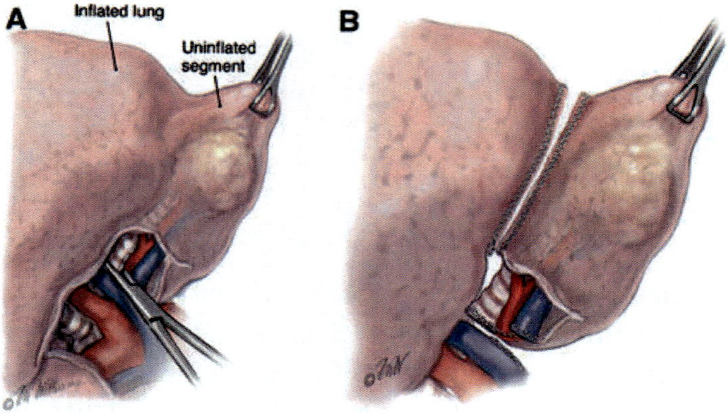

Figure 16-2 – Segmental vessels and bronchus are isolated (**A**) and divided (**B**) along with the corresponding lung parenchyma in a formal anatomic segmentectomy. *Reproduced with permission from Sugarbaker DJ, et al. Adult Lung Surgery. McGraw-Hill Medical, 2009. Copyright; Marcia Williams.*

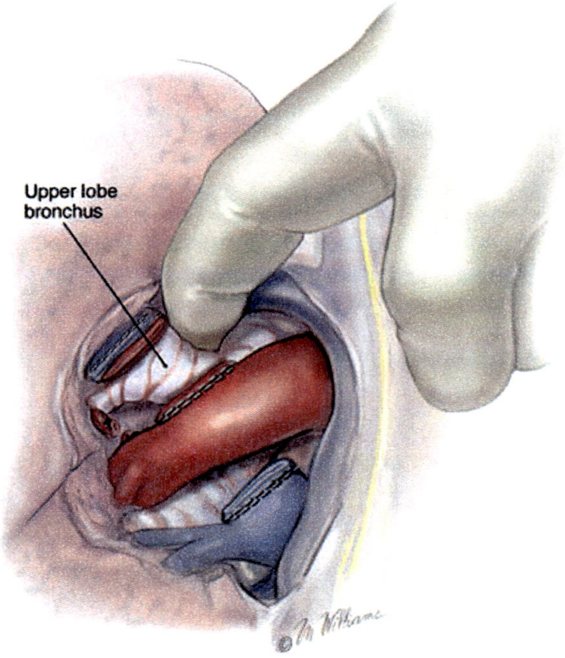

Figure 16-3 – Surgeon's view of a right upper lobectomy. Following division of lobar vessels (including bronchial), the right upper lobe bronchus is isolated by circumferential blunt dissection prior to application of stapling device. *Reproduced with permission from Sugarbaker DJ, et al. Adult Lung Surgery. McGraw-Hill Medical, 2009. Copyright; Marcia Williams.*

Box 16-2 – Overview: Anesthetic Considerations for Pulm. Resection

- General anesthesia tailored to immediate post-op extubation
- Pain management plan tailored to anticipated incision:
- Thoracic Epidural for large VATS or thoracotomy
- PCA for limited VATS incisions
- Invasive monitors and IVs tailored to extent of surgery and pathophysiology

(continued)

Box 16-2 – (continued)

- Lung isolation technique based on anatomy and planned resection
- Lateral decubitus position
- Satisfactory one-lung gas exchange
- Avoidance of lung injury
- Relatively restrictive fluid management
- Control of secretions
- Prevention of bronchospasm
- Detection of surgical air leaks
- Full recruitment of remaining lung following resection
- Safe tube exchange for terminal toilette bronchoscopy
- Rapid return of adequate spontaneous ventilation
- Immediate post-op extubation
- Aggressive control of acute postsurgical pain
- Possible mitigation of chronic postthoracotomy pain

Surgical Approach

The extent of the incision (rather than resection) is the most important determinant of postoperative pain.

Lobectomy and lesser resections may be performed by a video-assisted thoracic surgical (VATS) approach, full open thoracoctomy, or any intermediate, limited thoracotomy. The term "VATS" signifies the use of a camera, but does not guarantee that the incision will be small. The size of the utility port in a VATS resection is often dictated by the size of the specimen which must exit that wound, as well as other variables (surgeon's experience, adhesions, etc.) (see Chapter 7). The technical requirements of segmentectomies generally require mini-thoracotomy incisions comparable to that for lobectomy. Wedge resections are more often performed via porthole incisions only, depending on the size of the wedge. The anticipated extent of incision impacts preoperative decisions regarding pain control and invasive monitoring. Not uncommonly the extent of incision deviates from the original plan.

Immediate Preoperative Encounter

The formal preoperative evaluation often occurs days or weeks prior to surgery. Questions regarding *resectability* and *operability* should have been satisfied prior to this stage (Chapter 14). The immediate preoperative encounter is an opportunity to identify interval changes and potentially modify risk. Particular attention should be paid to pulmonary symptoms (wheezing, sputum production, dyspnea, positional symptoms). Unlike nonthoracic surgery, pulmonary complications outweigh cardiac as the most frequent cause of perioperative mortality (1). Lung cancer surgery is semielective, but risk reduction may occasionally justify modest postponements or interventions to treat acute processes such as pulmonary infections, bronchospasm, or effusions. For example, malignant pleural or pericardial effusions can accumulate rapidly, and increase induction risk. Hemodynamically significant effusions detected in the preoperative encounter can be drained under local prior to induction.

Prior to entering the operating room the team should have the clearest possible picture of the anticipated extent of the incision, and resection. Unambiguous "side-of-surgery" verification is now a universal institutional priority. The anesthesiologist should examine the chest CT to identify high risk inductions due to mass effects. Radiographic data will also provide insights into the size and accessibility of the lesion, and potential issues with lung isolation.

Monitors and Lines

Lobectomy and lesser resections are typically associated with limited blood loss. When hilar dissection is involved (lobectomy or greater), or adhesions exist from prior surgery, greater IV access and invasive arterial blood pressure monitoring is indicated. Severe pathophysiology or coexisting disease may also dictate invasive monitoring. One-lung anesthesia per se is not an indication for an arterial cannula.

Central venous pressure (*CVP*) monitoring and access is employed by some as an aid to assessment of intravascular volume and right heart function. In practice, CVP monitoring rarely influences intraoperative management decisions. Interpretation of CVP can be confounded by one-lung ventilation with an open chest and PEEP. Crossclamp of the pulmonary artery (or branch thereof) typically does not result in any change in CVP. There is no evidence that CVP monitoring prevents or predicts right heart failure following pulmonary resection. Nonetheless, it may be useful as a trend monitor to help assess intravascular volume, as a route for central drug delivery, or an aid to postoperative management in the patient with fragile cardiopulmonary status. If employed, the *central line is best placed on the side of surgery*, since an unrecognized pneumothorax in the contralateral chest would be particularly problematic during one-lung anesthesia.

Pulmonary artery catheters **(PACs)** are rarely employed due to the danger of entrapment in the surgical staple line, and the multiple pitfalls of interpretation imposed by thoracotomy physiology. Pulmonary artery occlusion pressures (PAOP) are spuriously depressed when the PA is crossclamped (2). The accuracy of PAOP during lesser resections is probably acceptable. If the tip of the PAC lies in the collapsed (operative) lung, PA pressures and cardiac output readings may be unreliable. PACs are principally employed in thoracic surgery when patients have significant pulmonary hypertension or severe left heart dysfunction. *Communication with the surgeon prior to PA crossclamp is essential to prevent entrapment of the catheter in the staple line.*

Cardiac monitoring is compromised by pulmonary resection. Left-sided surgery precludes proper lateral ECG lead placement. One-lung ventilation may alter the position of the heart relative to the chest wall leads. The prevalence of cardiac disease in thoracic patients, most of whom have smoking histories, is high. Transesophageal echocardiography (TEE) is recommended if myocardial ischemia or RV dysfunction is suspected.

Other Monitors: In addition to usual ASA monitors, increased attention is paid during thoracic surgery to the shape of the *capnograph* (obstructive disease, bronchospasm), the *volumes of ventilation* (especially during OLV), and to indicators of air trapping (*auto-PEEP*). If equipped with flow-volume loops, failure of flow to return to zero at end-expiration indicates air-trapping. A simple in-line circuit flow detector can manually perform the same function.

Orogastric tubes are useful to decompress the stomach and increase the room for maneuvering by surgeons during VATS resections. They also aid surgeons in identifying the esophagus.

Pain Management Decisions (Preoperative)

Which VATS Resections Require Epidural Catheters?

Lobectomies and segmentectomies generally warrant epidurals, while wedge resections generally do not. Thoracic epidurals are best placed in the awake patient prior to induction. Yet it can be challenging to predict which "VATS" resection will turn into a mini-thoracotomy and thus likely benefit from an epidural. One should consult the surgeon, consider the size, and position of the lesion, and the likelihood of adhesions or other factors complicating the procedure.

Even peripheral wedge resections may benefit from an epidural if they have severe pulmonary disease, opioid intolerance, sleep apnea, or other factors favoring a narcotic-sparing technique. There is evidence to suggest that thoracic epidural analgesia has cardio-protective effects (3–5), which may tip the balance in patients with unstable coronary disease (Chapter 37). There is also the suggestion that epidural analgesia may reduce the incidence of chronic post-thoracotomy pain syndrome, a problem which can occur with VATS approaches as well (Chapter 38).

Asleep Versus Awake Thoracic Epidurals:

Inevitably, on occasion, patients will receive unexpectedly large incisions. There is debate whether it is safe to place epidurals in anesthetized patients prior to emergence. In the USA, the predominant sentiment is against asleep epidurals in adults. The small but nonzero risk of nerve injury from asleep epidurals seems unjustified, given that comparable pain control can be achieved with intercostal blocks, paravertebral blocks, or moderate opioids +/− adjuncts (NSAIDS, ketamine, dexmetetomidine, etc.). In such a situation, those alternatives may be employed as a bridge to emerge the patient before placing an awake epidural in the PACU. Paravertebral catheters or pain pumps may achieve efficacy that is comparable to thoracic epidurals (Chapter 37).

Epidural Hematoma Risk Assessment: (see Chapter 37)

There is no universal agreement on clotting parameter thresholds for safe placement of epidural catheters. At the author's institution, neuraxial blockade is generally avoided when the INR > 1.3 international units, but the decision always requires a balancing of perceived benefits versus risks for the individual patient (6).

Confirmation of Catheter Position

A *test dose* prior to induction (e.g., 2% lidocaine with epinephrine [1:200,000]) should be used to rule out an intravascular/intrathecal catheter, and confirm an appropriate band of analgesia. It is important to be aware that an accidental intrapleural catheter will also produce a band of analgesia following a test dose, but the analgesia will be unilateral.

Epidural Management: Intraoperative

If significant bleeding is anticipated, or blood pressure is tenuous, further use of the epidural is best deferred to the latter stages of the case. If there is unstable coronary disease, there may be benefit to early use of TEA, so long as coronary perfusion pressure is not sacrificed in the process (3–5). Barring the above, it matters little when the epidural is begun, so long as a block is established in time for a comfortable emergence.

The epidural block may be established by boluses, a continuous infusion, or a combination of the two. In general, the sympathetic response to a bolus is fully expressed in about 10–15 min following bupivacaine. If this effect coincides with a bolus of anesthetic for the terminal tube exchange, there can be an inconvenient, additive hemodynamic effect. Incremental boluses of bupivacaine (0.125%) (total of 10–15 mg) or its equivalent in an adult, will generally establish an excellent block for emergence from a thoracotomy.

Special Induction Considerations in Thoracic Patients

Aside from the usual considerations for induction (drug effects, aspiration, airway securement, etc.), four issues deserve special consideration in thoracic patients with regard to risk of induction:

(1) Air Trapping

(2) Bronchospasm

(3) Mass Effect on Airway Patency

(4) Mass Effect on Cardiac Output

Patients at risk are those with severe obstructive lung disease, brittle or active bronchospasm, or symptomatic/radiographic evidence of mass effects on the airway, heart, or great vessels. As a rule, the wise thoracic anesthesiologist will at a minimum always know the symptomatology of the patient, their FEV_1, and will have examined the chest CT prior to induction.

Air Trapping: Failure to fully exhale the preceding inspiration leads to trapped air, auto-PEEP, dynamic hyperinflation, and potentially barotrauma or hemodynamic compromise from impaired venous return. The thoracic surgical population is particularly prone to this hazard. It is essential to compensate for expiratory flow limitation with longer expiratory time when converting such patients to controlled ventilation. Cardiac arrest has been reported in this scenario.

Bronchospasm: Airway hyperreactivity is increased in patients with a history of smoking, COPD, or certain other chronic lung diseases which are more prevalent among thoracic surgical patients. Laryngoscopy and intubation at induction can trigger bronchospasm in such patients. Adequate depth at the time of instrumentation is the most effective preventive measure. Preoperative bronchodilators and avoidance of histamine releasing agents may mitigate as well. The theoretical risks of beta-adrenergic blocking drugs are often overstated, and if indicated for cardiac reasons, such drugs should not be withheld for fear of bronchospasm.

Mass Effect on Airway Patency: Although generally applicable to patients with anterior mediastinal masses, large central tumors may also impinge on the caliber of airways. The decrease in FRC associated with induction may convert subcritical obstruction to complete airway obstruction. See full discussion in Chapter 20.

Mass Effect on Venous Return and Cardiac Output: Induction and conversion to positive pressure ventilation compromises venous return to the heart by several mechanisms (Chapter 3). Mass effects on the heart or great vessels accentuate the reduction of venous return during induction. Air trapping further exacerbates the decrease in venous return. Pericardial or large pleural effusions can also contribute to embarrassment of cardiac filling. Tension pneumothorax should be considered in patients with bullous emphysema who display recalcitrant hypotension following induction. Lower extremity IV access is essential for patients with SVC syndrome. Patients at risk should receive an arterial line prior to induction, and close attention to defending venous return during induction (IV fluids, vasopressors, long expiratory times, Trendelenberg, and possibly maintenance of spontaneous ventilation).

Surgical Bronchoscopy

Large (>8.0 mm OD) endotracheal tubes are necessary to accommodate the adult bronchoscope and allow for ventilation. Attention to the bronchial anatomy at this time will anticipate issues for lung isolation. In particular, the length of the right mainstem, or anomalies of the right upper lobe (Chapter 9) should be noted if a right-sided double lumen tube is planned. Other considerations for bronchoscopy are addressed in Chapter 18.

Lung Isolation Decisions

Left double-lumen endobronchial tubes (L-DLT) are most commonly used for any lobectomy or lesser resection of either side. If there is potential for a left pneumonectomy, a right DLT would be recommended (but not imperative), anatomy permitting. Bronchial blockers (BB) may be preferred for patients who are difficult to intubate, because they obviate the need for a tube exchange. Left-mainstem bronchial blockers are also useful for left pneumonectomies when anomalous right upper lobe anatomy makes a right-sided DLT problematic. For right-sided pulmonary resections, bronchial blockers may become dislodged due to the short right mainstem anatomy. The slower onset of atelectasis and the difficulty suctioning secretions from the operative lung to maximize lung collapse are potential disadvantages of bronchial blockers in VATS resections. Despite this, bronchial blockers have their advocates and often the differences are clinically insignificant (see Chapter 9).

Fiberoptic confirmation of DLT or BB position is now widely considered a standard practice.

Preparation for Incision

Attention to the following details should take place prior to incision:

- Secure DLT
- Place orogastric tube
- Reposition in lateral decubitus (see Chapter 7)
    - Axillary roll
    - Padding to all pressure points
    - Flex table to spread ribs
- Repeat bronchoscopic confirmation of DLT (or BB)
    - Assess need for clearance of secretions

    - Confirm absence of orogastric tube in operative airway
    - Confirm air seal at bronchial cuff
- Initiate one-lung ventilation and adjust ventilator accordingly (see below, and Chapters 5 and 6)

Ventilator Management

Initial Two-Lung Ventilation Phase:

The patient's pathophysiology dictates the ventilatory pattern during the two-lung phase. Patients with restrictive disease require higher pressures and PEEP. Those with obstructive disease will require longer expiratory times, and attention to minimize air-trapping (auto-PEEP). Hypoxia and hypercarbia are to be avoided in patients with pulmonary hypertension. Those with bullae require attention to avoid or detect a pneumothorax (tension pneumothorax if closed hemithorax). Those with large bullae, recent resections, or vulnerable staple lines (or bronchopleural fistula) may require immediate lung isolation to avoid disruption. If permissive hypercapnea is anticipated for the OLV phase, it is strategic to hyperventilate during initial two-lung ventilation phase.

One-Lung Ventilation Phase:

See Chapters 5 and 6 for details of the physiology of OLV and lung injury.

To summarize, one-lung ventilation strategies strive to strike a balance between adequate (not necessarily highest) oxygenation, CO_2 elimination, and avoidance of lung injury. Adequate oxygenation (>90%) is the first imperative. *Lung protective ventilatory strategies* (6 ml/kg ideal body weight with PEEP), when tolerated, are currently recommended to avoid lung injury (Chapter 6). In patients with severe obstructive disease, permissive hypercapnea may be employed, within limits. Barring contraindications (unstable coronary disease, cerebrovascular disease, increased intracranial pressure, pulmonary hypertension with right heart dysfunction, etc.), transient permissive hypercapnea is benign, and easily reversed with subsequent two-lung ventilation. Hypercapnea may be unavoidable in patients with severe obstructive disease during OLV. Default initial ventilatory parameters employed at the authors' institution during OLV are provided in Box 16-3, the basis of which was discussed in Chapters 5 and 6. Individualization should be made based on patient pathophysiology and surgical situation.

Box 16-3 – Initial One-Lung Ventilator Settings

Initial $FiO_2 = 1.0$

Initial VT = 6 ml/kg ideal body weight

Initial PEEP = 5 cmH_2O

Adjust RR & I:E Ratio for $ETCO_2 = 35$ or $PaCO_2 = 40$ mmHg (if possible)

Mode: Either Pressure Control or Volume Control

Adjust to minimize intrinsic PEEP and plateau pressures (maintaining satisfactory gas exchange)

Titrate down FiO_2 consistent with $SpO_2 > 90\%$

Intermittent recruitment maneuvers to dependent lung

Optimizing Operative Lung Collapse

Excellent atelectasis of the operative lung can be instrumental to surgical success in minimally invasive pulmonary resection, and to preventing the conversion to an open technique. As such, it may directly impact outcome.

Poor atelectasis of the operative lung should prompt several quick responses. First, observation of the lung should be performed to assess whether it is ventilating or just failing to collapse. The former suggests a misplaced DLT/BB, or insufficient air in the bronchial cuff for an effective air seal. Occasionally, high ventilation pressures (e.g., restrictive lung disease) may squeeze air past an otherwise reasonably inflated bronchial cuff. A ventilated lung must be distinguished from one which is moving from mediastinal shift. The latter is a failure of collapse rather than a failure to isolate.

Second, fiberoptic bronchoscopy of the operative lung should confirm proper DLT position and the absence of obstructions to air egress from a herniated cuff, secretions, or tube malposition. Active suctioning via the bronchoscope may encourage air egress, but the principal of flow limitation suggests that this will have limited impact after airways close in patients with significant obstructive disease. The time course of atelectasis following initiation of lung isolation depends in part on elastic recoil of the lungs, and suggests that earlier isolation leads to earlier atelectasis. However, little ground is gained until the pleural space is opened by the surgeon. Physical or pneumatic compression of the lung by the surgeon certainly accelerates atelectasis. Use of 100% FiO_2 prior to lung isolation has been associated with superior collapse through absorption atelactasis (7). Although it is widely assumed that the rate and degree of lung collapse are greater with DLTs than with bronchial blockers, the data on this are mixed (8, 9).

Treatment Strategies for Hypoxemia During One-Lung Ventilation

Common causes of hypoxemia during OLV are listed in Box 16-4.

Box 16-4 – Common Causes of Hypoxemia During OLV

- Malposition of DLT/BB
- Secretions
- Bronchospasm
- Excessive blood flow (shunt) to the nondependent lung
- Excessive atelectasis (shunt) in the dependent lung
- Excessive V/Q mismatch in the dependent lung

Treatment strategies which have been elaborated upon in Chapter 5 are briefly summarized in Box 16-5 below:

Box 16-5 – Treatment of Hypoxemia During OLV

1. *Treatment of hypoxemia during OLV should be individualized to the patient, the situation, and the most probable cause.*
2. Delivery of *100% oxygen* in adequate tidal volumes should be confirmed.
3. If the desaturation is abrupt, severe, or suspected of causing ischemia, the nondependent lung should be *reinflated* in coordination with the surgeon.
4. *If time* permits, *bronchoscopy* should be performed to rule out tube malposition, secretions, blood, kinks, etc.
   - *Pearl*: Check for secretions in the right upper lobe during left-lung surgery, as this lobe is directly dependent, and frequently collects secretions.
5. *CPAP* (5–10 cmH_2O) to the nondependent lung will reliably improve oxygenation (reduce nondependent lung shunt), but at the cost of partial reinflation of the lung.
   - CPAP is most effective if preceded by a partial recruitment maneuver.
   - Avoid CPAP if possible in VATS to avoid forcing the surgeon to extend the incision.
   - Patients with large % blood flow to the operative lung will benefit most from CPAP.
6. *PEEP* (5–12 cmH_2O) to the dependent lung may improve oxygenation in certain patients.
   - Young patients with good lung elastic recoil, and patients with restrictive physiology (pulmonary fibrosis, obesity, pressure on mediastinum, etc.) tend to develop more atelectasis in the dependent lung and tend to benefit from PEEP.
   - Excessive PEEP to the dependent lung redirects blood to nondependent lung, with net increase in shunt.

(continued)

Box 16-5 – (continued)

- Patients with obstructive lung disease tend to have intrinsic PEEP (auto-PEEP) at or beyond optimal PEEP, and fail to benefit from adding extrinsic PEEP.
  - Optimal PEEP is sought by titrating PEEP to SpO_2 or PaO_2.
  - Extrinsic PEEP in patients with intrinsic PEEP does not increase total PEEP until it exceeds approximately 75% of the pre-existing intrinsic PEEP.

7. *Surgical crossclamp (or compression) of the pulmonary artery* branch will reliably reduce nondependent lung shunt and improve oxygenation. When surgical crossclamp is planned and imminent, this is a useful strategy.

Choice of Anesthetics

There exists no acknowledged "best" anesthetic regimen for thoracic surgery. Pros and cons exist for TIVA and inhalation-based anesthetics (Table 16-1). Inhalation agents are best avoided in patients with severe obstructive pulmonary disease due to slow elimination. The argument that TIVA improves oxygenation during OLV because it preserves HPV is at best loosely supported in the literature.

Table 16-1 – Pros and cons of anesthetic techniques for thoracic surgery

	PRO	CON
Inhalational	Convenient (in-line)	Depends on lungs for elimination
	Easily titrated	May linger in Obstructive Dz
	Bronchodilator	Inhibits HPV
TIVA	No inhibition of HPV	Inconvenient
	Elimination independent of lung function	Risk of awareness

In clinically relevant doses (<1.5 MAC), one-lung oxygenation is roughly equivalent between TIVA and currently employed inhalational agents (10, 11) (Chapter 5).

Fluid Management and Postpneumonectomy Pulmonary Edema

Restrictive fluid management for pulmonary resection surgery is widely practiced. Published recommendations are for a target 24 h fluid balance of <20 ml/kg (11). Historically, this stems from concern that *postpneumonectomy pulmonary edema* (PPE) may be caused or exacerbated by excessive fluid administration.

Current consensus holds that PPE is a form of *acute lung injury* (ALI) of unknown etiology (see Chapter 6). As such, pulmonary capillary endothelial integrity, rather than intravascular volume, is the primary problem. However, should ALI occur, excessive fluid administration may impair gas exchange, reduce pulmonary compliance, and increase the work of breathing in the immediate postoperative period. Thus, while not directly causative, excessive fluid complicates management, should ALI occur.

Pulmonary resection patients are more vulnerable because of impaired lymphatic drainage (particularly after right pneumonectomy), and reduced pulmonary reserve. This rationale for restrictive fluid management of pulmonary resection patients should be individualized, and balanced against blood loss, and the imperative for sufficient intravascular volume to assure end-organ perfusion and tolerance of thoracic epidural sympathetic blockade (when applicable). See Chapter 6 for full discussion.

Division of the Bronchus

In the case of lobectomy, it may be helpful for the anesthesiologist to provide a bronchoscopic view of the stump during crossclamp in order to assure a short stump and patency of adjacent branches of the airway (Fig 16-4).

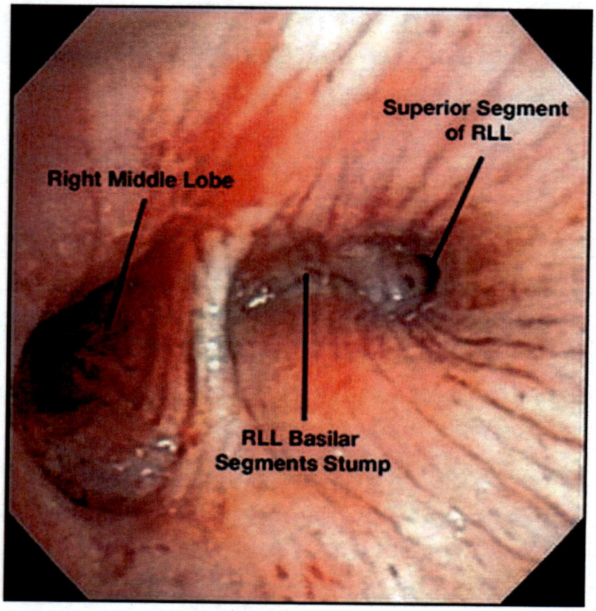

Figure 16-4 – Bronchoscopic view of the bronchus intermedius after division of the basilar segments of the right lower lobe. This confirms an appropriately short stump, and that the superior segment of the right lower lobe and middle lobe bronchus remain patent.

Leak Test

Following specimen removal, most surgeons will test the stump/staple line for air leaks by submerging the operative site with saline for a "leak test." Using manual ventilation, the anesthesiologist provides several seconds of progressively increasing positive pressure up to 25–30 cmH_2O, while the surgeon observes the field for air bubbles.

Recruitment/Re-expansion of Remaining Lung

Prior to chest closure, full recruitment of remaining lung is desirable to minimize airspace and atelectasis. Recruitment maneuvers resemble the leak test above, and may require several series of sustained (several seconds) positive pressure inspiratory "holds" at pressures between 20 and 35 cmH_2O. The anesthesiologist should observe the expanding lung while keeping an eye on the manometer. Sustained positive pressure can impair cardiac output, even with an open chest. Therefore, multiple, brief maneuvers are safer than long sustained ones. In theory, reinflation with a low FiO_2 may ameliorate ischemia reperfusion injury following prolonged lung collapse. This is most likely to be of clinical significance following lung transplantation.

Tube Exchange

The terminal exchange from a DLT to a single lumen endotracheal tube for bronchoscopy and emergence is a maneuver treated with great respect by the experienced thoracic anesthesiologist. Conditions for reintubation are seldom as favorable as during the initial intubation. Edema may have accumulated, and paralysis and depth of anesthesia are often lighter, in anticipation of emergence. Backup options for a lost airway should be immediately available. Use of a tube exchange catheter is wise when the initial intubation was difficult, or edema has become significant. Technical details in the use of tube exchange catheters are critical to its success (Chapter 10).

An underutilized alternative option is to exchange to an LMA instead of a SLT. Bronchoscopy can be performed through an LMA with ease (Fig 16-5), but laryngospasm and aspiration are possible.

If the airway is lost at this point, several options are available. If an LMA is in place, reintubation can be secured using an Aintree Catheter (Cook Medical, USA). Many other options for the lost airway now are available, including fiberoptic intubation, use of fiberoptic laryngoscopes, or other supraglottic devices. The choice should be dictated by the experience and comfort level of the anesthesiologist. Reversing paralysis and allowing the patient to emerge are sometimes appropriate as well.

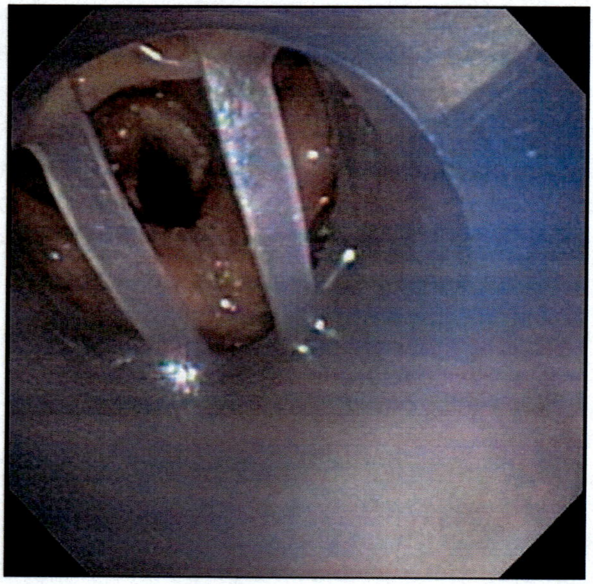

Figure 16-5 – Bronchoscopic view of the vocal cords and entire trachea is conveniently achieved via a laryngeal mask airway.

Emergence Strategies

Rapid emergence and extubation depend on the strategic use of short-acting anesthetic agents, limited narcotic use, full reversal of muscle relaxation, control of secretions, bronchospasm, and pain, and the return of airway reflexes, sensorium, and adequate respiratory efforts.

Brisk emergence requires foresight to turn off inhalational agents early in patients with obstructive lung disease. Ultrashort acting narcotic agents (remifentanil) are advantageous to supplement depth and blunt airway reflexes for the tube exchange while allowing for rapid emergence after a brief bronchoscopy. Attention to density of paralysis during the 30-min prior to tube exchange allows titration to a reversible but moderate degree of paralysis for the exchange. If the thoracic epidural had not been utilized previously, it may be necessary to establish a block during the final 30 min of the case with intermittent boluses. Generally, hemodynamics remain relatively stable as the onset of epidural boluses approximates the elimination of inhalational agents.

Attention to pattern and depth of breathing is the most important indicator of readiness for extubation, as this is often the limiting factor in thoracic patients. Raising the head of the bed improves the mechanics of breathing and often improves spontaneous tidal volumes.

Selected References

1. Nakahara K, Ohno K, Hashimotot J, et al. Prediction of postoperative respiratory failure in patients undergoing lung resection for cancer. Ann Thorac Surg. 1988;46:549–52.

2. Wittnich C, Trudel J, Zidulka A, Chiu R. Misleading "pulmonary wedge pressure" after pneumonectomy. Its importance in postoperative fluid therapy. Ann Thorac Surg. 1986;42:192.

3. Beattie WS, Badner N, Choi P. Epidural analgesia reduces postoperative myocardial infarction: a meta-analysis. Anesth Analg. 2001;93:853–8.

4. Vic-Mo H, Ottesen S, Renck H. Cardiac effects of thoracic epidural analgesia before and during acute coronary occlusion in open chest dogs. Scand J Clin Lab Invest. 1978;38:737–48.

5. Saada M, Catoire P, Bonnet F, Delaunay L, et al. Effect of thoracic epidural anesthesia combined with general anesthesia on segmental wall motion assessed by transesophageal echocardiography. Anesth Analg. 1992;75:329–35.

6. Horlocker T, Wedel D, Benzon H, Brown D, et al. Regional anesthesia in the anticoagulated patient: defining the risks. (The second ASRA consensus conference on neuraxial anesthesia and anticoagulation). Reg Anesth Pain Med. 2003;28(3):172–97.

7. Ko R, McRae K, Darling G, et al. The use of air in the inspired gas mixture during two-lung ventilation delays lung collapse during one-lung ventilation. Anesth Analg. 2009;108(4):10926.

8. Narayanaswamy M, McRae K, Slinger P, Dugas G, et al. Choosing a lung isolation device for thoracic surgery: a randomized trial of three bronchial blockers versus double-lumen tubes. Anesth Analg. 2009;108(4):1097–101.

9. Campos J, Kernstein K. A comparison of the left-sided Broncho-Cath with the torque control blocker Univent and the wire-guided blocker. Anesth Analg. 2003;96:283–9.

10. Schwarzkopf K, Schreiber T, Preussler N, Gaser E, Huter L, Bauer R, et al. Lung perfusion, shunt fraction, and oxygenation during one-lung ventilation in pigs: the effects of desflurane, isoflurane, and propofol. J Cardiothorac Vasc Anesth. 2003;17(1):73–5.

11. Saito M, Cho S, Morooka H, Hasuo H, Shibata O, Sumikawa K. Effects of sevoflurane compared with those of isoflurane on arterial oxygenation and hemodynamics during one-lung ventilation. J Anesth. 2000;4(1):1–5.

12. Slinger PD. Perioperative fluid management for thoracic surgery: the puzzle of post-pneumonectomy pulmonary edema. J Cardiothorac Vasc Anesth. 1995;9(4):442–51.

Further Suggested Reading

Hartigan PM. Anesthesia management. Chapter 5. In: Zellos L, Sugarbaker DJ, Bueno R, Krasna MJ, Mentzer SJ, editors. Adult chest surgery. New York: McGraw-Hill Co., Inc.; 2009. p. 44–59.

Hartigan PM, Body SC, Sugarbaker DJ. Pulmonary resection. Chapter 11. In: Kaplan JA, Slinger PD, editors. Thoracic anesthesia. 3rd ed. Philadelphia, PA: Churchill Livingstone; 2003. p. 213–42.

Chapter 17
Management of Common Complications Following Thoracic Surgery

Andrew D. Friedrich

Keywords Mechanical and hypoxic respiratory failure • Acute lung injury and pneumonia atrial fibrillation • Myocardial infarction • Bronchopleural fistula • Hylothorax • Anastamotic leak • Vocal cord paralysis • Lobar torsion • Atelectasis • Air leaks • Subcutaneous emphysema • Chylothorax

Introduction

Epidemiological studies of thoracic surgical procedures have demonstrated three broad categories of postoperative complications that occur most commonly. They are

Pulmonary: Examples include mechanical and hypoxic respiratory failure, acute lung injury (ALI), and pneumonia.

Cardiac: Examples include atrial fibrillation, myocardial infarction, and heart failure.

Technical: Examples include bronchopleural fistula, chylothorax, anastamotic leak after esophagectomy, vocal cord paralysis, and lobar torsion following lobectomy.

It is important to recognize that a patient's risk of developing one of these complications is related both to the severity of the patient's underlying comorbidities and to the level of invasiveness of the surgical procedure. Preoperative risk assessment is discussed elsewhere in this text. The purpose of this section is to discuss the management of the most common thoracic surgical complications, with an emphasis on their prevention.

P.M. Hartigan (ed.), *Practical Handbook of Thoracic Anesthesia*,
DOI 10.1007/978-0-387-88493-6_17,

Pulmonary Complications

Thoracic surgery is unique in that pulmonary complications represent the predominant cause of perioperative morbidity and mortality. Although standardized definitions of postoperative pulmonary complications do not exist, those most commonly reported are *atelectasis, respiratory failure, pneumonia*, and *ALI*.

While it is convenient to discuss each of these entities separately, in reality they are interrelated and mutually reinforcing. For example, atelectasis may lead to pneumonia, which then leads to respiratory failure; alternatively, *ALI* may be the cause of acute respiratory failure, which predisposes to pneumonia.

The key clinical principle is that each of these pathologic entities can lead to a vicious cycle of progressive pulmonary compromise and death: respiratory failure requiring intubation is a severe complication following lung resection, and is associated with a mortality rate of 60–80% (1). Optimal management of postoperative pulmonary complications, therefore, requires an understanding of the pathophysiology of each of these conditions and the simultaneous utilization of strategies for both their prevention and management.

Pathophysiology of Pulmonary Complications

Respiratory Failure: Generally defined, respiratory failure is a condition in which the respiratory system fails in one or both of its gas exchange functions: oxygenation and/or elimination of carbon dioxide (2). Postoperative respiratory failure has been more specifically categorized as a condition requiring postoperative mechanical ventilation for >24 h, or postoperative reintubation (3). The thoracic surgical population is predisposed to postoperative respiratory failure, owing to the high prevalence of tobacco abuse and chronic obstructive pulmonary disease (COPD). The main pathophysiologic etiology of respiratory failure in COPD patients is expiratory flow limitation, which predisposes to the development of auto-PEEP, increased work of breathing, and ultimately respiratory muscle fatigue. Patients with compensated COPD are vulnerable to the effects of anesthesia, surgery, infection, and lung edema, which create an imbalance in the supply–demand energetics of the respiratory muscles.

Atelectasis: Atelectasis is a common postoperative condition that results from the combined effects of lung compression, gas resorption, and impaired surfactant production. The consequences of atelectasis are increased shunt and predisposition to *ALI* (4). Although the consequences of atelectasis are minor in many post-operative patients, they can be clinically significant in patients with limited pulmonary reserve.

Idiopathic ALI: Multiple insults are recognized triggers of the *ALI* syndrome, including but not limited to pneumonia, sepsis, gastric acid aspiration, lung contusion, and ventilator associated lung injury (VALI). Pulmonary resection patients (principally pneumonectomy patients) are unique in that a proportion of them (2–4%) develop early ALI with no readily recognized etiology.

The search for a novel cause of idiopathic ALI initially focused on fluid overload, leading to the term "postpneumonectomy pulmonary edema." More recent evidence, including autopsy findings, indicates an endothelial injury and capillary leak as the principal lesion (see Chapter 6). Postulated causes and/or contributing factors to post lung resection idiopathic ALI include:

- Injurious ventilation during one-lung anesthesia
- Ischemia reperfusion injury and oxidative stress
- Blood flow-related stress injury to the endothelium following crossclamp of the pulmonary artery
- Inflammatory response to surgery
- Surgical disruption of lymphatic drainage
- Unrecognized known triggers of ALI (occult aspiration, transfusion-related lung injury, etc.)

The result of this endothelial lesion is the accumulation of extravascular lung fluid resulting in diffuse pulmonary infiltrates, impaired gas exchange ($PaO_2/FiO_2 < 300$ mmHg), reduced lung compliance, and increased work of breathing. The diminished cardiopulmonary reserve, due to underlying disease as well as pulmonary resection, impedes recovery in this patient population, and it is important to emphasize that 25–50% of patients with this condition progress to ARDS and death. Idiopathic ALI is emerging as the principal cause of perioperative mortality following pneumonectomy, and is discussed in more detail in Chapter 6.

Pneumonia: Postoperative pneumonia has a mortality rate of 20–30%, and results from the combined effects of preoperative colonization with bacterial pathogens and the impaired cough, mucociliary clearance, and diminished pulmonary neutrophil function that result from anesthesia and surgical trauma. The major risk factors for development of postoperative pneumonia are COPD and the extent of pulmonary resection. The most common bacterial pathogens are those implicated in community-acquired pneumonia: *Haemophilus* and *Streptococcus*. However, a significant percentage of cases are caused by polymicrobial infection or resistant infection with Gram-negative organisms such as *Pseudomonas*, *Serratia*, or *Enterobacter*, and typical surgical antibiotic prophylaxis with first or second-generation cephalosporins is inactive against many of these strains (5).

Prevention of Pulmonary Complications

The effectiveness of several strategies for preventing pulmonary complications after pulmonary resection has been suggested by the publication of successful fast-tracking protocols that incorporate them into routine patient care (6).

Ambulation: An intervention that has been reported to attenuate the development of muscle weakness, delirium, and atelectasis, postoperative ambulation is a simple and safe strategy that offers multiple benefits for patients at risk of developing pulmonary complications.

Analgesia: Thoracic incisional pain causes voluntary limitation of respiratory muscle activity and subsequent atelectasis. Thoracic epidural analgesia has been shown to improve tidal volumes following thoracic incisions, and to decrease the incidence of pulmonary complications in patients with COPD when compared with other analgesic modalities (7) (see Chapter 37).

Fluid Restriction: Although research supporting the standard practice of perioperative fluid restriction and diuresis is both limited and conflicting, two lines of evidence support a conservative fluid management strategy. First, studies of diuresis and fluid restriction in nonthoracic surgical patients with ALI have shown improved oxygenation and reductions in the need for mechanical ventilation and intensive care (8). Second, the lowest reported incidences of post-lung resection ALI have occurred in centers where fluid restriction is standard. In clinical situations where clinically significant hypotension or signs of shock are preventing fluid restriction, it is appropriate to utilize echocardiography and/or invasive hemodynamic monitoring to define the etiology of hemodynamic compromise. Thus, while a state of euvolemia to moderate hypovolemia is a reasonable management goal with possible pulmonary benefit, it must be emphasized that iatrogenic severe hypovolemia and shock is not an acceptable clinical tradeoff.

Lung Expansion Maneuvers: In addition to ambulation, interventions such as incentive spirometry, intermittent positive-pressure breathing, chest physiotherapy, and deep-breathing exercises have been shown to be equally effective in decreasing the incidence of postoperative pulmonary complications. More important than the specific intervention is the need to ensure that one or more of them is utilized multiple times a day in the postoperative period.

Bronchodilator Therapy: For patients with COPD and expiratory flow limitation, combination bronchodilator therapy with a beta-agonist and an anticholinergic agent should be given every 6 h and as needed to limit the development of auto-PEEP and the associated increase in work of breathing.

Management of Pulmonary Complications

Although outcomes are worse when primary prevention measures have failed, effective management of pulmonary complications can prevent their progression to atelectasis, pneumonia, or respiratory failure.

Atelectasis: If clinically significant atelectasis is present and has not responded to the measures listed above, mask CPAP should be utilized, as it has been shown to significantly improve atelectasis-induced hypoxia and reduce the likelihood of intubation in postoperative patients. If this is ineffective, the possibility of postobstructive collapse should be considered, and awake bronchoscopy should be performed in order to remove obstructing mucous plugs.

Pneumonia: When pneumonia is suspected, it is imperative that adequate antimicrobial therapy be instituted immediately; outcomes are worse when therapy is delayed. The choice of antibiotic should be based upon the probability that the patient has been colonized with antibiotic-resistant organisms and upon the gravity of the clinical situation.

If a patient has had previous nosocomial exposure or has been in the hospital for 5 days or more, the probability of infection with methicillin-resistant *Staph aureus* or multidrug-resistant Gram-negative organisms such as *Pseudomonas*, *Enterobacter*, or *Acinetobacter* is increased. In this situation or in cases where a patient is clinically decompensating, initial therapy should include Vancomycin for Gram-positive organisms and two antibiotic classes against potentially resistant Gram-negative organisms; cefepime, piperacillin–tazobactam, an aminoglycoside, or a carbepenem are all appropriate choices.

If a patient is clinically stable and is unlikely to have been exposed to resistant organisms, then initial antibiotic therapy should be directed against community-acquired organisms such as *Haemophilus* or *Streptococcus*. Antibiotics such as ceftriaxone, azithromycin, and moxifloxacin are all appropriate choices.

Ideally, bronchoalveolar lavage (BAL) specimens should be obtained and sent for quantitative culture prior to instituting antibiotic therapy. If the culture result is $<10^4$ colony-forming units (cfu)/mL, it is unlikely that the patient has pneumonia and strong consideration should be given to stopping antibiotics. If the culture result is $>10^4$ cfu/mL and clinical signs of pneumonia are present, the diagnosis of pneumonia is likely, and the therapeutic regimen should be narrowed to the antibiotic sensitivities of the isolated organisms.

If BAL is not feasible because of the clinical situation, empiric therapy should be instituted according to the principles outlined above.

Most cases of pneumonia can be adequately treated with 7–10 days of therapy. Complicated cases, such as empyema or pseudomonal infections, may require a longer therapeutic course. If the patient is not clinically improving after several days of antibiotic therapy, it is reasonable to repeat BAL, obtain CT imaging of the chest, or consider alternative sources of infection. *A cardinal rule of critical care medicine is that patient recovery will not occur unless infectious source control is achieved.*

Respiratory Failure: A recent randomized trial demonstrated that nasal-mask noninvasive positive-pressure ventilation (NPPV) decreased the need for endotracheal intubation and conferred a significant survival advantage to patients with acute hypoxemic respiratory insufficiency following lung resection (9). Although this modality may not be appropriate in certain settings, such as obstructed or unprotected airways or hemodynamic instability, it is a reasonable first approach in patients with acute respiratory failure. If clinical improvement is not seen within the first several hours of NPPV, endotracheal intubation is warranted. If clinical improvement is observed, NPPV may be continued for several days as long as it is clinically tolerated. Importantly, the application of NPPV is a temporizing measure; it does not correct the underlying problem. Aggressive efforts to diagnose and treat the etiology of respiratory failure are paramount once the patient is stabilized on noninvasive ventilation.

For patients who require endotracheal intubation, evidence-based management of sedation and mechanical ventilation can improve outcome.

Sedation: For most intubated patients, sedation is both humane, and necessary to prevent self-injury (self-extubation, self-removal of lines and drains). However, over-sedation is associated with an increased duration of mechanical ventilation and length of ICU stay. The goal therefore is a calm, comfortable, easily arousable patient whose separation from the ventilator is not postponed by the sedation regimen. This clinical goal can be achieved most readily by tailoring the pharmacologic regimen to independent and objective assessments of analgesia, delirium, and depth of sedation. For example, a narcotic analgesic such as fentanyl is titrated to the Visual Analogue Scale (VAS) score, a neuroleptic agent such as haloperidol is titrated to the Confusion Assessment Method for ICU (CAM-ICU) score, and anxiolytics/hypnotic agents such as lorazepam or propofol are titrated to the Richmond Agitation and Sedation Scale (RASS) (10). As discussed in the next section, sedation management and ventilator weaning should be thought of as tightly linked clinical entities.

Mechanical Ventilation: There are two goals of mechanical ventilation: the correction of mechanical respiratory failure and the achievement of an adequate level of oxygen saturation. Ventilator settings such as mode, tidal volume, and PEEP level must be tailored to the individual patient, and although this is a daunting prospect for many clinicians, strategies for setting the ventilator appropriately are described in detail by several excellent review articles (11, 12). Particularly important considerations for mechanical ventilation in thoracic surgical patients are the implications of COPD and the presence of a new bronchial stump for the ventilator strategy. Consequently, the use of pressure-limited modes of ventilation such as pressure control or pressure support should be given preference over volume/flow-controlled modes.

Perhaps more important than the choice of ventilator mode upon patient outcome are the use of complementary interventions that can hasten recovery from respiratory failure. Specifically, a strategy of daily lightening of sedation for the purpose of performing a spontaneous breathing trial (13) and for the provision of physical therapy (14) has been shown to decrease the duration of mechanical ventilation.

For patients who do not manifest clinical improvement within the first few days on mechanical ventilation and who are felt to be at significant risk for >14 days of mechanical ventilation, strong consideration should be given to the performance of tracheostomy early in the course of respiratory failure. The use of this strategy has been associated with improved outcomes, perhaps because it allows for less sedation and greater provision of physical therapy (15).

Cardiovascular Complications

Unlike other areas of noncardiac surgery, the most common postoperative cardiovascular complications following thoracic surgery are not myocardial ischemia and infarction, but atrial fibrillation and hypotension. Perioperative myocardial ischemia and infarction (MI) occur following thoracic surgery, but the pathophysiology and management are not different from other noncardiac surgeries. Strategies for risk stratification and prevention of MI are discussed in Chapter 14. Accordingly, this section focuses on the pathophysiology, prevention, and management of postoperative atrial fibrillation (PAF) and hypotension. In addition, despite its rarity, right heart failure is briefly discussed because of its clinical importance.

Pathophysiology of Postoperative Atrial Fibrillation

The mechanism of atrial fibrillation is multiple re-entrant electrical circuits ("circulating wavelets") that conduct around areas of functional block. These areas of block and re-entry are the result of abnormal dispersion of refractoriness of atrial myocardium. Although the precise mechanisms for dispersion of the atrial refractory period are unknown, this electrophysiologic state is associated with age >60 years, inflammation, and increased adrenergic output, all of which are common in the thoracic surgical population (16). Identification of patients at risk for abnormal atrial refractoriness and utilization of pharmacologic treatments directed toward the atrial refractory period are thus cornerstones of perioperative management.

Prevention and Management of Postoperative Atrial Fibrillation

PAF is of clinical concern because it predisposes patients to hypotension and stroke. At increased risk for hypotension are patients with evidence of diastolic dysfunction on preoperative echocardiographic exam (who have greater dependence upon atrial contribution to ventricular filling), patients receiving epidural analgesia, and patients who are managed with intravascular volume restriction. At increased risk for stroke are patients with previous transient ischemic attack or stroke, hypertension, age^{3}75 years, heart failure, and diabetes mellitus (17). In these high-risk patient groups, it is reasonable to consider initiation of prophylactic therapy with either diltiazem or beta-blockers (18), both of which have been shown to be moderately effective in reducing the incidence of PAF. In addition, Vaughan-Williams class 1c drugs such as flecainide and propafenone or class III drugs such as amiodarone or sotalol can be utilized, and are attractive because of their ability to prolong the electrical refractory period. Although these agents have been shown to be the most effective at maintaining and restoring sinus rhythm in the nonperioperative setting and after cardiac surgery, there is insufficient data in the thoracic surgical population. Whether amiodarone is associated with an increased incidence of pulmonary toxicity after thoracic surgery is controversial.

For patients who develop PAF following thoracic surgery, it is important to keep several facts in mind when formulating a management strategy. First, the majority of cases of PAF resolve prior to hospital discharge, and 98% resolve by 4–8 weeks after surgery. Second, the risk of thromboembolic stroke becomes clinically significant approximately 48 h after the onset of PAF. Finally, the risk/benefit analysis for any therapy must occur in the context of the individual patient. Thus, a general approach of rate-controlling patients with beta-blockers or diltiazem for the first 48 h after onset of PAF is reasonable, with "rhythm management" reserved for hypotensive patients and patients in whom the risk of anticoagulation is prohibitive.

Hypotension

Relative hypotension following thoracic surgery is extremely common. Restrictive fluid management predisposes most patients, but is rarely the only factor. In addition to the usual suspects, thoracic patients have several thoracic-specific etiologies, with treatment implications, that one must be aware of (Table 17-1).

Table 17-1 – Causes of hypotension following thoracic surgery

Impaired Pump Function

- Myocardial ischemia/infarction
- Right ventricular failure
- Impaired contractility from thoracic epidural

Rhythm Disturbance

- Atrial fibrillation
- Other atrial/ventricular dysrhythmias

Decreased Preload

- Hypovolemia (restrictive fluid management)
- Hemorrhage
- Lost atrial kick (see Atrial Fibrillation above)
- Pericardial tamponade
- Tension pneumothorax
- Large pleural effusion/hemothorax with tamponade effect
- Cardiac herniation (torsion of great vessels) following pneumonectomy
- Mediastinal shift following pneumonectomy resulting in partial cardiac herniation
- Tight pericardial patch following intrapericardial pneumonectomy
- Stenosis/torsion of pulmonary vein anastomosis following lung transplantation

Decreased Peripheral Vascular Tone

- Sepsis
- Thoracic epidural sympathetic block
- Surgical disruption of sympathetic chain
- Paraneoplastic effect (e.g., carcinoid syndrome)

(continued)

Table 17-1 – (continued)

Increased Right Ventricular Afterload
▪ Lack of sufficient remaining recruitable vascular capacitance for the amount of lung resected
▪ Pulmonary emboli

Those relatively specific or frequent to thoracic surgery are in *bold*.

Management should ideally address the causes, preserving interventions (such as thoracic epidural analgesia) which are beneficial if possible.

Right Ventricular Failure

Acute right ventricular (RV) failure following pulmonary resection is a rare but ominous complication. Etiologies are listed in Table 17-2, most of which are specifically applicable to thoracic surgical patients. Early recognition and prompt treatment of reversible factors is essential. Maximal medical treatment usually includes mechanical ventilation with 100% oxygen, inodilator therapy (milrinone, with vasopressin as needed for systemic tone), inhaled nitric oxide (vs. prostaglandin), and optimal intravascular fluid resuscitation. The last item is challenging, and often requires guidance with a pulmonary artery catheter or echocardiography. Suboptimal intravascular volume forfeits preload-dependent cardiac output, while excessive volume dilates the RV, exacerbates ischemia, and impairs LV function through septal shift and ventricular interdependence.

Prevention of irreversible RV failure by excessive pulmonary resection is based on rough estimates of cardiopulmonary reserve (Chapter 14). Response to temporary balloon occlusion of PA is sometimes measured in marginal surgical candidates, but the predictive value of this is not well established. Echocardiographic RV evaluation during intraoperative test clamp of the PA has also been attempted without established predictive value.

Table 17-2 – Causes of RV failure following thoracic surgery

Irreversible:

- Surgical resection of excessive lung tissue relative to pulmonary vascular reserve
- Right ventricular infarction

Medically Reversible:

- Reactive Pulmonary Vasoconstriction
  - Hypoxia
  - Hypercarbia
  - Elevated sympathetic tone (pain, anxiety)

Surgically Reversible:

- Saddle pulmonary embolus
- Pulmonary artery stenosis from pneumonectomy staple line
- Pulmonary vein stenosis following lung transplantation
- Tight pericardial patch over right heart following right pneumonectomy

Technical Complications

Despite continual improvements in surgical technique and technology, technical complications are destined to be an inevitable consequence of thoracic surgical procedures. Although the most commonly encountered technical complications are discussed in detail, this section begins with an overview of the essential features and functions of chest tube drainage systems, as they are a critical component of the management of the majority of these complications.

The Three-Bottle Chest Tube Drainage System

The traditional chest tube drainage system is depicted in Fig 17-1, and consists of three bottles connected in series. The first is

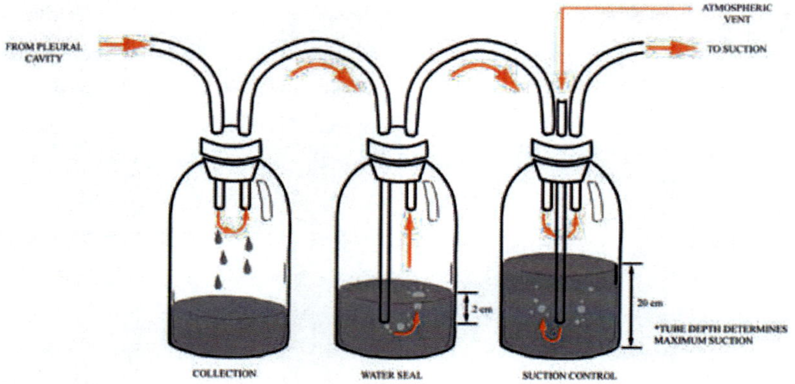

Figure 17-1 – Simple three bottle drainage system illustrates principles of collection chamber, water seal, and suction control. See text for explanation.

the *collection bottle*, into which flows any drainage from the chest cavity. The second bottle is the *water seal bottle*, the principal function of which is to act as a one-way valve and prevent air from re-entering the pleural space during inspiration. This is accomplished by submerging the tip of the tube that connects the collection bottle with the water seal bottle. The final bottle is the *suction control bottle*, which allows the drainage system to maintain a constant negative pressure and prevent possible complications related to malfunction of the vacuum source. It is the depth of the atmospheric vent tube below water that determines the negative pressure of suction control bottle. For example, if the tip of the vent tube is 20 cm below water and the wall suction is set to −30 cm H_2O, the "excess" −10 cm H_2O of negative suction will cause air to be entrained through the vent and bubbles will be observed in the suction control bottle. *It is important to understand that with this type of system, the "extra" suction from the wall will not be transmitted to the patient*; the bubbles will disappear once wall suction is reduced to the level of negative suction imparted by the submerged vent tube (in this case −20 cm H_2O). To alter the level of negative pressure transmitted to the patient, adding water will increase the level of transmitted negative pressure and removing water will decrease the level of transmitted negative pressure. The first commercially available version of an integrated disposable chest drainage unit based on three-bottle system was introduced by Deknatel in 1967, and is depicted in Fig 17-2.

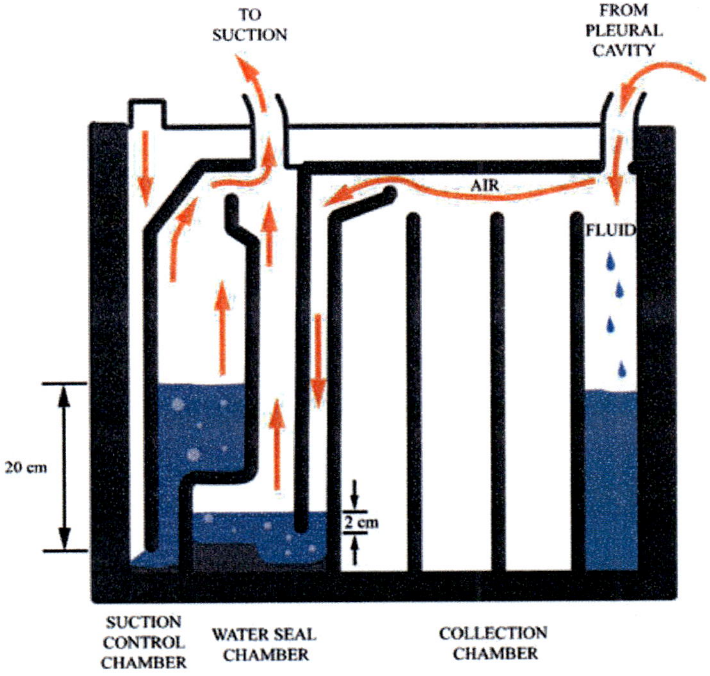

Figure 17-2 – Integrated chest drainage unit modeled on the three-bottle drainage system.

The New Generation: Dry Suction Drainage Systems

Currently, most commercially available chest tube drainage systems do not use a column of water to regulate suction. Instead, the level of transmitted negative pressure is controlled by a self-compensating regulator, and set by the clinician via a suction control dial. Other features of modern chest tube drainage systems include (see Fig 17-3):

Suction control regulator

Vacuum indicator

Air leak monitor

Suction monitor bellows

Manual high negativity vent

Positive pressure release valve

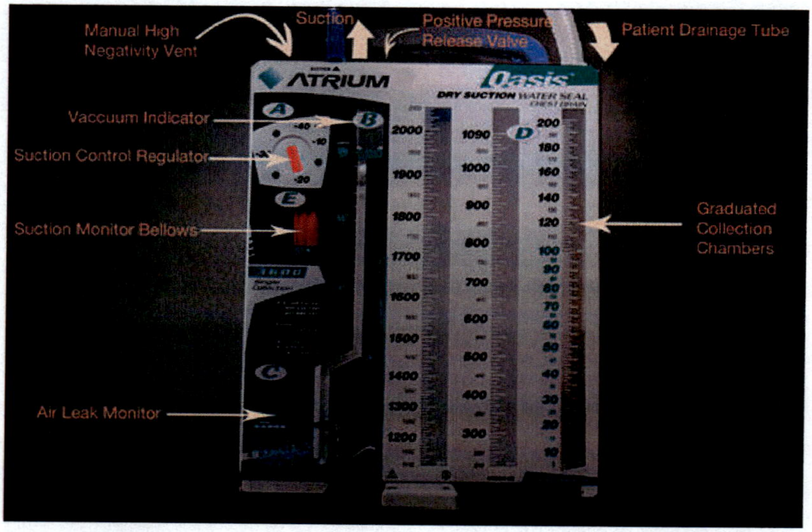

Figure 17-3 – Modern generation dry suction chest drainage system. Extent of air leak is indicated by the number of columns (chambers) with bubbles in the air leak monitor at *bottom left*. Positive pressure release valve and manual high negativity vent are on top surface of the system (not shown).

Common Technical Complications

1. *Air Leaks*: Despite being one of the most common complications after pulmonary resection, studies on the management of air leaks were not conducted until relatively recently. Work by Cerfolio et al. has produced a scientific approach to management of air leaks, which is notable for several principles:

   (a) Most air leaks, except those >4/7 chambers in size, will resolve faster on water seal than they will on suction (19).

   (b) The majority of chest tubes can be removed on postoperative day 2 after lobectomy, or on postoperative day 1 after wedge resection, provided the drainage is less than 450 cc per day, and there is not an expanding pneumothorax or development of subcutaneous emphysema on water seal (20). Patients with persistent air leaks and pneumothoraces on postoperative day 3 or 4, who are otherwise ready for discharge, can be sent home on an outpatient suctionless device, provided they tolerate water seal for 24 h (21). The majority of these patients can have their chest tubes removed uneventfully at follow-up visit 2 weeks postdischarge.

(c) Patients who fail water seal should be placed on $-10\ cmH_2O$ suction, which should be increased if the pneumothorax or subcutaneous emphysema does not improve (22).

2. *Subcutaneous Emphysema*: Although most cases of subcutaneous emphysema can be managed with increased levels of chest tube suction, a significant number, especially in the setting of lobectomy, fail to respond to this management strategy. Treatment of these recalcitrant cases of subcutaneous emphysema by video-assisted thoracoscopic surgery (VATS), with pneumolysis between the leaking lung, has been demonstrated to be highly effective (23).

3. *Chylothorax*: Although chylothorax occurs in less than 1% of thoracic procedures, it is worth mentioning because of its high morbidity, causing nutritional deficiencies, respiratory insufficiency, and immunosuppression in patients who develop this complication. The mortality rate is high, approaching 50% if left untreated. Conservative treatment is often effective, and consists of drainage and a medium-chain tryglyceride diet. It has been suggested that the majority of patients who fail conservative therapy can be successfully treated by VATS exploration and repair of the thoracic duct laceration by suture, clipping, or fibrin glue and/or talc application (24).

4. *Intrathoracic Anastamotic Leak after Esophagectomy*: This complication is relatively rare, occurring in approximately 5% of patients who undergo esophagectomy with intrathoracic anastamosis. Although older studies quoted a mortality of 70% with this complication, modern management techniques have decreased the associated mortality to 3% (25). It is important to emphasize that the clinical approach

to intrathoracic leaks should be individualized (26). Asymptomatic patients or those with small, contained leaks can usually be managed conservatively with drainage of extraluminal fluid collections and restriction of oral intake. In contrast, symptomatic and/or noncontained leaks warrant prompt surgical intervention. Common surgical techniques for dealing with this complication include esophageal diversion, anastamotic repair with tissue flap reinforcement, or deployment of a temporary esophageal stent (27).

5. *Lobar Torsion*: This is an extremely rare complication after lung resection that is caused by rotation of the bronchovascular pedicle and results in airway obstruction and vascular compromise. The diagnosis should be considered when complete atelectasis on the operative side is observed on chest X-ray, and must be confirmed by bronchoscopy. Treatment is surgical, and involves resection of the nonviable lobe(s) (28).

6. *Vocal Cord Paralysis*: A common complication after thoracic surgery, vocal cord paralysis occurs as a consequence of surgical injury to the recurrent laryngeal nerve. The diagnosis is made by fiberoptic laryngoscopy. Early treatment with vocal cord medialization is advisable, as it has been shown to decrease the incidence of postoperative pneumonia, need for bronchoscopy, and median length of stay when compared with late vocal cord medialization (29).

Selected References

1. Kutlu CA, Williams EA, Evans TW, et al. Acute lung injury and acute respiratory distress syndrome after pulmonary resection. Ann Thorac Surg. 2000;69:376–80.

2. Roussos C, Koutsoukou A. Respiratory failure. Eur Respir J. 2003;22 Suppl 47:3S–14.

3. Stephan F, Boucheseiche S, Hollande J, et al. Pulmonary complications following lung resection: a comprehensive analysis of incidence and possible risk factors. Chest. 2000;118:1263–70.

4. Duggan M, Kavanagh BP. Pulmonary atelectasis: a pathogenic perioperative entity. Anesthesiology. 2005;102:838–54.

5. Schussler O, Dermine H, Alifano M, et al. Should we change antibiotic prophylaxis for lung surgery? Postoperative pneumonia is the critical issue. Ann Thorac Surg. 2008;86:1727–34.

6. Cerfolio RJ, Pickens A, Bass C, Katholi C. Fast-tracking pulmonary resections. J Thorac Cardiovasc Surg. 2001;122:318–24.

7. Licker MJ, Widikker I, Robert J, et al. Operative mortality and respiratory complications after lung resection for cancer: impact of chronic obstructive pulmonary disease and time trends. Ann Thorac Surg. 2006;81:1830–8.

8. The National Heart, Lung and Blood Institute Acute Respiratory Distress Syndrome Clinical Trials Network. Comparison of two fluid-management strategies in acute lung injury. N Engl J Med. 2006;354:2564–75.

9. Auriant I, Jallot A, Herve P, et al. Noninvasive ventilation reduces mortality in acute respiratory failure following lung resection. Am J Respir Crit Care Med. 2001;164:1231–5.

10. Jacobi J, Fraser GL, Coursin DB, et al. Clinical practice guidelines for the sustained use of sedatives and analgesics in the critically ill adult. Crit Care Med. 2002;30:119–41.

11. Tobin MJ. Advances in mechanical ventilation. N Engl J Med. 2001;344: 1986–96.

12. Tobin MJ. Mechanical ventilation. N Engl J Med. 1994;330:1056–61.

13. Girard TD, Kress JP, Fuchs BD, et al. Efficacy and safety of a paired sedation and ventilator weaning protocol for mechanically ventilated patients in intensive care (Awakening and Breathing Controlled trial): a randomized controlled trial. Lancet. 2008;371:126–34.

14. Schweickert WD, Pohlman MC, Pohlman AS, et al. Early physical and occupational therapy in mechanically ventilated, critically ill patients: a randomized controlled trial. Lancet. 2009;373:1874–82.

15. Rana S, Pendem S, Pogodzinski MS, et al. Tracheostomy in critically ill patients. Mayo Clin Proc. 2005;80:1632–8.

16. Amar D. Perioperative atrial tachyarrhythmias. Anesthesiology. 2002;97: 1618–23.

17. Amar D. Postthoracotomy atrial fibrillation. Curr Opin Anaesthesiol. 2007;20: 43–7.

18. Jakobsen CJ, Bille S, Ahlburg P, et al. Perioperative metoprolol reduces the frequency of atrial fibrillation after thoracotomy for lung resection. J Cardiothorac Vasc Anesth. 1997;11:746–51.

19. Cerfolio RJ, Bass C, Katholi CR. Prospective randomized trial compares suction versus water seal for air leaks. Ann Thorac Surg. 2001;71:1613–7.

20. Cerfolio RJ, Bryant AS. Results of a prospective algorithm to remove chest tubes after pulmonary resection with high output. J Thorac Cardiovasc Surg. 2008;135:269–73.

21. Cerfolio RJ, Minnich DJ, Bryant AS. The removal of chest tubes despite an air leak or a pneumothorax. Ann Thorac Surg. 2009;87:1690–6.

22. Cerfolio RJ, Bryant AS, Singh S, et al. The management of chest tubes in patients with a pneumothorax and an air leak after pulmonary resection. Chest. 2005;128:816–20.

23. Cerfolio RJ, Bryant AS, Maniscalco LM. Management of subcutaneous emphysema after pulmonary resection. Ann Thorac Surg. 2008;85:1759–65.

24. Fahimi H, Casselman FP, Mariani M, et al. Current management of postoperative chylothorax. Ann Thorac Surg. 2001;71:448–51.

25. Martin LW, Swisher SG, Hofstetter W, et al. Intrathoracic leaks following esophagectomy are no longer associated with increased mortality. Ann Surg. 2005;242:392–402.

26. Crestallano JA, Deschamps C, Cassivi SD, et al. Selective management of intrathoracic anastamotic leak after esophagectomy. J Thorac Cardiovasc Surg. 2005;129:254–60.

27. Freeman RK, Ascioti AJ, Wozniak TC. Postoperative esophageal leak management with the Polyflex esophageal stent. J Thorac Cardiovasc Surg. 2007;133:333–8.

28. Cable DG, Deschamps C, Allen MS, et al. Lobar torsion after pulmonary resection: presentation and outcome. J Thorac Cardiovasc Surg. 2001;122:1091–3.

29. Bhattacharyya N, Batirel H, Swanson SJ. Improved outcomes with early vocal fold medialization for vocal fold paralysis after thoracic surgery. Auris Nasus Larynx. 2003;30:71–5.

IV

Specific Thoracic Surgical Procedures: Surgical and Anesthetic Management Essentials

Chapter 18
Flexible Bronchoscopy

Philip M. Hartigan

Keywords Bronchoscopy • Flexible bronchoscopy • Anesthesia for bronchoscopy • General endotracheal anesthesia • Awake flexible bronchoscopy • Endobronchial ultrasound

Introduction

Bronchoscopy is the visual inspection of the tracheobroncheal tree using a scope inserted into the airway.

In the context of thoracic surgery, flexible bronchoscopy is most commonly performed to stage lung cancer, but has many other applications in and out of the operating room (Table 18-1).

Anesthesia for bronchoscopy is tailored to the situation and pathophysiology. Often, bronchoscopy is coupled with another procedure (e.g., mediastinoscopy) which requires general anesthesia.

P.M. Hartigan (ed.), *Practical Handbook of Thoracic Anesthesia*,
DOI 10.1007/978-0-387-88493-6_18,

Definitions

Flexible Fiberoptic Bronchoscopy: Image is viewed directly through the proximal lens of a flexible scope. Light and image are transmitted by fiberoptics.

Flexible Videobronchoscopy: Image is projected to a monitor from a camera at the tip of a flexible scope. Light is transmitted by fiberoptics.

Rigid Bronchoscopy: Long, tubular, rigid scope inserted through glottis to directly view and access trachea (see Chapter 26).

Endobronchial Ultrasound (EBUS): Combines ultrasound with videobronchoscopy to guide transbronchial biopsies.

Electromagnetic Navigational Bronchoscopy™: Proprietary technology (superDimension inReach System®) for distal navigation of the tracheobronchial tree using a steerable extension of the flexible bronchoscope, guided by a GPS-like electromagnetic system for tracking its real-time location (see below).

Table 18-1 – Surgical indications for flexible bronchoscopy[a]

- Staging of lung cancer
- Evaluation of:
  - Tracheobroncheal stenoses
  - Intrinsic airway obstruction
  - Extrinsic airway obstruction
  - Hemoptysis
  - Persistent, unexplained cough
  - Persistent, localized wheeze

(continued)

Table 18-1 – (continued)

- Broncho-alveolar lavage, brushings, biopsies
- Deployment, evaluation, or adjustment of stents
- Guide to transbronchial biopsy
- Retrieval of foreign bodies of the airway
- Airway balloon dilatation
- Delivery of laser therapy, brachytherapy, or photodynamic therapy
- Placement of brachytherapy cannullae
- Evaluation of suspected aspiration or burn/chemical injury to airway
- Evaluation and potential treatment (adhesives, etc.) of bronchopleural or tracheoesophageal fistulae
- Surveillance evaluation of lung transplant recipients (infection vs. rejection)
- Delivery of agents or devices for bronchoscopic lung volume reduction surgery

[a] Partial list. Does not include supraglottic indications, or anesthetic use as an aid to intubation or lung isolation.

Surgical Considerations for Flexible Bronchoscopy

There are very few surgical considerations specific to flexible bronchoscopy, per se.

- Biopsy via bronchoscopes may cause tracheobronchial disruption or bleeding.
- Laser via bronchoscopes may cause airway fires (Chapter 27).
- Manipulation of stents or foreign bodies may result in airway obstruction (Chapter 28).
- Malfunctioning bronchoscopes may rarely become overheated at the tip.
- Postbronchoscopy pneumonia is a relatively rare complication of bronchoscopy performed in the OR.

Anesthetic Considerations for Flexible Bronchoscopy

The anesthetic requirements for bronchoscopy, itself, are limited to blunting or ablating the airway reflexes, as well as the powerfully noxious affective response to airway instrumentation. This may be accomplished through general anesthesia or topical anesthesia with sedation. The latter is often preferable for patients with advanced pulmonary disease or significant airway obstruction.

General Endotracheal Anesthesia

When general endotracheal anesthesia (GETA) is appropriate, the principal anesthetic issues are related to the obstruction to airflow and air return, due to the presence of the bronchoscope and the use of suction. Because bronchoscopy is often brief and can easily be interrupted if problems occur, there is typically limited risk to the procedure. Nonetheless, attention should be paid to compliance, airflow, chest rise, and the amount of suctioning being performed by the surgeon.

Frequent, prolonged *suctioning leads to*:

- Reduced "return" to the ventilator.
- Inaccurately measured tidal volumes.
- Inaccurately measured end-tidal CO_2 and anesthetic gasses.
- Atelectasis and impaired delivery of O_2 and anesthetic gasses.

These issues are *mitigated by*:

- Use of a large (>8.0 O.D.) endotracheal tube or laryngeal mask airway (LMA).
- Use of high FiO_2 (unless history of Bleomycin, or planned use of laser).
- Use of TIVA if procedure becomes prolonged.
- Use of high fresh gas flows.
- Hand ventilation with attention to chest rise and compliance.

Conversely, *infrequent use of suction may lead to air trapping* (auto-PEEP) due to expiratory airflow obstruction (by bronchoscope). Exacerbating factors include obstructive pulmonary disease, a small endotracheal tube, and short expiratory times. In practice, this is rarely an issue due to the brevity of the procedure, and the usually frequent use of suctioning.

General Anesthesia Without Intubation

Avoiding intubation obviates the airflow obstruction issues and reduces airway stimulation and anesthetic requirements, but does not protect against aspiration or laryngospasm. An advantage is that the entire trachea can be viewed. An LMA or other supraglottic device provides a convenient conduit to the larynx (Fig 18-1).

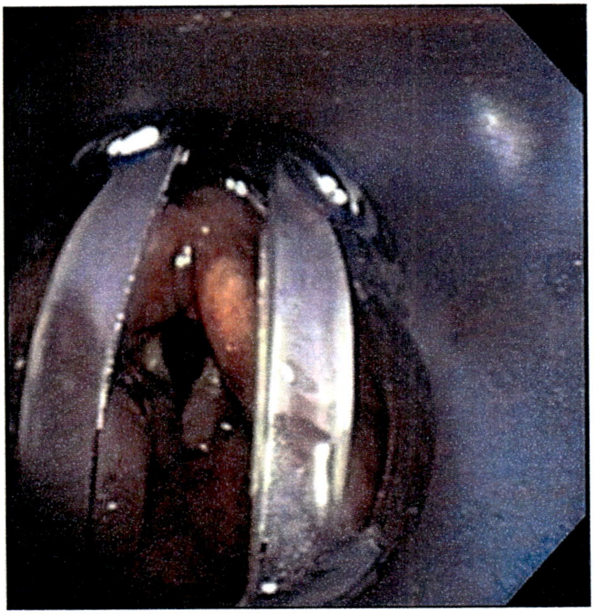

Figure 18-1 – Bronchoscopic view of vocal cords via laryngeal mask airway (LMA). This approach allows visualization of the entire trachea. The LMA also helps stent open soft tissue or edematous airways as in this example. The vertical struts may also be cut out for an even less obstructed view of the larynx.

Sedation for Awake Flexible Bronchoscopy

Avoidance of general anesthesia and preservation of spontaneous ventilation are indicated for patients with critical airway obstruction (1) (Chapter 20). Flexible bronchoscopy in such patients is often best performed with topical anesthesia and judicious sedation, in the sitting or semisitting position.

- Sedation should be tailored to the reserves, requirements, and response of the individual patient.
- Thorough topical anesthesia minimizes sedation requirements.
    - Nebulized or atomized local anesthetic for the posterior pharynx and vocal cords.
    - "Spray-as-you-go" via bronchoscope for distal trachea and carinal anesthesia.
    - Beware of local anesthetic toxicity (rapid mucosal absorption).
- Dexmedetomidine has the advantage of relative preservation of ventilatory drive.
- An antisialagogue such as glycopyrolate aids in control of secretions.
- A bite block will protect teeth and bronchoscopes.

Endobronchial Ultrasound-Guided Transbronchial Biopsy

EBUS uses a small ultrasound probe mounted on a videobronchoscope. With the bronchoscope, the operator navigates to the target region of the tracheobroncheal tree, and the EBUS provides an "ultrasound view" of the tissue beneath the surface. A biopsy probe or needle is then passed through the working port of the bronchoscope for transbronchial biopsy of nodes or masses, guided by EBUS (Fig 18-2).

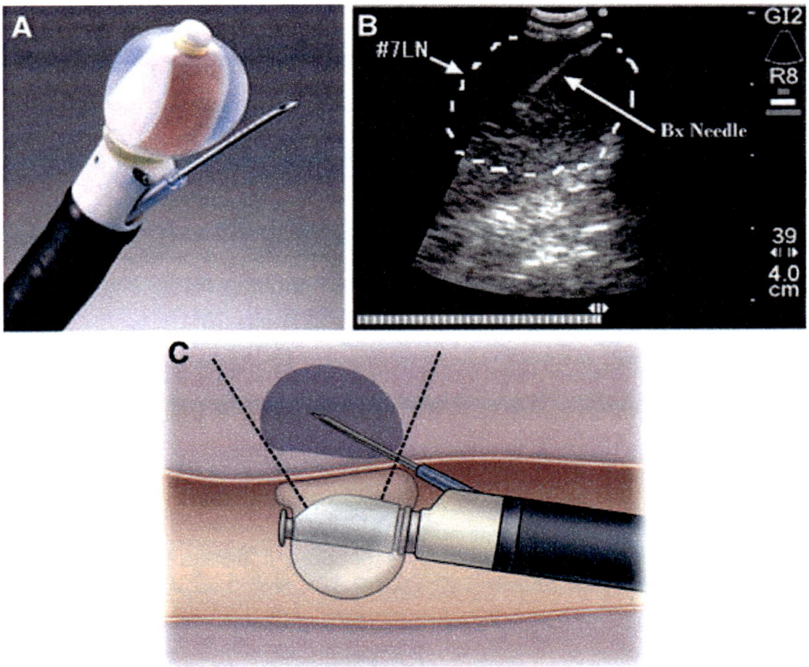

Figure 18-2 – (**A**) Endobronchial ultrasound (EBUS) probe with fluid-filled balloon to improve acoustic contact, and fine biopsy needle emerging from the working port for transbronchial biopsy. (**B**) Ultrasound image of transbronchial needle biopsy of lymph node. (**C**) Schematic demonstrating EBUS transbronchial needle biopsy. Images provided by Olympus Corp.

Surgical Considerations for EBUS

EBUS provides greater access than cervical mediastinoscopy, including paratracheal, subcarinal, hilar, and interlobar lymph node stations (see Fig 18-3) (2). EBUS-guided transbronchial needle aspiration (EBUS-TBNA) to stage lung cancer patients, whose mediastinum was negative by CT and PET, was found to compare favorably to mediastinoscopy, with a sensitivity and specificity of 89% and 100%, respectively (3). Bleeding complications are rare because the needle diameter is small, and doppler helps identify blood vessels.

Anesthetic Considerations for EBUS

Anesthetic considerations for EBUS-TBNA are largely similar to those for bronchoscopy. The principal issues include the following (4):

- There is *potential for hemoptysis or tracheobronchial disruption* following biopsy.
- A *motionless field* during biopsy is important. Most favor *General Anesthesia* for this reason.
- *Large ETT* (>8.5 O.D.) required to accommodate probe and ventilate adequately.
- *LMA* allows improved access to high paratracheal nodes, and reduces airflow obstruction issues (see above).
- *TIVA* obviates obstruction of gas delivery and elimination.

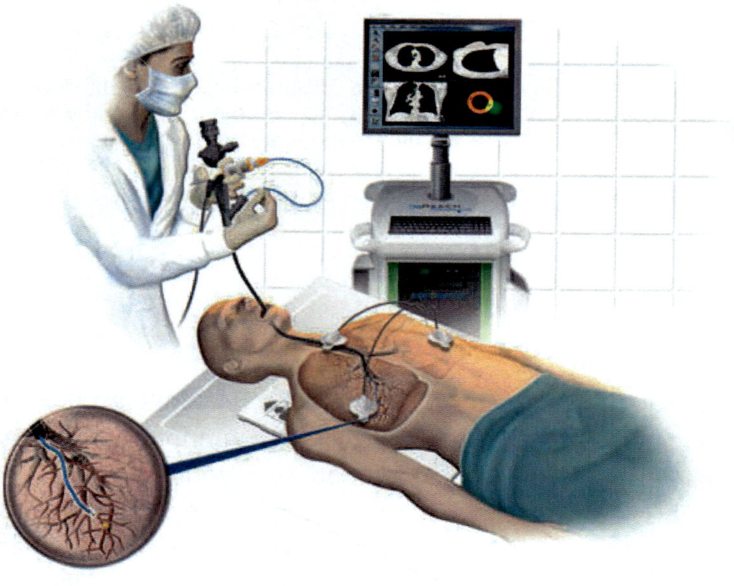

Figure 18-3 – *Electromagnetic navigational bronchoscopy* employs a navigable catheter (*blue*) passed through a bronchoscope to reach more peripheral lesions. Navigation system merges GPS-like system with CT scan data. See text for explanation. Image provided by superDimension, Inc.

- Post-op pain is minimal (minor sore throat).
- Suitable for out-of-OR procedure room, on outpatient basis.
- A fluid filled balloon over the transducer tip is needed to overcome the ultrasound interference from the air-filled trachea.
- There is *potential for tracheal or bronchial obstruction* when the balloon tip is inflated (this may require intermittent apnea).

Electromagnetic Navigation Bronchoscopy

Peripheral lesions outside the reach of conventional bronchoscopes or EBUS may potentially be biopsied by Electromagnetic Navigation Bronchoscopy™ (superDimension inReach System®) (Fig 18-3). This system uses a navigable extension for the working port of the bronchoscope, with a sensor at the distal tip to aid navigation. Rather than directly "seeing" where it navigates, the sensor's position appears on a screen which merges preoperative CT scan data with real-time GPS-like technology to locate the sensor's position within the chest.

When the extended working port is sited at the target lesion, the sensor is withdrawn, and a biopsy instrument is inserted to sample the lesion. Thus, the biopsy is made with the sensor out of place (blind). The patient should not move appreciably relative to the extended working port during this time or the biopsy may be off target. Aside from this, there are no anesthetic implications of this procedure that differ from any bronchoscopic biopsy.

Selected References

1. Neuman GG, Weingarten AE, Abramowitz RM, Kushins LG, Abramson AL, Ladner W. The anesthetic management of the patient with an anterior mediastinal mass. Anesthesiology. 1984;60:144–7.

2. Kennedy MP, Shweihat Y, SarkissM EGA. Complete mediastinal and hilar lymph node staging of primary lung cancer by endobronchial ultrasound: moderate sedation or general anesthesia? Chest. 2008;134(6):1350–1.

3. Herth FJ, Eberhardt R, Krasnik M, Ernst A. Endobronchial ultrasound-guided transbronchial needle aspiration of lymph nodes in the radiologically and

positron emission tomography normal mediastinum in patients with lung cancer. Chest. 2008;133(4):887–91.

4. Sarkiss M, Kennedy M, Riedel B, Norman P, Morice R, Jimenez C, et al. Anesthesia technique for endobronchial ultrasound-guided fine needle aspiration of mediastinal lymph node. J Cardiothorac Vasc Anesth. 2007;21(6):892–6.

Further Suggested Reading

Soodan A, Pawar D, Subramanium R. Anesthesia for removal of foreign bodies in children. Paediatr Anaesth. 2004;14(11):947–52.

Chapter 19
Mediastinoscopy

Philip M. Hartigan

Keywords Intraoperative hemorrhage • A-Med • C-Med • Mediastinum • Mediastinoscopy • Cervical mediastinoscopy • Anterior mediastinoscopy

Introduction

Mediastinoscopy involves the surgical insertion of a scope into the mediastinum to examine or biopsy tissue. It is principally performed to sample lymph nodes for diagnosis or staging of lung cancers.

Definitions

Cervical Mediastinoscopy (C-Med), the most common approach, provides access to the majority of mediastinal lymph nodes through a small incision above the manubrium (Fig 19-1).

Anterior Mediastinoscopy (A-Med), generally performed through a small left parasternal incision, allows sampling of nodes inaccessible from the cervical approach (Fig 19-2). A-Med is also performed to biopsy anterior mediastinal or hilar masses.

P.M. Hartigan (ed.), *Practical Handbook of Thoracic Anesthesia*,
DOI 10.1007/978-0-387-88493-6_19,

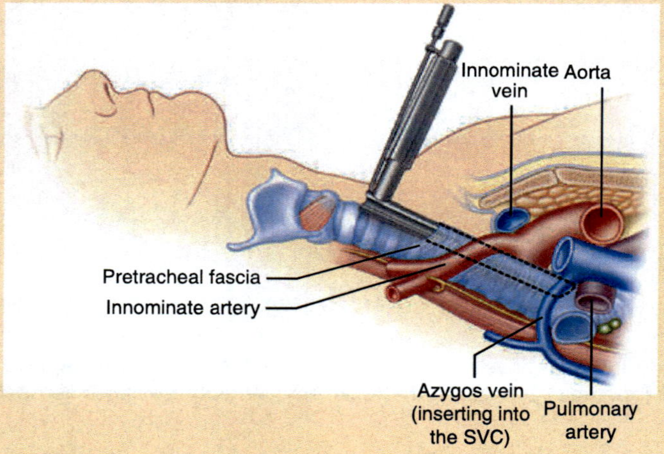

Figure 19-1 – The cervical mediastinoscope is advanced through a potential plane between the trachea and pretracheal fascia, dorsal to the innominate artery. Vulnerable adjacent structures are depicted. *(Modified with permission from Kaplan and Slinger (Editors), Thoracic Anesthesia (3 rd edition), Churchill Livingstone 2003. pp187).*

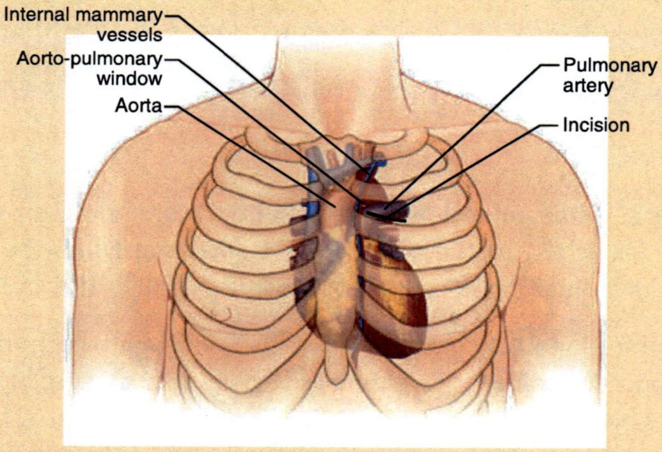

Figure 19-2 – A left parasternal approach for anterior mediastinoscopy provides access to aortopulmonary window lymph nodes. Note vulnerable adjacent structures.

Staging mediastinoscopy is often coupled with bronchoscopy as a day surgical procedure, or combined with subsequent pulmonary resection. Compression of vital structures by large mediastinal masses imparts additional significant risk and is discussed separately in Chapter 20. Barring such mass effects or significant comorbidity, mediastinoscopy is typically a low-stress procedure, but takes place in a potentially treacherous territory.

Surgical Considerations

The principal surgical concerns of mediastinoscopy are to obtain sufficient tissue for accurate staging or diagnosis, and to avoid hemorrhage.

Accurate staging is critical to treatment decisions for lung cancer (Chapter 15). Despite advances in less invasive approaches (e.g., PET-CT), surgical staging (usually by mediastinoscopy) remains the gold standard. Lymph nodes of the aortopulmonary window (level 5) or preaortic station (level 6) are not normally accessible by C-Med (Fig 19-3). These drain from the left lung and can be reached by left A-Med. Extended cervical mediastinoscopy is an alternative route to access level 5 and 6 nodes through a cervical incision and a more superficial, substernal plane (Fig 19-4) (1). Extended c-med involves greater manipulation of the aorta and innominate artery, and may have a higher risk of stroke than anterior mediastinoscopy.

Significant intraoperative hemorrhage, although rare, is the major risk. Access is difficult, and vision is quickly obscured by blood. Often, the source must be inferred from the location. Typical sources include bronchial or innominate arteries, or azygous vein. Bronchial artery bleeding tends to arise from the subcarinal space and may be difficult to control with electrocautery, but rarely requires thoracotomy. Azygous vein bleeding can generally be controlled with packing, allowing for calm preparation and positioning for a right thoracotomy. Azygous tears, however, may extend into the superior vena cava. Because different exposures are required for different

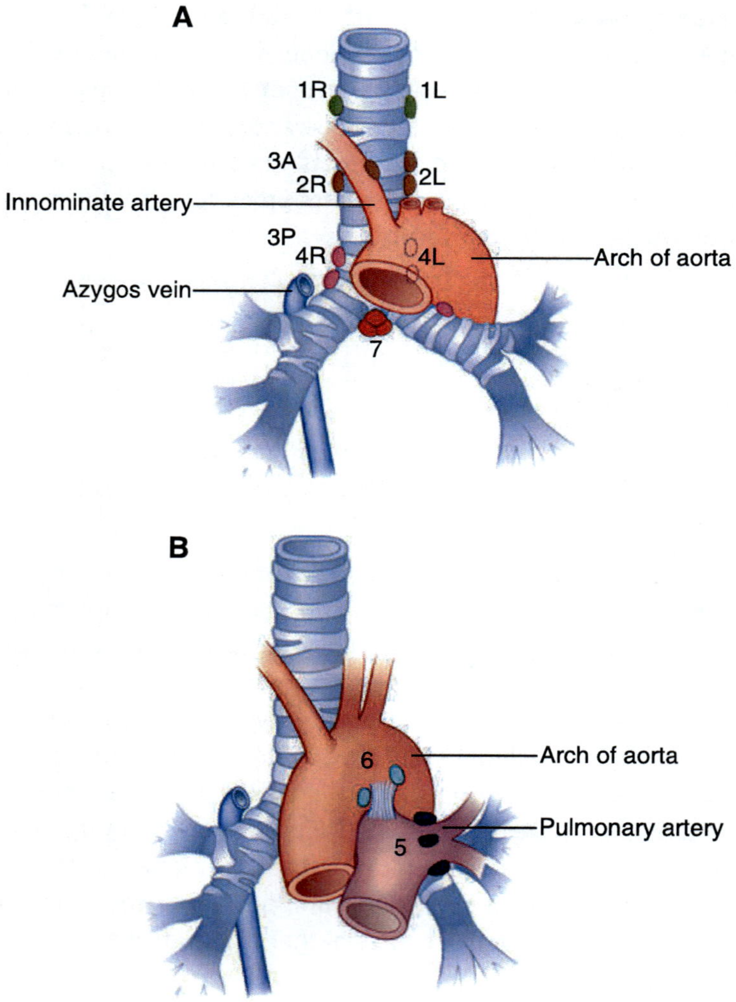

Figure 19-3 – Lymph node stations of the mediastinum typically targeted for staging.

sources of bleeding, it is important to establish the source when possible. Sternotomy provides ready access to the innominate artery, but limited visualization of the azygous. Pulmonary artery (PA) bleeds are rare, often a result of avulsion injuries from harvesting adherent lymph nodes. Because the PA is usually a low-pressure

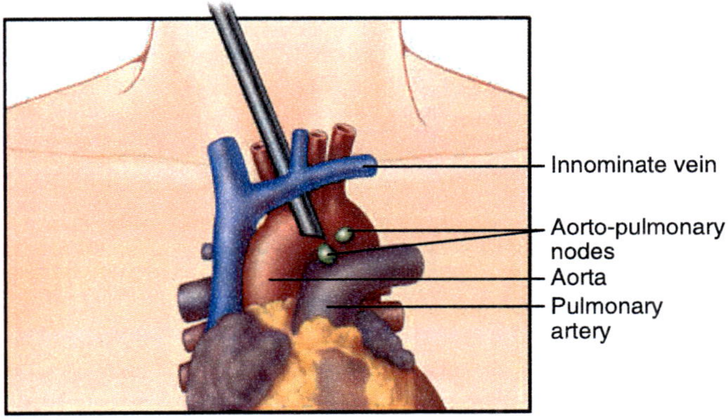

Figure 19-4 – Extended mediastinoscopy offers a cervical approach to aortopulmonary nodes via a more superficial path, anterior to the aorta and innominate arteries.

vessel, small injuries can be controlled with packing. Large PA bleeds require immediate sternotomy.

Delayed postoperative bleeding into the mediastinum can lead to airway or cardiac compression. The surgical team should be confident about hemostasis at the conclusion of the procedure because CXR and physical exam are notoriously misleading in the evaluation of mediastinal hematoma. An end-inspiratory hold maneuver can help evaluate potential venous bleeding. At minimum, the patient with potential mediastinal hematoma should be observed overnight.

Other complications relate to the other structures in the vicinity (Table 19-1). Left paratracheal adenopathy, left hilar mass, or biopsy/electrocautery in the vicinity of the recurrent laryngeal nerve may lead to vocal cord paresis. Evaluation of the patient's voice prior to surgery and assessment of vocal cord symmetry at the time of intubation can be useful for postoperative management. Small pneumothoraces (<10%) are not uncommon, particularly after anterior mediastinoscopy, but generally resolve with conservative management. *Relative contraindications* to cervical mediastinoscopy are summarized in Table 19-2.

Table 19-1 – Complications of cervical mediastinoscopy

Hemorrhage

- Major
  - Azygous vein
  - Bronchial artery
  - Pulmonary artery
  - Innominate artery or vein
  - Aorta (extremely rare)
  - SVC (extremely rare)
- Minor
  - Small disruptions of above vessels
  - Inferior thyroid vessels
  - Potential delayed bleeding

Non-hemorrhage-related complications (*Extremely Rare*)

- Nerve injury
  - Recurrent laryngeal n.
  - Vagus n.
  - Phrenic n.
- Injury to tracheobronchial tree
- Innominate artery compression-related stroke
- Pneumothorax
- Position-related cervical neck injury
- Thoracic duct injury
- Esophageal injury
- Cardiac dysrhythmias
- Air embolus

Table 19-2 – Relative contraindications to cervical mediastinoscopy

- Coagulopathy
- Prior cervical mediastinoscopy
- SVC syndrome
- Ascending thoracic aneurysm
- Severe kyphosis
- Tracheostomy
- Prior radiotherapy to region
- Severely enlarged goiter

Anesthetic Considerations for Cervical Mediastinoscopy

Anesthesia for C-Med typically requires general endotracheal anesthesia with muscle relaxation, tailored for same-day discharge. Barring significant coexisting disease or mass effects (see Chapter 20), anesthetic issues are largely intuitive, directed by an awareness of the potential complications (Table 19-3).

Hemorrhage: The response depends on its magnitude, and ranges from packing and observation, to emergent sternotomy, thoracotomy, or cardiopulmonary bypass (2). The preferred surgical approach depends on the source (see Sect. "Surgical Considerations", above).

Massive Hemorrhage: It is immediately evident that the bleeding will not abate with surgical packing, and the patient is hemodynamically unstable. This usually calls for immediate sternotomy, volume resuscitation, and vasopressors. Blood products, invasive monitoring, supplemental IV access, and warming maneuvers are established as the situation permits, without delaying surgical control of the bleeding source (usually PA, SVC, or innominate artery).

Intermediate Hemorrhage: The bleeding is at least temporarily controllable by packing the wound, and hemodynamics are

Table 19-3 – Anesthetic considerations for cervical mediastinoscopy

- Exclude significant mass effect
- GETA tailored to same day discharge
- Motionless field (bleeding risk)
- Innominate artery compression
  - Right hand pulse detector
  - Screen for cerebrovascular disease
- Limit nitrous oxide use (pneumothorax potential)
- Cervical neck positioning considerations
- Avoid exacerbation of bleeding (NSAIDS, Hypertension)
- Be prepared for sternotomy/thoracotomy/transfusion/bypass
  - Initial IV access ^{3} 18 guage
  - Cross-matched blood available
  - Available helping hands for:
    - Supplemental IV access
    - Arterial line
    - Rapid transfusion
    - Efficient lung isolation

acceptable. Discussion should take place with the surgeon regarding suspected source, surgical approach, and need for lung isolation. There is time to establish extra IV access and invasive monitoring, and to set up blood products for rapid, warm resuscitation. If the innominate vein is suspected, lower extremity IV access is needed.

Options for efficient *lung isolation* include advancing the SLT into the left mainstem over a bronchoscope, or use of a bronchial blocker in the right mainstem if the patient is a difficult intubation. One can exchange to a DLT if the mediastinoscope is not in place. Edema from massive transfusion may make a tube exchange at the end of the case problematic. Azygous repairs via right thoracotomy can be performed with packing or retraction of the lung and judicious timing of low volume ventilations by the anesthesiologist without formal lung isolation.

Minor Hemorrhage: The bleeding is resolved by a period of packing, electrocautery, Surgicel®, or other maneuvers performed through the mediastinoscope. This is the most common scenario and results from limited injury to low-pressure vessels. Preventing hypertension, coughing, and bucking on the ventilator may aid efforts to establish hemostasis.

Delayed Hemorrhage: Insidious bleeding into the mediastinum following discharge with potential airway compression or tamponade is a concern, since patients are usually discharged to home. Any coagulopathy should be corrected prior to surgery, and many would advocate avoidance of NSAIDS.

Position: Patients are generally supine with arms tucked at their sides, a transverse roll under the shoulders, and the *neck maximally extended*. The patient's head should be at the very head of the bed to provide good mechanics for the surgeon. Lines and monitors should be arranged to allow the surgeon access to the head of the bed, or alternatively, the bed may be rotated 90 °. Patients with cervical disk disease should be positioned while awake to establish maximal tolerated neck extension. The chest is prepped to prepare for the rare sternotomy. The patient's head and endotracheal tube are draped and are often inaccessible for evaluation or monitoring.

Motionless Field: Patient movement during mediastinoscopy may cause mishap and hemorrhage. Sufficient anesthetic depth and paralysis consistent with a motionless field and brisk emergence can be a challenge. The level of surgical stimulation is mercurial, the duration is unpredictable, and access to the patient is limited for monitoring neuromuscular blockade. Moderate paralysis and deep anesthesia using short or ultrashort acting agents is a widely employed strategy.

Innominate Artery Compression: The mediastinoscope passes dorsal to the innominate artery and often results in partial or complete innominate artery compression. Logically, patients with left carotid stenosis or cerebrovascular disease would be at increased risk of stroke in this scenario. Anectodally, the author has observed transient EEG flatline during cervical mediastinoscopy which resolved with removal of the mediastinoscope in a patient with an occluded left carotid artery.

Placement of a pulse detector (arterial line or pulse oximeter) in the right hand is widely advocated to detect innominate artery compression, but its value in prevention of stroke is undocumented. EEG monitoring should be considered in the patient with suspected poor collateral cerebral perfusion. Stroke following C-Med is rare, possibly owing to the generally transient and incomplete nature of innominate artery compression. Measurement of blood pressure in the right upper extremity may be spurious due to innominate artery compression.

Postoperative Considerations: Pain following C-Med is mild, and well managed with low doses of narcotics. Patients should be screened for complications prior to discharge. A *CXR* may reveal an expanding mediastinum, elevated hemidiaphragm (phrenic n. injury), or very rarely a pneumothorax, pneumomediastinum, or subcutaneous emphysema (tracheal injury). Stridor, hoarseness, or dyspnea may signal recurrent laryngeal nerve injury, tracheal injury, or an expanding hematoma in the neck.

Anesthetic Considerations for Anterior Mediastinoscopy

Considerations for A-Med are identical to those for C-Med with the exception that the vessels at risk are different, the risk of pneumothorax is higher, and the innominate artery is not compressed.

Consider Mass Effects: Always distinguish the high risk patient with mediastinal mass effects on the airway, heart, or great vessels prior to induction. In general, positional respiratory symptoms, stigmata of SVC syndrome, or CT scan evidence of a large mass effect will identify such patients (see Chapter 20). *A-Med may be performed under local anesthesia in high risk patients.*

Hemorrhage: While the azygous vein and innominate artery are less vulnerable, the pulmonary artery and aorta are perhaps more vulnerable during A-med compared to C-Med. Should massive hemorrhage occur, sternotomy would be the approach of choice. As with C-Med, a motionless surgical field is important, and coagulopathies are to be avoided.

Lung Isolation: Some surgeons will prefer one-lung anesthesia (usually left lung deflated) to improve visualization and preempt the consequences of a pneumothorax during A-Med. One-lung oxygenation in the supine position is less effective than in the lateral decubitus position due to greater blood flow (shunt) to the deflated lung by gravity.

Selected References

1. Bocage J-P, Mackenzie J, Nosher J. Invasive diagnostic procedures. Chapter 17. In: Shields TW, LoCicero J, Ponn RB, editors. General thoracic surgery. 5th ed. Lippincott, Williams and Wilkins; 2006. p. 273–84.

2. Lohser J, Donington J, Mitchell JD, et al. Anesthetic management of major hemorrhage during mediastinoscopy. J Cardiothorac Vasc Anesth. 2005;19(5): 678–83.

Further Suggested Reading

Plummer S, Hartley M, Vaughan RS. Anaesthesia for telescopic procedures of the thorax. Br J Anaesth. 1998;80:223–34.

Park B. Management of major hemorrhage during mediastinoscopy. J Thorac Cardiovasc Surg. 2003;726:31–5.

Foster ED, Munro DD, Dobell ARC. Mediastinoscopy: a review of anatomical relationships and complications. Ann Thorac Surg. 1972;13:273–8.

Vaughn RS. Anaesthesia for mediastinoscopy. Anaesthesia. 1978;33:195–9.

Chapter 20
Anterior Mediastinal Mass

Ju-Mei Ng and Philip M. Hartigan

Keywords Anterior mediastinal mass • AMM • Airway compression • Mediastinoscopy

Introduction

Anesthesia for biopsy or excision of an anterior mediastinal mass (AMM) has the potential for life-threatening or fatal events as a result of airway occlusion, tamponade, pulmonary outflow obstruction, and/or loss of venous return. General anesthesia may convert such mass effects from subcritical to critical.

The central concept of this chapter is that *anesthetic management depends on the perceived risk* (extent of mass effect). Guidelines must err on the conservative, due to the absence of well-defined predictors, or thresholds for high risk. The usefulness of clinical signs and symptoms, radiologic evaluation and pulmonary function tests in the determination of the perioperative risk are discussed, including some general principles of safe anesthesia for these patients.

P.M. Hartigan (ed.), *Practical Handbook of Thoracic Anesthesia*,
DOI 10.1007/978-0-387-88493-6_20,

Mechanisms

The hazards associated with AMM include extrinsic compression of the airway, pulmonary artery (PA), right ventricular outflow tract (RVOT), heart, and superior vena cava (SVC). More than one may apply to a given patient. Although it is well known that general anesthesia exacerbates mass effects within the chest, there are limited data regarding the precise mechanism(s).

The term "general anesthesia" is often loosely employed to include all of the following transitions:

- Upright posture to supine position
- Awake state to anesthetized state
- Spontaneous negative pressure ventilation to positive pressure mechanical ventilation
- Unparalyzed to paralyzed muscular tone

Supine Position. In the supine position, functional residual capacity (FRC) and thoracic volume are reduced, thus increasing any thoracic mass effect. In addition, the vector of gravitational forces from an AMM will be more likely to compress airways, vessels or the heart when compared to the upright position. High-risk patients will generally be symptomatic or intolerant of lying flat supine while awake.

General Anesthesia. General anesthesia (GA) imposes an additional loss of FRC and thoracic volume (Chapter 4). This occurs independent of the induction agents (excepting ketamine), method of ventilation (spontaneous or positive pressure), or state of muscle paralysis. The magnitude is variable but significant, averaging 16–20% beyond that in the awake, supine state (1). This volume loss translates to reduced caliber of airways and exacerbates mass effects on vascular structures within the chest.

Mode of Ventilation. Classic teaching emphasizes that maintenance of spontaneous ventilation offers some protection from airway compression by AMM (2). This is based on a number of case reports in pediatric patients. One such case, for example, described an intubated 16 year old with a large mediastinal mass whose right lung could not be ventilated by positive pressure, whereas ventilation was restored after resumption of spontaneous efforts (3). The mechanism by which spontaneous ventilation might protect airway patency is unclear, but this conviction is deeply rooted among pediatric anesthesiologists. This may be a reflection of different practice patterns, and the different respiratory mechanics of children.

Airflow velocities tend to be faster with positive pressure ventilation (PPV), which predisposes to conversion of laminar to turbulent flow through a stenosis (4). Whether it is the positive pressure aspect of mechanical ventilation, or the airflow velocity profile which disrupts ventilation is unclear. Case reports exist of successful induction and maintenance using spontaneous ventilation, followed by airway obstruction during emergence, postulated to be caused by the more rapid breathing pattern (4).

Importantly, AMM may obstruct *expiration* as well as inspiration. Forceful positive pressure ventilation may force air past obstructions which subsequently becomes trapped because expiration is passive. The resulting dynamic hyperinflation and elevated airway pressures (auto-PEEP) may impair venous return, exacerbate mass effects or tamponade.

Paralysis. Use of neuromuscular blocking agents is classically thought to further exacerbate airway obstruction and thoracic mass effects from an AMM (2). Direct evidence for this is lacking. The FRC effect of GA is no different with paralysis compared to without (1). In case reports, it is difficult to separate the transition to the paralyzed state from the transition to PPV. If one performs a staged induction and safely transitions to the supine position, general anesthesia, and PPV, it is unclear whether paralysis would then add additional risk. Pending clarification, caution is recommended.

Surgical Considerations

While diagnostic biopsies may be carried out via mediastinoscopy (cervical or anterior) or video-assisted thoracoscopic surgery (VATS), the approach for therapeutic surgery varies with size, location and pathology of the AMM. These include median sternotomy, anterior thoracotomy, clamshell incision, or VATS. Involvement of major vessels or cardiac structures may necessitate vascular repair, graft replacement surgery, or even cardiopulmonary bypass.

When perceived anesthetic risk is high, the least invasive route to diagnosis should be pursued under local anesthesia if possible. These include image-guided needle biopsy and palpable lymph node biopsy. In children or adolescents, bone marrow biopsy, thoracentesis, or even peripheral blood smear may provide sufficient diagnostic certainty to initiate therapy (5). Empiric treatment with steroids or radiation can dramatically reduce mass effects for certain tumors, but has the potential to confound histologic architecture and diagnostic certainty. In extremely high-risk patients, however, this may be justified.

Surgeons must recognize that the principal risk with AMM is often anesthetic rather than surgical. A joint team review of the Computed Tomography (CT) scan (Fig 20-1) and plan prior to induction is prudent. While rigid bronchoscopy is considered a rescue maneuver for collapsed airways, anesthesiologists in turn must understand that placement of a rigid bronchoscope takes time and may be technically challenging. Tracheal distortion may make it difficult to see and navigate, and the absence of a cuff makes positive

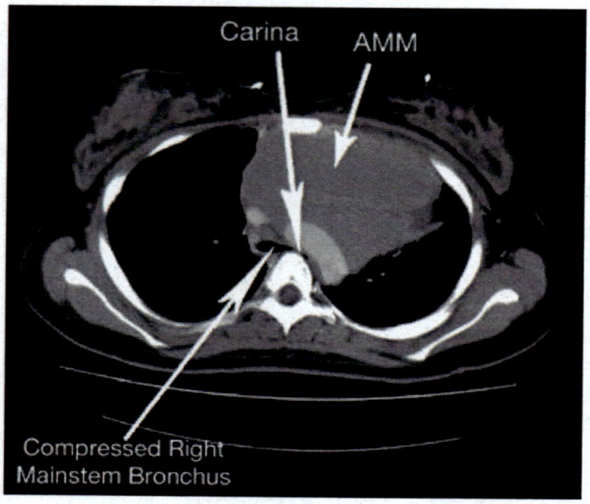

Figure 20-1 – Chest CT scan of large anterior mediastinal mass with airway compression at the level of the carina and mainstem bronchi.

pressure ventilation difficult until the stenotic portion is bridged. An alternative rescue maneuver is to advance a stenting endotracheal tube over a flexible bronchoscope.

Risk Assessment

The main aims are to

- Delineate the extent of encroachment on other structures
- Quantify any functional cardiorespiratory compromise caused by such encroachment
- Estimate the risk of general anesthesia (supine position/induction/PPV/paralysis)

Symptoms

Signs and symptoms (Table 20-1) are related to mass effect on or invasion of surrounding structures. Most adult mediastinal tumors are asymptomatic or associated with vague complaints such as chest pain, dyspnea, and cough. Orthopnea is the single most important symptom, and may be due to airway obstruction or compression of RVOT or PA. Cough may be due to apposition of tracheal mucosal surfaces. Presyncope suggests impaired cardiac output from compression of heart or vessels. By contrast, mediastinal masses are symptomatic in 70% of children. Increased perioperative risk in children has been associated with dyspnea (orthopnea) or cough when supine (increased risk of airway complications) and presyncopal symptoms or pericardial effusion (increased risk of cardiovascular complications). Any intolerance of the supine position should prompt caution, and any preference for lying on one side or the other should be noted as a potential rescue maneuver for patients with an eccentric AMM.

The presence of positional symptoms is clearly nonreassuring, but the relationship between the severity of symptoms and the degree of risk of perioperative complications appears to be soft (8). Orthopnea may be the exception, and severe orthopnea with an AMM suggests high risk of GA.

Table 20-1 – Clinical presentation of anterior mediastinal masses

COMPRESSION OR INFILTRATION OF ADJACENT STRUCTURES	SYMPTOMS/SIGNS
Tracheobronchial tree	Cough
	Stridor
	Wheeze
	Dyspnea
	Recurrent pulmonary infections
	Hemoptysis
Esophagus	Dysphagia
Right ventricular outflow tract	Dyspnea
	Syncope
Recurrent laryngeal nerve	Hoarseness
	Vocal cord paralysis
Sympathetic chain	Horner's syndrome
Phrenic nerve	Elevated hemidiaphragm
Superior vena cava	Dyspnea
	Cough
	Syncope
	Orthopnea
	Stridor
	Headache
	Decreased mentation
	Venous engorgement
	Upper body edema
	Plethora
	Cyanosis

It is controversial whether the asymptomatic adult with AMM is at increased risk of cardiorespiratory complications of anesthesia. Pediatric case reports exist describing presumed airway obstruction (inability to ventilate intubated patients) in previously asymptomatic children (6, 7). Because the reports were retrospective, and involved children, the quality of the history may be questioned. Shamberger, et al., found that orthopnea predicted severe tracheal compression (>50% predicted) by CT scan in children (8). It is apparent that symptoms triggered or exacerbated by the supine position should increase concern, but the degree to which the absence of postural symptoms should be reassuring is unclear. The answer may be different for adults than children.

The authors agree with Bechard, et al., who have suggested that GA can be induced safely in the asymptomatic adult with AMM, if the results of the radiographic and bronchoscopic evaluations are reassuring (9).

Radiologic Data

A chest CT is indicated in all patients. This helps identify the location of the mass, delineate margins, define its relationship to adjacent structures and determine the extent of tracheal or vascular compression. The tracheal cross-sectional area (TCA) at the narrowest point can also be measured by planimetry and expressed as a percentage of age/gender predicted values. It must be remembered that CT scans are obtained at attempted total lung capacity, when airways are maximally "tethered open." Magnetic resonance imaging (MRI) shows more extensive disease than CT in 25% of patients and aids assessment of tumor involvement of cardiac structures. Three dimensional reconstructions may prove helpful for tortuous, complex tracheal stenoses.

A few studies have attempted to define the TCA that represents the threshold for excessive risk of GA. Patients with TCA > 50% predicted generally tolerate GA well, (10, 11) barring other indicators of risk. Since most patients with TCA < 50% predicted were empirically treated more conservatively, it is unclear whether this threshold is too restrictive. Similar studies have not been performed in adults.

Other radiologic data besides TCA impact risk assessment. A large, low, central AMM compressing the distal trachea and carina is the greatest risk. High (cephalad) masses (e.g., intrathoracic thyroid) are less concerning because there is room to position an ETT to stent open the trachea. Intuitively, large masses impose greater risk than small (6). Mid-sagittal masses are greater risk than eccentric ones which are more easily "off-loaded" by tilting the patient "mass-side down." The coexistence of a pericardial effusion has been associated with increased risk with induction (9). Extrinsic compression of the PA or RVOT is easily overlooked by the anesthesiologist who might be overly focused on assessment of tracheal compression (Fig 20-2). A chest CT with contrast also allows assessment of the patency of the superior vena cava, which has obvious implications for volume resuscitation. A pericardial effusion is important to note as a potentially modifiable factor (pericardiocentesis) that clearly increases the risk of induction.

Pulmonary Function Testing and Postural Flow-Volume Loops

Postural spirometry has traditionally been part of the preoperative assessment of patients with AMM. Truncation of expiratory flow (mid-expiratory plateau), when changing from the upright to the

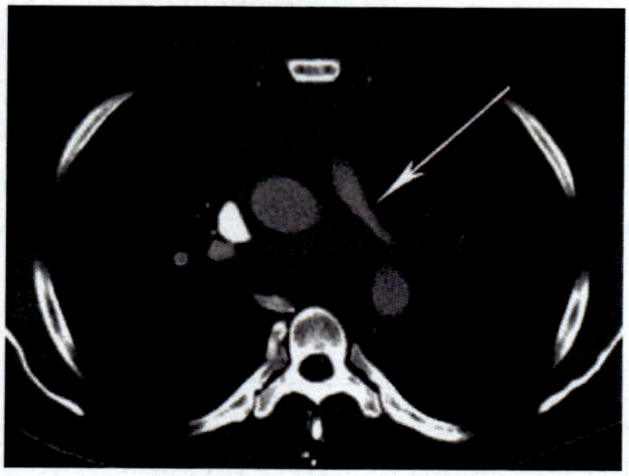

Figure 20-2 – Contrast chest CT scan at level just above the carina demonstrates large anterior mediastinal mass compressing the left main pulmonary artery (*arrow*).

supine position, is thought to be pathognomonic for a variable intrathoracic airway obstruction. In practice, flow-volume loops tend to demonstrate limitation of both inspiratory and expiratory flow with airway obstruction from an AMM, though the expiratory limb tends to be more severely affected.

Pulmonary function testing gives information about functional impairment but data do not predict airway morbidity and do not describe anatomic abnormality. Moreover, studies of flow-volume loops have shown poor correlation with the degree of airway obstruction and may not be any better at predicting perioperative complications than symptoms and CT scan. In clinical practice, postural spirometry probably does not offer any additive benefit in predicting perioperative complications in a minimally symptomatic population beyond that which is obtained from history and chest imaging. In part, this may be due to the effort dependence of pulmonary function tests.

Peak Expiratory Flow Rate

The risk of perioperative complications was increased more than tenfold when the peak expiratory flow rate (PEFR) was <40% of predicted. In a prospective evaluation of 31 children before 34 procedures, all patients did well under general anesthesia if their TCA and PEFR were >50% of predicted (10). Functionally important bronchial compression, which is more difficult to quantify by CT scan, may be uncovered by PEFR.

Echocardiography

Patients with cardiovascular symptoms, or those unable to give an adequate history, should also undergo trans-thoracic echocardiography to assess for cardiac, systemic or pulmonary vascular compression. Echocardiography reliably identifies pericardial thickening, effusion, and masses adjacent to the pericardium and can help evaluate myocardial dysfunction due to tumor compression or infiltration.

Anesthetic Considerations

The anesthetic considerations for patients with AMM vary according to the individual anatomy, pathology, the proposed surgical procedure, and most importantly, the perceived risk (extent of mass effect). Assessment of risk (see above) is principally determined by symptoms and radiographic data. Experience level by the anesthesia team may also influence decisions, and it is appropriate that less experienced teams adopt a more conservative approach, given the imprecision of risk assessment.

Acute Management

When a patient presents with acute symptoms, it is important to maintain the sitting posture (or most comfortable position) and provide humidified oxygen. Heliox may help reduce the work of breathing, but the lower FiO_2 of heliox may not be tolerated. Steroids have been used successfully to decrease tumor size without affecting the accuracy of histologic diagnosis postadministration. The use of steroids, radiation, or chemotherapy in advance of diagnosis is controversial and must be weighed against the individual risk of obtaining tissue for diagnosis without empiric treatment.

Heliox

Heliox is provided in tanks with oxygen–helium ratios of approximately 21%:79%, depending on suppliers. The FiO_2 can be adjusted by blending with oxygen from other sources (Fig 20-3). The lower density of helium permits more laminar gas flow across a stenosis (Fig 20-4), and decreased resistance to flow (decreased work of breathing).

Diagnostic Procedures Under Local Anesthesia

When risk profile is high, and only biopsy is required, the least invasive route to diagnosis should be sought (see Sect. "Surgical Considerations," above). Often in adults, a large AMM is readily

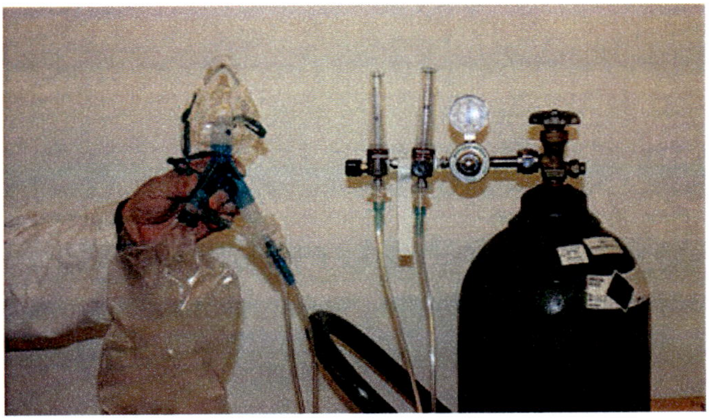

Figure 20-3 – Heliox H cylinder is shown connected to a facemask with a "Y" connector which allows coadministration of nebulized medications. With both lines connected to heliox, the FiO_2 is fixed by the tank concentration (usually 0.21). Connecting one line to wall oxygen allows titration to a higher FiO_2, but sacrifices the flow advantages of heliox correspondingly.

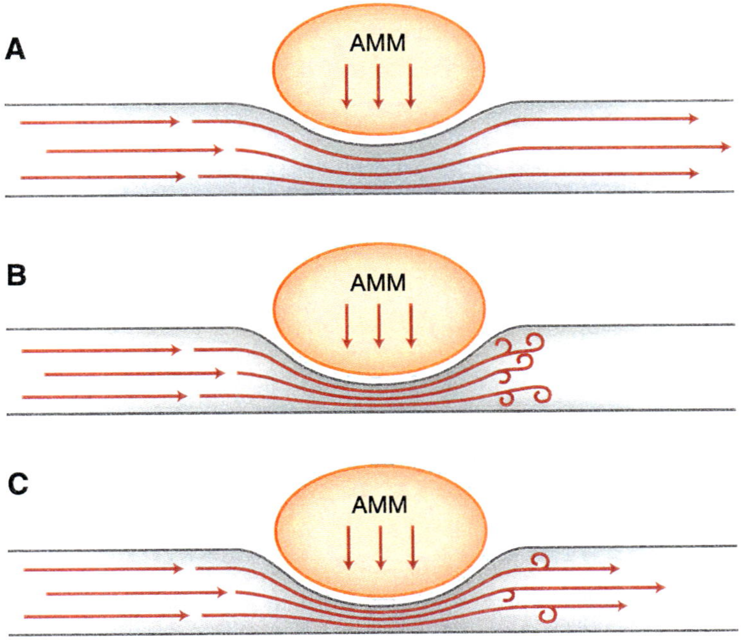

Figure 20-4– Laminar gas flow through a stenotic region (**A**) becomes turbulent at a critical velocity or cross-sectional area (**B**). Reduction of velocity or density restores more laminar flow at the same degree of stenosis (**C**).

accessed by anterior mediastinoscopy under local anesthesia in the semi-sitting position.

Avoiding GA is not a guarantee of safety. Anxiety and pain may increase ventilatory demand and worsen airflow dynamics by inducing turbulent flow across the obstruction. A variety of techniques have been used to mitigate this. Ketamine has been shown to preserve chest wall tone and FRC. Anxiolytics and narcotics have obvious potential hazards and must be titrated with caution. Heliox may reduce anxiety by reducing work of breathing. Backup equipment (for distal intubation, rigid bronchoscopy, etc.) must be available.

Strategies for General Anesthesia in the Patient with an AMM and Airway Compression

When general anesthesia is required, anesthetic strategy hinges on the perceived risk and is summarized in Fig 20-5. It is acknowledged that the perceived risk exists along a spectrum, and that it is an imprecise estimate. For the purposes of a simplified algorithm, the spectrum of risk may be divided into three subsets: 1) High, 2) Intermediate, and 3) Low Risk (Table 20-2 and Fig 20-5).

Low Perceived Risk

At the extreme low-risk end of the spectrum, a routine intravenous induction and intubation can be performed in patients with no symptomatic, radiologic, or bronchoscopic evidence of airway obstruction.

High Risk of Airway Obstruction

Symptomatic patients who are intolerant of the supine position and have large AMM compression of the distal trachea/carina are at high risk. If GA cannot be avoided, induction should be preceded by awake, fiberoptic bronchoscopy (thorough airway topicalization vital) in the sitting position with a tube sheathed over the bronchoscope. If bronchoscopy is nonreassuring, the tube should be advanced to stent open the airway prior to induction. With carinal masses, endobronchial intubation may be necessary. (To intubate the left main bronchus over a bronchoscope, rotate the ETT 180° to orient the bevel toward the left). Reinforced tubes are frequently

Table 20-2 – Risk stratification for Airway obstruction from AMM

RISK	PREOPERATIVE EVALUATION
Low	Asymptomatic supine TCA >> 50% predicted AMM is small, eccentric, or proximal PEFR >> 50% predicted
Intermediate (mixed picture)	Asymptomatic, but large, distal AMM with TCA < 50% Large, eccentric AMM severely obstructing one bronchus >> other Borderline CT scan (TCA approx 50%) but decreased PEFR and equivocal symptoms.
High	Symptomatic (especially orthopnea) Intolerant of supine position TCA < 50% predicted PEFR < 50% predicted Large, mid-sagittal mass compressing distal trachea and/or carina

recommended, but rarely necessary. Double-lumen tubes (DLT) serve as excellent stents and allow ventilation of both lungs even with carinal compression, but require pediatric bronchoscopes and are more stimulating to place in awake patients.

Should the airway become completely obstructed, and the ETT cannot be advanced as a stent, other backup plans should be employed (Table 20-3).

At the extreme high risk end of the spectrum, surgery may be performed under local anesthesia and/or cardiopulmonary bypass (CPB) or extracorporeal membrane oxygenation (ECMO) may be required to maintain circulation or oxygenation. The institution of

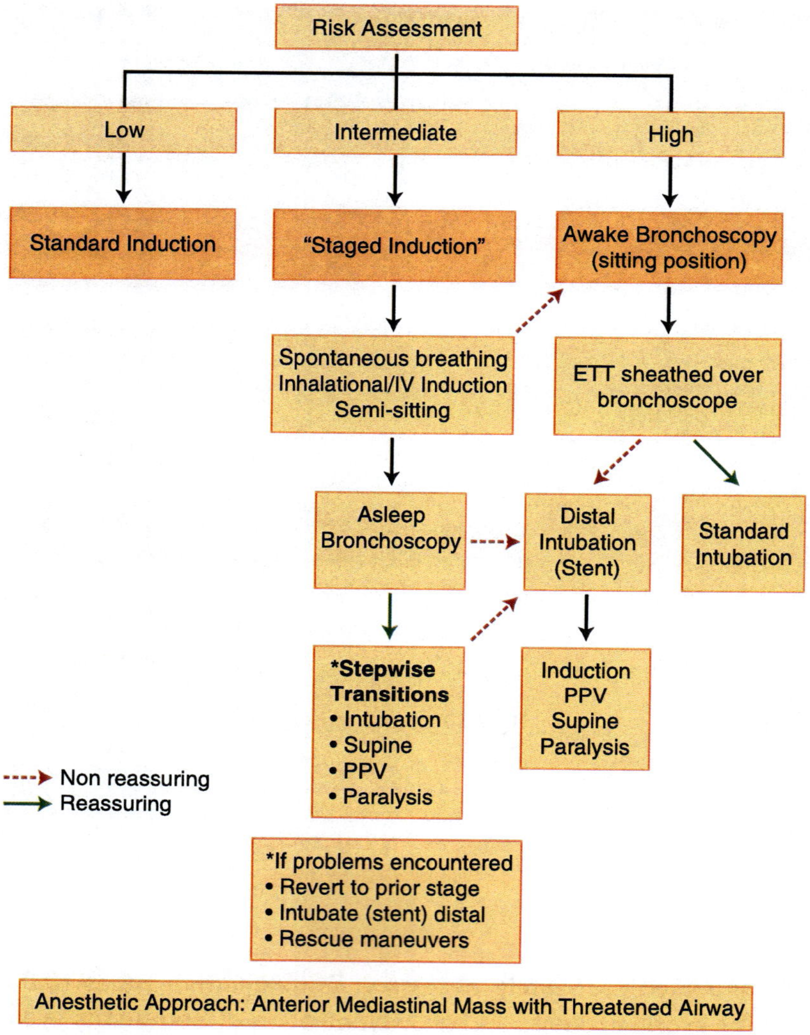

Figure 20-5 – Algorithm for the anesthetic approach to the patient with an AMM and threatened airway. See text for explanation. *Dashed red lines* indicate response to a nonreassuring finding (such as difficulty ventilating, or worrisome finding on bronchoscopy). *Green solid lines* indicate response to reassuring findings. Staged induction implies the stepwise progression through each potentially exacerbating transition. Imprecision in risk assessment is acknowledged. Therefore, rescue maneuvers (Table 20-3) should be readily available.

Table 20-3 – Rescue options for Airway obstruction from an AMM

Advance ETT to stent airway open. (Endobronchial intubation for carinal masses)
Revert to prior anesthetic stage (Resume spontaneous ventilation, upright position, lighten anesthesia, etc.)
Lateral position (If eccentric mass, turn patient "mass-side-down")
Rigid bronchoscopy
CPB or ECMO if preemptively cannulated

CPB by femoral cannulation prior to induction of anesthesia has been successful in adult patients, but its use is limited as a "standby" technique because of the necessary delay in its establishment.

Intermediate Risk

When the perceived risk of anesthesia is intermediate, (Table 20-2), the authors recommend a "staged approach" to general anesthesia (Fig 20-5).

The principle behind a staged approach is to engage each transition (asleep → awake, spont vent → PPV, etc.) in a controlled, stepwise fashion, preserving the option of rapidly reversing any step that triggers problems. Thus, a staged induction might proceed as follows:

- Spontaneously breathing inhalation or IV induction in semi-sitting position
    - Asleep fiberoptic bronchoscopy via ETT or LMA
    - Intubation
- Gradual transition to supine position
- Trial of PPV (manual bag ventilation)
- Trial of short-acting paralytics (succinylcholine)

Generally, the bronchoscopic view of the threatened region of the trachea is either alarming or reassuring (most often the latter). If nonreassuring (Fig 20-6), or if difficulties arise in ventilation, the

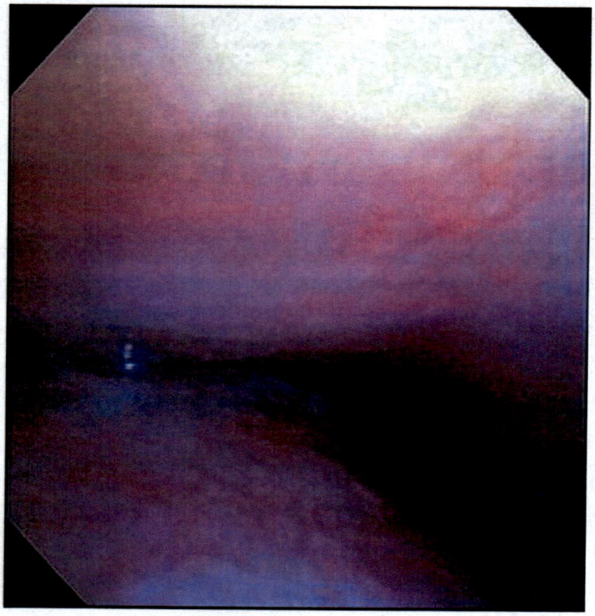

Figure 20-6 – Bronchoscopic view of carina, extrinsically compressed by AMM.

patient should be returned to the prior stage, and if needed, rescue options should be employed (Table 20-3). Tolerance of the staged induction is reevaluated at each transition.

Since the line between intermediate and high risk is indistinct, and since the benefits of spontaneous ventilation are questionable (at least in the adult), when in doubt, it is prudent to have a low threshold to manage patients as described for high risk (i.e., start with an awake bronchoscopy).

Emergence/Extubation

Emergence is another critical point, particularly when the AMM has only been biopsied, and still exerts a mass effect. Rapid ventilatory rates during emergence may cause turbulence and obstruction. Sufficient narcotic analgesia to control respiratory rate, and optimal positioning help prevent this. The backup rescue plans must remain at the ready. Even when the AMM is removed, airway obstruction may occur following emergence if tracheomalacia has occurred. Care should be taken to differentiate central airway obstruction (wheezing) from extrathoracic, upper airway obstruction (stridor). In the postoperative period, corticosteroids, racemic epinephrine, or Heliox may be useful.

Strategies for General Anesthesia for the Patient with AMM and Cardiovascular Compression

If the principal threat is to *venous return* or *cardiac output* (compression of heart, RVOT, PA, SVC), induction should be performed with augmentation of preload (fluids and mixed alpha-beta adrenergic agonists), and positioning to minimize compression of heart/vessels. Generous IV access and invasive arterial blood pressure monitoring are indicated. Lower extremity IV access is imperative if SVC compression is a risk. If a large pericardial effusion is present and accessible, percutaneous drainage should be performed prior to induction. Spontaneous ventilation augments venous return and should be preserved in high risk patients. Sevoflurane induction is most commonly used, with or without IV supplements. Vasodilating agents are to be avoided. Ketamine and etomidate are preferred.

Risk assessment for cardiovascular complications is less well defined. The multiple mechanisms by which an AMM may cause cardiovascular collapse with anesthesia preclude a neat algorithm. Coexisting pericardial effusion clearly increases risk, as does tamponade physiology (pulsus paradoxicus). Cardiovascular compression may coexist with airway compression with a large AMM.

Should cardiovascular collapse occur, repositioning lateral may help to off-load the heart/vessels. Standard pharmacologic resuscitation should be instituted. Returning to spontaneous ventilation may help (if possible). In extremis, emergent sternotomy will reduce compression. As mentioned, preemptive awake, femoral cannulation for CPB is a very conservative approach, but reliance on emergent cannulation as a rescue maneuver is not recommended.

SVC Syndrome

SVC obstruction may result in severe hypotension when the impairment in venous return is coupled with pharmacologic vasodilation

Table 20-4 – Perioperative concerns with SVC syndrome

Airway	Edema
	Airway congestion and hemorrhage
Venous access	Lower extremity
	Potential for massive hemorrhage

from induction drugs. Nonetheless, there is no data to support any particular induction and intubation technique. Airway edema may make intubation difficult. Anesthetic concerns for SVC syndrome are summarized in Table 20-4.

Coughing, straining, supine or Trendelenberg positioning all exacerbate SVC syndrome. The use of an antisialagogue, bronchodilators, racemic epinephrine and maintenance of the sitting position appear to be helpful. As mentioned, lower extremity IV access is imperative.

Selected References

1. Lumb AB, editor. Nunn's applied respiratory physiology. 6th ed. Italy: Elsevier, Ltd.; 2005. p. 302.

2. Neuman GG, Weingarten AE, Abramowitz RM, Kushins LG, Abramson AL, Ladner W. The anesthetic management of the patient with an anterior mediastinal mass. Anesthesiology. 1984;60:144–7.

3. Bittar D. Respiratory obstruction associated with induction of general anesthesia in a patient with mediastinal Hodgkin's disease. Anesth Analg. 1975;54: 399–403.

4. Sibert KS, Biondi J, Hirsch N. Spontaneous respiration during thoracotomy in a patient with a mediastinal mass. Anesth Analg. 1987;66:904–7.

5. Perger L, Lee E, Shamberger R. Management of children and adolescents with a critical airway due to compression by an anterior mediastinal mass. J Pediatr Surg. 2008;43:1990–7.

6. Piro AJ, Weiss DR, Hellman S. Mediastinal Hodgkin's disease: a possible danger for intubation anesthesia. Int J Radiat Oncol Biol Phys. 1976;1:415–9.

7. Bray RJ, Fernandes FJ. Mediastinal tumour causing airway obstruction in anaesthetized children. Anaesthesia. 1982;37:571–5.

8. Shamberger RC, Holzman RS, Griscom NT, et al. CT quantification of tracheal cross-sectional area as a guide to the surgical and anesthetic management of children with anterior mediastinal masses. J Pediatr Surg. 1991;26:138–42.

9. Bechard P, Letourneau L, Lacasse Y, Cote D, Bussieres JS. Perioperative cardiorespiratory complications in adults with mediastinal mas. Anesthesiology. 2004;100:826–34.

10. Shamberger RC, Holzman RS, Griscom NT, Tarbell NJ, Weinstein HJ, Wohl ME. Prospective evaluation by computed tomography and pulmonary function tests of children with mediastinal masses. Surgery. 1995;118:468–71.

11. Azizkhan RH, Dudgeon DL, Buck JR, et al. Life threatening airway obstruction as a complication of the management of mediastinal masses in children. J Pediatr Surg. 1985;20:816–22.

12. Azarow KS, Pearl RH, Zurcher R, et al. Primary mediastinal masses: a comparison of adult and pediatric populations. J Thorac Cardiovasc Surg. 1993;106:67–72.

13. Torchio R, Gulotta C, Perbondi A, et al. Orthopnea and tidal expiratory flow limitation in patients with euthyroid goiter. Chest. 2003;124:133–40.

Chapter 21
Lung-Sparing Pulmonary Resections: Bronchoplastic/Sleeve Resection

Philip M. Hartigan

Keywords Bronchoplastic resection • Sleeve resection • Sleeve lobectomy • Lung isolation • One-lung ventilation • Anastomosis phase

Introduction

Lesions involving or encroaching upon main bronchi preclude clean resection by traditional lobectomy. Options for complete resection then include proximal mainstem transection (pneumonectomy or bilobectomy), or a bronchoplastic resection vs. sleeve resection with preservation of distal parenchyma. There is confusion and inconsistency in the terminology of such parenchymal-sparing techniques.

Bronchoplastic Resection is a general term encompassing a variety of techniques in which a portion of the bronchial wall is excised, followed by closure of the defect (Fig 21-1).

Sleeve Resection implies removal of a portion of large airways, by proximal and distal division (transection of a segment of airway), followed by anastomosis (Fig 21-2). Strictly speaking, simple sleeve resection does not involve removal of lung parenchyma, but in common vernacular, it is often used interchangeably with sleeve lobectomy.

Sleeve Lobectomy implies resection of a lobe together with a "sleeve" of its mainstem bronchus, with anastomosis of the remaining mainstem bronchus (Fig 21-3).

P.M. Hartigan (ed.), *Practical Handbook of Thoracic Anesthesia*,
DOI 10.1007/978-0-387-88493-6_21,

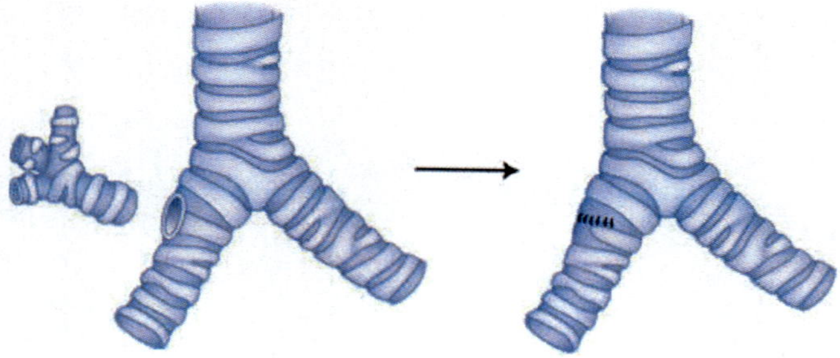

Figure 21-1 – Right upper lobectomy with "wedge bronchoplasty."

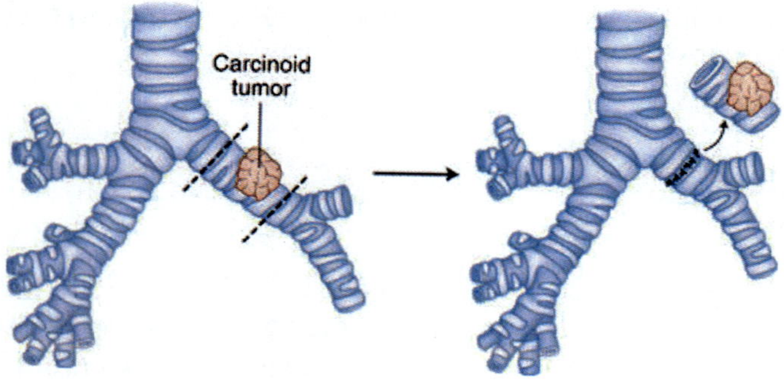

Figure 21-2 – Left mainstem simple sleeve resection for carcinoid.

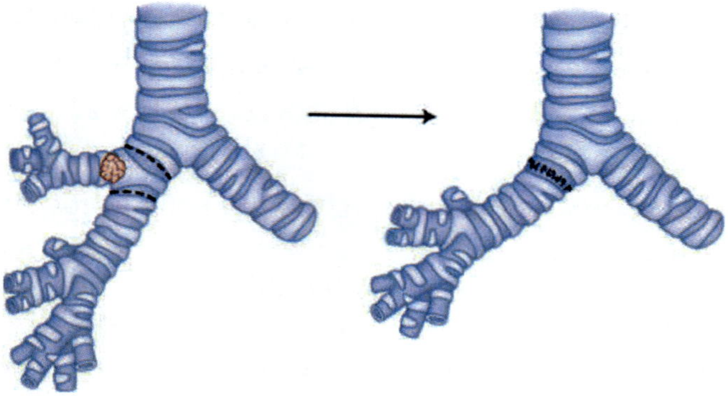

Figure 21-3 – Right upper lobe sleeve lobectomy.

The most common parenchymal-sparing pulmonary resection is "right upper lobe sleeve lobectomy" (because of its favorable anatomy). Such a sleeve lobectomy provides conservation of remaining lobes in situations where simple staple division of the lobar bronchus at its mainstem origin (traditional lobectomy) would have resulted in positive margins. The technical challenges of a hand-sewn anastomosis and its risk of failure must be weighed against the benefits of preserved pulmonary function.

Surgical Considerations

The patient undergoing sleeve resection provides both intraoperative and perioperative challenges. The technical challenges in the operating room center on obtaining negative margins and reconstructing the airway. In many cases, the potential anastomotic sites can be biopsied prior to definitive surgery – thereby providing detailed histologic evaluation of the margins. In other patients, the margins may require time-consuming frozen section evaluation during the operation. During these periods, the airway should be carefully monitored by both the surgical and anesthesia teams to prevent blood contamination of the dependent lung as well as airborne bacterial contamination of the pleural space.

Once the tumor is resected, the reconstruction of the airway must compensate for varying degrees of airway size "mismatch." The size of the airway, the interrupted bronchial circulation, and the potential for tumor recurrence are all factors that must be considered during the construction of an airtight anastomosis.

The postoperative course after sleeve resection is notable for the marked decrease in compliance of the reconstructed lung parenchyma. Presumably, a result of impaired lymphatic clearance, the remaining lung is prone to increasing interstitial edema and volume loss over the first 3–4 days after surgery. Because sleeve resections are commonly performed in patients with emphysema, the compliance difference between the remaining lung parenchyma and the contralateral hypercompliant lung can present management problems. The judicious use of intravenous fluids both intraoperatively and postoperatively can help maintain relatively normal lung compliance, lung volumes, work of breathing, and airway clearance. Major airway dehiscence is a rare complication; the major morbidity associated with sleeve resections involves volume loss, poor mucociliary clearance and pneumonia in the reconstructed lung.

Anesthetic Considerations

While the conduct of an anesthetic for bronchoplastic resections is minimally different from those of lobectomy previously described in Chapter 16, several points deserve emphasis.

Preoperative Planning

The technical challenges of a hand-sewn anastomosis/bronchoplasty generally require at least a muscle-sparing limited thoracotomy. Thus, a thoracic epidural is generally indicated to facilitate immediate extubation. Anticipated blood loss and access/monitoring requirements are no different from a lobectomy.

Lung Isolation

A DLT inserted into the contralateral, nonoperative bronchus is frequently the best choice for lung isolation. This provides the surgeon the greatest latitude to manipulate and operate on the mainstem bronchus. It also largely obviates the issue of a suture catching or deflating the bronchial balloon. While distal left mainstem bronchoplastic/sleeve resections can be performed with a left-sided DLT, the stiffness imposed by the presence of the bronchial lumen is disadvantageous.

In the case of a left-sided sleeve resection, if a right-sided DLT is not practical due to anomalous right-upper lobe anatomy, a proximally situated bronchial blocker in the left mainstem can be workable. However, the possibility that it might become displaced (tracheal occlusion) or allow air leakage into the operative field are high. Often, a right-sided DLT, even with an imperfect fit and incomplete RUL ventilation is workable, and preferable in this situation.

One-Lung Ventilation

Often, patients for parenchymal-sparing resection are selected because they have compromised cardiopulmonary reserve which precludes the technically simpler pneumonectomy or bilobectomy. If desaturation occurs during OLV, CPAP to the operative lung is not an option during the phase that the bronchus is open to atmosphere. Assuming other options have been exhausted (100% oxygen, optimal dependent-lung PEEP, bronchoscopic confirmation of tube position and clearance of secretions, dependent-lung recruitment), there are limited means to improve oxygenation. The yield from the minor variables discussed in Chapter 5 is limited or negligible (inhaled nitric oxide, TIVA, manipulation of cardiac output, etc.).

As a temporary maneuver to allow completion of the anastomosis/bronchoplasty, the introduction of oxygen into the operative lung distal to the surgical resection can be accomplished by several techniques, including the following (analogous to techniques described in tracheal resection/reconstruction surgery – see Chapter 30):

- Jet ventilation/air insufflation through a small bore catheter temporarily inserted "over-the-field."
- Jet ventilation/air insufflation through a catheter inserted via the airway with tip distal to surgical site.
- Temporary intubation of the distal airway with a small, cuffed, reinforced ETT "over the field" for delivery of CPAP or partial ventilation.
- Temporary partial occlusion (or compression) of the operative-side pulmonary artery by the surgeon.

Extracorporeal oxygenation (ECMO, cardiopulmonary bypass) is also an option, but is rarely employed due to the associated complications.

Anastomosis Phase

Technical issues with the anastomosis/bronchoplasty leading to airleak, breakdown, stenosis, kinking, torsion, failure to heal, etc. are among the most dire complications. Optimal surgical conditions for this phase of surgery are outcome-relevant. A motionless field is obviously important. Air leaks past the bronchial balloon blowing into the field can be avoided by adding air to the bronchial cuff, lowering airway pressures or PEEP, or by timing hand ventilations to the surgical events.

Passing a videobronchoscope during this phase can guide or provide an inside view for surgeons as the bronchus is closed to rule out stenosis, kinking, torsion, or other technical problems with the anastomosis, or with other lobes. The appearance can be misleading when deflated, and airways generally appear more patent when ventilated.

Lung Recruitment and Leak Test

Providing 20–35 cmH_2O positive pressure hold maneuvers for 3–5 s intervals will recruit the operative lung and rule out anastomotic air leaks by the absence of bubbles in the saline-submerged surgical field. The importance of minimizing positive pressure stress to the anastomosis may be more important for these hand-sewn closures. Therefore, the lowest effective recruitment pressures should be employed, and the field should be observed during recruitment. Once recruited, positive pressure ventilation to the operative lung should be limited to the lowest practical degree.

Nonetheless, full terminal recruitment is important for several reasons. Residual air space collects fluid with risk of pleural infection. Atelectasis impairs gas exchange and also may promote infection. Torsion or rotation may not be apparent until the lung is reinflated, and must be recognized prior to closure. Bronchoscopy should be performed by the anesthesiologist to clear secretions, and examine the anastomosis prior to terminal reinflation.

Emergence Strategies

Immediate postoperative extubation is desirable. Toward that end, aggressive narcotic-sparing pain control (thoracic epidural), and appropriate timing of agents and dosages is important. There is generally a desire by surgeons to repeat the bronchoscopy through a single-lumen endotracheal tube for formal evaluation of the anastomosis/bronchoplasty with full lung inflation. If the tube exchange requires a tube exchange catheter, the potential to damage the surgical repair with the catheter is a danger to be cognizant of.

Further Suggested Reading

Murthy S. Sleeve resection/bronchoplasty for lung cancer. Chapter 66. In: Sugarbaker DJ et al., editors. Adult chest surgery. New York: McGraw-Hill Medical; 2009. p. 567–74.

Ng JM. Hypoxemia during one-lung ventilation: jet ventilation of the middle and lower lobes during right upper lobe sleeve resection. Anesth Analg. 2005;101(5): 1554–5.

Newton JR, Grillo HC, Mathison DJ. Main bronchial sleeve resection with pulmonary conservation. Ann Thorac Surg. 1991;52(6):1272–80.

Hess DR, Gillette MA. Tracheal gas insufflation and related techniques to introduce gas flow to the trachea. Respir Care. 2001;46(2):119–29.

Murakami S, Watanabe Y, Kobayashi H. High frequency jet ventilation in tracheobronchoplasty. An experimental study. Scand J Thorac Cardiovasc Surg. 1994; 28(1):31–6.

Chapter 22
Pneumonectomy

Ju-Mei Ng

Keywords Pneumonectomy • Considerations for pneumonectomy • Posterolateral incision • Mediastinal shift • Cardiac herniation • Transesophageal echocardiography • Pulmonary artery catheters • Lung-protective ventilation • Hilar dissection

Introduction

Standard pneumonectomy involves the removal of an entire lung and its visceral pleura, stapling the bronchus close to the carina, and the pulmonary artery (PA) and pulmonary veins close to their entry into the pericardium. Variations on this theme are shown in Table 22-1.

Anesthetic considerations for pulmonary resection in general have been discussed in Chapter 16. This chapter highlights essential considerations for pneumonectomy with emphasis on aspects particular to pneumonectomy as opposed to pulmonary resection in general.

P.M. Hartigan (ed.), *Practical Handbook of Thoracic Anesthesia*,
DOI 10.1007/978-0-387-88493-6_22,

Table 22-1 – Types of pneumonectomy

Completion	Removal of the entire remaining lung after some other portion of that lung has been removed at a previous operation
Extrapleural	Removal of the entire lung along with the ipsilateral pleura, hemidiaphragm, and hemipericardium
Intrapericardial	Removal of the entire lung with ligation of pulmonary vessels within the pericardium
Carinal	Removal of an entire lung and the carina; this requires an anastomosis with the remaining mainstem bronchus and the distal trachea

Surgical Considerations

Indications for pneumonectomy are summarized in Table 22-2.

Exclusions

Assessment of cardiorespiratory reserve remains an inexact science (see Chapter 14). Widely employed exclusion criteria for pneumonectomy include predicted postoperative forced expiratory volume in 1 s ($ppoFEV_1$) <0.8 L, diffusing capacity for carbon monoxide (DLCO) <40% predicted, or maximal oxygen consumption (VO_2 max) <15 mL/kg/min. Functional capacity may be the best reflection of cardiopulmonary reserve sufficient to tolerate a pneumonectomy. The ability to climb two flights of stairs or walk 2,000 ft in 6 min without a 4% or greater fall in SpO_2 roughly correlates to an adequate VO_2 max and functional reserve. Considerable emphasis is particularly placed on $ppoFEV_1$. Patients with FEV_1 <2 L should undergo quantitative ventilation/perfusion (V/Q) scintigraphy to more accurately assess $ppoFEV_1$. Often, this reveals pathology-related reductions in perfusion to the operative lung, which can be used to proportionally correct the $ppoFEV_1$. Advanced age and comorbidities must also be taken into account, though improvements in

Table 22-2 – Indications for pneumonectomy

Malignancy (most common)	Bronchogenic carcinoma centrally located, adherent to hilar structures or large parenchymal tumors that violate the fissures or invade the interlobar vessels
	Pulmonary metastases
Benign disease	Inflammatory lung disease, e.g., tuberculosis and fungal infections
	Trauma
	Congenital lung disease

operative and perioperative care appear to be expanding the envelope of operability even for pneumonectomy.

Surgical Technique (1, 2)

A standard *posterolateral incision* or limited variation (see Chapter 7) is typically utilized. The pleural space is entered, and chest and mediastinal structures evaluated to establish local-regional disease (≤ stage IIIa).

The sequence of *ligation of the hilar structures* is dependent on the position of the lesion and the surgeon's preference. Some advocate test occlusion of the PA for 1–2 min, and assessment of hemodynamic stability, for physiological tolerance of pneumonectomy. Hard evidence that this predicts right heart tolerance of pneumonectomy is currently absent. The *bronchus* is commonly *taken last*, most favoring stapler closure over hand sewn. Long stumps are prone to collect secretions and are more prone to failure than short (flush) bronchial stumps. It is thought that this is because the tenuous (watershed) perfusion of the bronchus is better preserved by short stumps than long. A *leak test* is then performed and the bronchial stump is often buttressed with a vascularized pedicle such as pericardial fat pad or intercostal muscle flap.

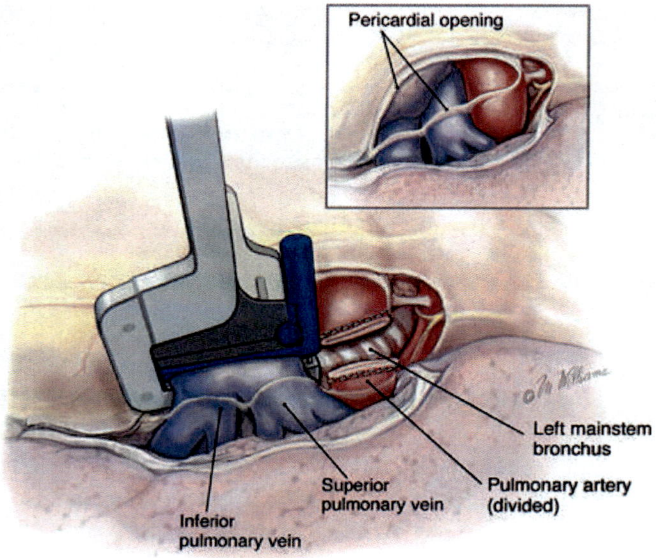

Figure 22-1 – View of the hilum during left pneumonectomy. The surgeon's access to hilar structures is more limited than for right pneumonectomy. Intrapericardial access (*inset*) is even more challenging. From Adult Chest Surgery. Sugarbaker DJ, et al., New York, McGraw-Hill, with permission. Copyright, Marcia Williams, 2009.

Left pneumonectomy has a lower mortality than right because less parenchyma is removed. However, left pneumonectomy is technically more challenging due to the confined anatomy and the location of the bronchus relative to the proximal pulmonary artery (Fig 22-1). Vocal cord paralysis from recurrent laryngeal nerve injury is more frequent with left pneumonectomy, and results in a weak cough and increased risk of aspiration. Intrapericardial left pneumonectomy can leave the right ventricular outflow tract narrow or less elastic. RV outflow tract obstruction may not be evident under anesthesia, but may become apparent with exercise.

Mediastinal Shift

Because of the weight of the mediastinum in the lateral decubitus position, and the relatively low (protective) lung volumes, the mediastinum is displaced toward the contralateral lung during pneumonectomy. To medialize the mediastinum after chest closure, air can be removed using a small catheter (usually 1–1.2 L) followed by withdrawal of the catheter. Alternatively, an indwelling catheter can be left in the chest (*no suction*) to allow passive medialization of the mediastinum when the patient has returned to the neutral position. Such a drainage catheter may also be useful to assess bleeding, but precautions should be exercised to prevent inadvertent application of suction. Even a "watersealed" chest drainage system can result in progressive mediastinal displacement in an awake patient as forced exhalation (e.g., cough) will expel air that cannot be reequilibrated.

Cardiac Herniation

When a pericardial defect is present after right pneumonectomy (intrapericardial or extrapleural pneumonectomy with inadequate pericardial reconstruction), the heart may herniate into the right hemithorax with torsion of the great vessels and abrupt cardiovascular collapse. The appropriate reflex response is to abruptly turn the patient left lateral decubitus to reduce the cardiac herniation. Closed chest cardiac massage is of no value when the heart lies in the empty right hemithorax, and venous return is cut off by torsion of the vena cavae. If turning the patient on his left side fails to restore stability, the thoracotomy should be re-opened with expediency.

Anesthetic Considerations

Anesthetic priorities for pneumonectomy include aggressive pain control, invasive monitors, lung isolation, and prompt emergence and postoperative extubation. Most centers employ *thoracic epidurals or paravertebral catheters* placed preoperatively, as the magnitude of the surgery usually requires a thoracotomy incision.

Although blood loss is generally low, the potential for major bleeding exists, especially for completion pneumonectomy (s/p chemo/radiation) and extrapleural pneumonectomy (Chapter 23). *Generous intravenous access* and *invasive monitors* (usually arterial line and central venous catheters) are thus widely employed, even in the absence of comorbidity.

In other respects, the conduct of anesthesia preparation and induction is similar to that for lesser resections (Chapter 16).

Lines and Monitors

Arterial catheters are almost universally employed for pneumonectomy surgery due to the magnitude of the surgical trespass and potential need for blood gas analysis intra- and postoperatively.

Central venous pressure monitoring is controversial. The relationship between intravascular volume and CVP is poor during OLV with an open chest. Nonetheless, the premium on tight fluid management argues for a potential advantage of CVP trends in the postoperative period. In theory, an abrupt rise in CVP with test clamping of the PA might signal right heart intolerance of the additional afterload. Absence of a spike in CVP, however, provides no assurance against impending right heart failure.

Pulmonary artery catheters are rarely used for pneumonectomies due to potential complications and interpretation pitfalls. If the PA catheter floats to the operative lung, its accuracy will be impaired by disrupted flow to the thermister and surgical manipulations of the collapsed lung. Even when it floats to the nonoperative lung, PA occlusion pressures after the operative PA is clamped may be spuriously low (3). Embolic or hemorrhagic events related to the PA catheter, particularly in the nonoperative lung, can be devastating.

PA catheters are most useful for following PA pressures in patients with reactive pulmonary hypertension. The relationship between PA pressures or "wedge" pressures to ventricular function or volume is likely tenuous in the setting of OLV, lateral decubitus position, open hemithorax, surgical pressure on the mediastinum, and PEEP (intrinsic and extrinsic). If a PA catheter is used, great care must be taken to exclude its presence from the operative PA during crossclamp. This is probably best assured by withdrawal of the PA catheter to the right ventricle prior to crossclamping the PA.

Transesophageal echocardiography (TEE) is a powerful and reliable monitor of ventricular volume and function, even in the lateral, one-lung situation. Reasonable images to assess right ventricular response to PA crossclamp can generally be obtained, however, the predictive value of this has not been validated. As a monitor for myocardial ischemia, TEE can be valuable, particularly during left pneumonectomy where the surgery precludes diagnostic EKG lead placement.

Lung Isolation and OLV

Lung isolation is best accomplished by intubating the nonoperative bronchus with an appropriately sized double-lumen endobronchial tube (DLT) (see Chapter 9). Bronchial blockers may be useful in patients with difficult airway anatomy. However they are more likely to become dislodged with surgical manipulation when used for right pneumonectomy due to the short right main bronchus.

For left pneumonectomies where a right-sided DLT is impractical (either because of anomalous anatomy or practitioner inexperience), a left-sided DLT may be employed. However, it must be withdrawn above the carina prior to bronchial crossclamp, and great care must be taken to prevent its inadvertent advancement to disrupt the stump thereafter. A bronchial blocker in the left mainstem is another option for such situations. Just prior to bronchial crossclamp, with the ventilator off and open to atmosphere, the balloon is collapsed and the bronchial blocker is withdrawn without inflating the operative lung. This brief window in lung isolation is an opportunity for blood or secretions to cross contaminate.

Equipment in the operative bronchus can easily become caught in the stable line or interfere with surgery. Ipsilateral bronchial blockers, double-lumen tubes, temperature probes, nasogastric tubes, etc. must be definitively excluded. Direct observation by videobronchoscopy prior to crossclamp is the most reliable for this.

Lung-protective ventilation (tidal volumes 5–6 mL/kg) should be employed with dependent lung PEEP in patients without intrinsic PEEP, limiting plateau, and peak pressures to less than 25 cm H_2O and less than 35 cm H_2O, respectively (4). Profound atelectasis is less important for pneumonectomy than video-assisted surgery due to the maneuvering room afforded by the thoracotomy incision.

Judicious continuous positive airway pressure (CPAP) can generally be employed without overinflating and interfering with surgical exposure.

Hypoxemia during OLV (prior to division of the PA) does not necessarily predict failure to tolerate pneumonectomy. Shunt to the nondependent lung will be eliminated when the PA is divided, predictably improving oxygenation, so long as cardiac reserve is adequate.

Hilar Dissection and Division of the PA

Division of the pulmonary vessels may occasionally result in moderate blood loss when staple guns misfire. Division of the PA should result in improved oxygenation (eliminates nondependent lung shunt), and rarely causes noticeable perturbations of the CVP. However, this depends on the amount of blood flow to the operative lung, the reserve of the right heart, and the capacity of recruitable pulmonary vessels in the nonoperative lung. If a PA line is employed, it must be excluded from entrapment in the PA stump by palpation (by the surgeon), withdrawal, or observation of the tracing during test clamp of the PA.

Division of the Bronchus

Technical issues with this predict stump-related complications. If video bronchoscopy is available, there may be benefit to visualizing the stump prior to firing staples. This reliably serves to confirm that the stump length is short (Fig 22-2), and that there is no equipment in the staple line. Observing unchanged compliance in the nonoperative lung excludes inadvertent inclusion or impingement of that bronchus by the staple gun.

Following removal of the specimen, a *leak test* is commonly employed with incremental increases in positive pressure (≤35 cm H_2O) ventilation to the submerged stump, while the surgeon looks for bubbles.

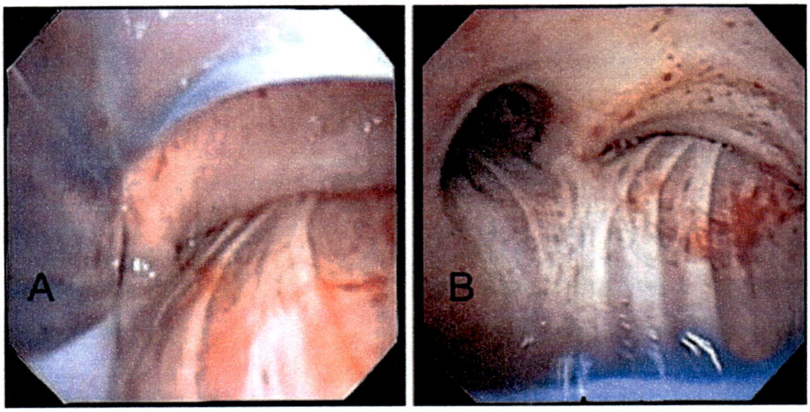

Figure 22-2 – Bronchoscopic view of right pneumonectomy stump via double-lumen tube at the time of crossclamp (**A**), and with an adult bronchoscope at the end of the case (**B**). Note the desirable short (shallow) nature of the stump for reference.

Fluid Management and Acute Lung Injury Following Pulmonary Resection

Fluid management aims to maintain hemodynamic stability and end organ perfusion (urine output) as well as sufficient intravascular reserve to tolerate thoracic epidural analgesia (TEA) postoperatively.

The incidence of postlung resection acute lung injury (ALI) following pneumonectomy is dramatically higher than for lesser resections (5) (Chapter 6). Although not causally related to postpneumonectomy pulmonary edema, excessive crystalloid administration potentially complicates management of ALI, should that occur. Because pneumonectomy blood loss is generally under 500 mL, fluid requirements for hemodynamic stability are not high, and excessive fluid is to be avoided. Studies indicate that positive fluid administration under 20 mL/kg in the first 24 h following pneumonectomy had no relationship to the development of postpneumonectomy pulmonary edema (6). Clearly fluid itself is a nonprimary cause. Improved or adapted alveolar water clearance following pneumonectomy appears to require roughly 6 weeks. During that time period (at least), an increased circulating blood volume results in increased lung water. Gas exchange, pulmonary compliance, work of breathing, and tolerance of challenges such as arrhythmias, aspiration, or pulmonary emboli will be accordingly compromised.

Thoracic Epidural Analgesia

TEA is widely employed intraoperatively to facilitate extubation at the conclusion of surgery by providing dense analgesia without depression of sensorium or respiratory drive. The risks and benefits of TEA and choice of epidural solutions are discussed in Chapter 37.

Closure, Repositioning, and Tube Exchange

Following closure, the patient is turned supine, the DLT is exchanged for a single-lumen ETT, and a fiberoptic bronchoscopic evaluation of the stump and clean-out of the remaining lung are performed. Care must be exercised to avoid disruption of the stump with deep intubation or tube exchange catheters. An LMA can also be used for the terminal bronchoscopy, and to examine the vocal cords for recurrent laryngeal nerve damage.

Embarrassment of venous return from mediastinal shift may cause hypotension at the terminus of the case which is relatively refractory to vasopressors. A shift of the trachea could suggest which direction, and whether to add or remove air from the chest drain (see section "Surgical Considerations" above). A portable chest radiograph is usually helpful in guiding medialization of the mediastinum. Abrupt cardiovascular collapse with repositioning (particularly, following right pneumonectomy) suggests cardiac herniation, requiring immediate reduction by returning the patient to the previous lateral position (see above).

Patients are routinely extubated and monitored in the ICU postoperatively. Table 22-3 provides a brief summary of acute postpneumonectomy complications.

Table 22-3 – Immediate/early complications of pneumonectomy

Mediastinal shift/ cardiac herniation	Change in patient position, coughing, extubation, or connection of the chest drain to negative pressure can cause a mediastinal shift or cardiac herniation (right pneumonectomy)
Supraventricular arrhythmias	Sinus tachycardia and atrial fibrillation and/or flutter are frequent after pneumonectomy
Postpneumonectomy pulmonary edema	Incidence ranges from 2 to 4% of pneumonectomy patients with a mortality in excess of 50%
	Right pneumonectomies at significantly higher risk than left
	Associated with low PAOP and high protein edema fluid suggesting endothelial damage (see Chapter 6)
Hemorrhage	
Vocal cord dysfunction	
Chylothorax	Usually seen in patients who have undergone extensive lymph node dissection
Bronchopleural fistula empyema	2–16% incidence after pneumonectomy with high mortality
Pulmonary embolism	Patients at high risk of deep venous thrombosis and thromboembolic events
	Thrombi can form in the PA stump and embolize to the contralateral lung

Selected References

1. Cerfolio R. Pneumonectomy. In: Kaiser LR, Kron IL, Spray TL, editors. Mastery of Cardiothoracic Surgery. 2nd ed. Philadelphia, Pa: Lippincott Williams & Wilkins; 2006. p. 53–63.

2. Roberts JR. Pneumonectomy. Chapter 64. In: Sugarbaker DJ et al., editors. Adult Chest Surgery. New York: McGraw-Hill; 2009. p. 552–60.

3. Wittnich C, Trudel J, Zidulka A, Chiu RC. Misleading "pulmonary wedge pressure" after pneumonectomy: its importance in post-operative fluid therapy. Ann Thorac Surg. 1986;42:192–6.

4. Slinger P. Pro: Low tidal volume is indicated during one-lung ventilation. Anesth Analg. 2006;103:268–70.

5. Waller DA, Gebitekin C, Saunders NR, Walker DR. Noncardiogenic pulmonary edema complicating lung resection. Ann Thorac Surg. 1993;55:140–3.

6. Turnage WS, Lunn JL. Post-pneumonectomy pulmonary edema. A retrospective analysis of associated variables. Chest. 1993;103:1646–50.

Chapter 23
Extrapleural Pneumonectomy

Ju-Mei Ng

Keywords Extrapleural pneumonectomy • Surgical technique EPP • Intraoperative intracavitary chemotherapy • EPP-specific anesthetic concerns

Introduction

Extrapleural pneumonectomy (EPP) differs from standard pneumonectomy in that the lung is removed en bloc, together with its associated visceral and parietal pleurae, ipsilateral hemidiaphragm and pericardium, as well as mediastinal lymph nodes. EPP is a radical and aggressive surgery, most commonly performed for treatment of malignant pleural mesothelioma (MPM).

Surgical Considerations

Perioperative morbidity and mortality for EPP is greater than for standard pneumonectomy due to greater blood loss, extent of incision and dissection, and disruption of mechanics (diaphragm removal) and autonomics (sympathetic chain), as well as the requirement for pericardotomy and intrapericardial division of vessels.

P.M. Hartigan (ed.), *Practical Handbook of Thoracic Anesthesia*,
DOI 10.1007/978-0-387-88493-6_23, © Springer Science+Business Media, LLC 2012

Patient Selection

The general exclusion criteria utilized by the surgical group with the most favorable published survival statistics (1) are listed in Table 23-1. To be considered resectable, the tumor must be limited to the ipsilateral hemithorax, with no significant invasion of the diaphragm, pericardium, or chest wall.

Surgical Technique (2)

1. Incision and exposure of the parietal pleura: An extended posterolateral thoracotomy with resection of the sixth rib is the most common approach.
2. Extrapleural dissection to separate the tumor from the chest wall.
3. En bloc resection of the lung, pleura, pericardium, and diaphragm with division of the hilar structures.

    A combination of blunt and sharp extrapleural dissection is initiated anterolaterally, and advanced to and over the apex, to bring the tumor down from the posterior and

Table 23-1 – Suggested exclusion criteria for EPP

Karnovsky performance status <70%
Abnormal creatinine
Abnormal liver function tests
Evidence of unresectability by CT, MRI, echocardiogram
Room air $PaCO_2 > 45$ mmHg
Room air $PaO_2 < 65$ mmHg
Left ventricular ejection fraction < 45%
Predicted postoperative $FEV_1 < 1$ L[a]

[a] Patients with predicted postoperative $FEV_1 < 2$ L are recommended to undergo quantitative radionuclide ventilation–perfusion scanning.

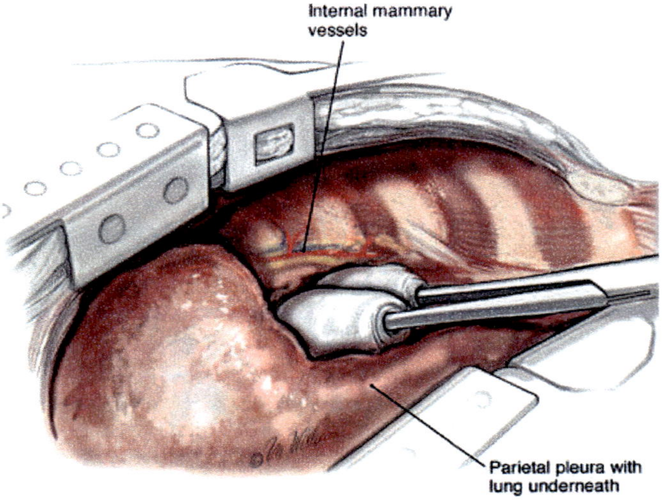

Figure 23-1 – Blunt anterior parietal dissection with identification of the internal mammary vessels. From Adult Chest Surgery, Sugarbaker DJ, et al., New York, McGraw-Hill, with permission. Copyright, Marcia Williams, 2009.

superior mediastinum (Fig 23-1). Beware of injury to the internal mammary vessels/grafts and subclavian vessels during dissection anteriorly and at the apex respectively, as well as traction injury to the azygous vein and superior vena cava in the superior mediastinum.

Posterior dissection is then performed and the esophagus dissected away from the tumor. The diaphragm is excised circumferentially (Fig 23-2) and the pericardium is opened. During division of the medial aspect of the diaphragm, the inferior vena cava may be injured or torsed. The main pulmonary artery (PA) and pulmonary veins are then dissected, isolated, and stapled intrapericardially. After the main bronchus is dissected as far as the carina, the bronchial stapler is fired under direct visualization with the fiberoptic videobronchoscope to assure a short bronchial stump.

Bleeding from numerous exposed vessels on the inner thoracic cavity is temporized by packing, but definitive hemostasis is not sought until the specimen is removed.

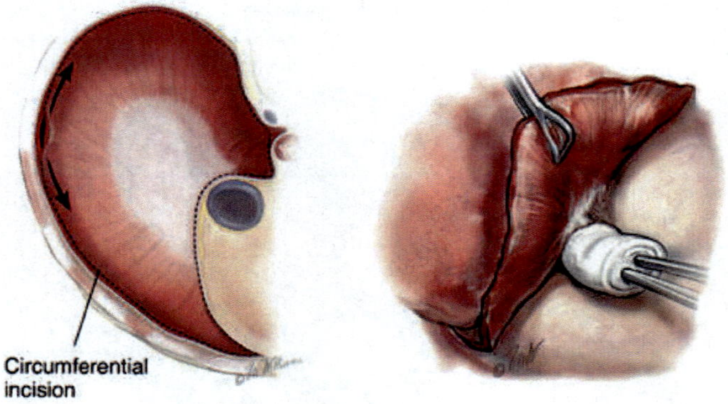

Figure 23-2 – The diaphragm is incised circumferentially (*left*) and dissected bluntly form the underlying peritoneum (*right*). From Adult Chest Surgery, Sugarbaker DJ, et al., New York, McGraw-Hill, with permission. Copyright, Marcia Williams, 2009.

4. Radical lymph node dissection: Radical mediastinal lymph node dissection is performed, followed by reinforcement of the bronchial stump. The hemithorax is then irrigated with warm saline and water (wash phase) to remove and osmotically lyse residual microscopic tumor.

5. Reconstruction of the diaphragm and pericardium: The last step is reconstruction of the diaphragm and pericardium using a prosthetic such as Gore-Tex DualMesh (W.L. Gore and Associated, Inc., Flagstaff, Arizona). These patches prevent subsequent herniation of abdominal contents and cardiac herniation into the empty hemithorax (Fig 23-3). The diaphragm patch also provides stability for cough and minimizes paradoxical ventilation (pendaluft).

Intraoperative Intracavitary Chemotherapy

No standard approach has been established in the treatment of MPM. Treatment options for MPM include chemotherapy, radiotherapy, surgery, and combinations of these modalities. Intraoperative administration of heated chemotherapy (e.g., Cisplatin ± Gemctabine) has been utilized in an effort to achieve cytoreduction with maximal cytotoxic effect, while minimizing the toxicity associated with systemic administration (3). The accompanying renal

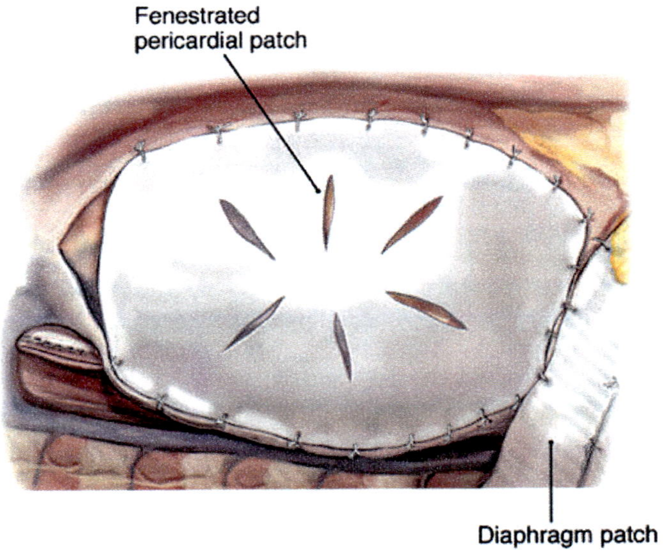

Figure 23-3 – Reconstruction with diaphragmatic and fenestrated pericardial patches. From Adult Chest Surgery, Sugarbaker DJ, et al., New York, McGraw-Hill, with permission. Copyright, Marcia Williams, 2009.

toxicity associated with cisplatin has implications for fluid management and other renal protective strategies which have been reviewed previously (4).

Anesthetic Considerations

Beyond standard anesthetic management issues for pneumonectomy (Chapter 21), there exist a number of important "EPP-specific" anesthetic concerns (Table 23-2).

Preoperative Patient Preparation

Cardiopulmonary Assessment

History, physical examination, and echocardiography will reflect cardiac functional status, but may not predict the response to the stress of pneumonectomy in the setting of major fluid shifts (5).

Table 23-2 – Anesthetic issues for extrapleural pneumonectomy

Significantly greater blood loss compared to pneumonectomy (due to parietal pleurectomy)
More delicate management of intravascular fluid and blood components
Greater operative impairment of venous return
Greater danger of surgical disruption of major vascular structures
More complex and variable physiology of the nonoperative lung (generally obstructive at baseline, but intermittently restrictive with surgical pressure during dissection)
High probability for disruption of internal mammary artery coronary grafts (if present) (note, coronary grafts may have tumor involvement)
High probability of dysrhythmias
Frequent "pseudo-ischemic" ST changes on EKG during wash phase, and greater axis shift
Greater potential for hemodynamic instability related to pericardial window and its patch
Greater postoperative pain and pulmonary dysfunction related to the larger incision, excision of diaphragm, and more extensive dissection

Invasive monitors (arterial and central venous lines) are routine; PA catheters may be employed for postoperative fluid and right heart management issues. Patients with a history of recent myocardial infarction in the last 3 months or life-threatening arrhythmias would be considered for pleurectomy/decortication rather than EPP.

Radiologic Studies

Computed tomography (CT) and magnetic resonance imaging (MRI) of the chest is important in assessing tumor invasion of the chest wall, vertebrae, diaphragm, and mediastinal structures. The anesthetic implications include safe placement of epidural catheters at the thoracic region, level of intravenous access, quantity of blood and blood products available, and the potential necessity for cardiopulmonary bypass during resection.

Thoracic Epidural Analgesia

Thoracic epidural analgesia (TEA) is widely used for intra- and postoperative analgesia. However, the sympatholytic effects of TEA may complicate hemodynamic management if dense blockade is imposed during or prior to the dissection phase of EPP.

Gastric Decompression

Work on the diaphragm is facilitated by efforts to minimize air insufflation. The presence of a nasogastric tube is important for this intra- and postoperatively and also aids surgeons in identification of the esophagus.

Lung Isolation and One-Lung Ventilation

Factors governing method of lung isolation are similar to that for pneumonectomy (see Chapter 22). EPP patients, during one-lung ventilation (OLV) in the lateral decubitus position, often exhibit an element of restrictive physiology in the dependent lung imposed by the weight of the tumor and surgical pressure during dissection. Lung-protective (5–6 ml/kg) ventilation with dependent lung positive end-expiratory pressure (PEEP) with the intention of limiting dependent lung volutrauma and atelectasis is important (6).

Frequent large changes in compliance require vigilance to prevent high airway pressures or volumes (depending on the mode of ventilation). Hypoxemia during OLV for EPP is unusual, as the best predictor of oxygen desaturation during OLV is increased (>55% of cardiac output) blood flow to the operative lung, which is seldom the case in MPM (7).

Hemodynamic Management

Hypertension

Hypertension should be avoided as it will greatly exacerbate bleeding from the innumerable avulsed chest wall vessels during the dissection phase. Hypertension may be an issue when the specimen is removed, and venous return to the heart is suddenly unimpeded.

Hypotension

Hypotension is more common, and its treatment should reflect its etiology whenever possible (Table 23-3).

Reduced venous return is by far the most common mechanism, caused by blood loss, mechanical pressure on the mediastinum during dissection, or torsion of great vessels. Critical phases of surgery when venous return is most threatened include the induction, dissection, and terminal repositioning phases (Table 23-4).

Fluid Management

The average estimated intraoperative blood loss during EPP in the best of surgical hands is approximately 0.5–1.5 L. Most of this occurs in a gradual, continuous fashion during the processes of blunt separation of the parietal pleura from the chest wall. Absent a coagulopathy, or difficulty with control of major vessels, blood loss is usually minor after argon beam coagulation of the of the chest wall. Nevertheless, catastrophic bleeding can occur from central vessels, particularly during dissection of the hilum.

Monitoring of the extent of blood loss requires vigilance and communication with the surgeons. Central venous pressure measurements, pulmonary artery occlusion pressures, or observance of respiratory variation on arterial line tracings may be unreliable barometers of intravascular volume during manipulation of weighty tumors, with the chest open to atmosphere. Much stock is placed on urine output as an indicator of end organ perfusion.

Table 23-3 – Causes of hypotension during EPP

Common	Compression of heart or great vessels by tumor or surgical pressure/retraction
	Blood loss/inadequate fluid resuscitation
	Thoracic epidural sympathetic blockade
Uncommon	Air-trapping (auto-PEEP)
	Tension pneumothorax
	Drugs (vasodilators/negative inotropes)
	Right heart dysfunction/failure
	Cardiac herniation
	Tight pericardial patch
	Shifted mediastinum following closure
	Myocardial ischemia
	Dysrhythmias
	Embolic events
	Transfusion reactions (more likely to transfuse EPP)
	Drug reactions
	Sepsis

Communication with the surgeon, judicious use of fluids and blood, and temporizing use of vasopressors usually allow for forward progress through the dissection phase with acceptable hemodynamics, without excessive administration of crystalloid.

Dysrhythmias

The incidence of supraventricular dysrhythmias (SVD) after EPP is higher (44%) than for standard pneumonectomy (20%) (1).

Table 23-4 – Hypotension during critical phases of surgery

PHASE	MECHANISM	MANAGEMENT STRATEGY
Induction	Reduced venous return – Vasodilation (induction agents, epidural) – Exacerbation of tumor compressive effects by the decrease in FRC – Loss of "thoracic pump" of spontaneous ventilation – Positive pressure ventilation	Preemptive vasoconstricting agents and judicious selection of induction agents/doses are particularly indicated for patients with large tumor burdens, large effusions, or radiographic evidence of cardiac or major vessel impingement
Dissection	– Blood loss – Insensible losses – Variable degrees of compression from the tumor, retractors, and blunt dissection pressure	Communication with the surgeon is paramount, and a coordinated effort is necessary to maintain forward progress with acceptable hemodynamics. Emphasis is placed on judicious use of vasopressors and a low threshold for administration of blood and products when appropriate When the specimen is removed, venous return, hemodynamics, and respiratory compliance should normalize. Persistent hypotension at this stage suggests hypovolemia

(continued)

Table 23-4 – (continued)

PHASE	MECHANISM	MANAGEMENT STRATEGY
Repositioning and emergence	Circulatory arrest – Herniation of the heart (particularly with right EPP), with torsion of the SVC and IVC	Immediate return to the lateral position
	Moderate hypotension – Partial cardiac herniation (loose or partially ruptured pericardial patch) – Tamponade (tight pericardial patch) – Hypovolemia – Deviated mediastinum – Aggressive bolus dosing of the epidural in anticipation of emergence	Attempts to medialize the mediastinum prior to turning supine are made by withdrawal of air from the chest drain. A sluggish response to fluid boluses and vasopressors suggest that mechanical impediments to venous return should be ruled out. A portable chest radiograph is usually helpful in ruling out partial cardiac herniation, or guiding medialization of the mediastinum

It is uncommon for routine prophylaxis against SVD, but important to avoid withdrawal of beta-adrenergic blocking drugs, if they are in use. Intraoperative dysrhythmias are generally triggered by mechanical irritation, and do not appear to predict postoperative SVD. EKG leads should be attached to a ready defibrillator to provide the capability of synchronized electrical cardioversion intraoperatively.

Myocardial Ischemia and Cardiac Function

Myocardial ischemia may be difficult to detect during EPP as alterations in the position of the heart relative to the surface EKG lead positions would be expected to alter their sensitivity. During left-sided thoracotomies, it is not practical to monitor lead V-5. When myocardial ischemia is suspected, TEE should be employed. TEE may also help in early detection of a tight pericardial patch (impaired diastolic filling), or signs of right ventricular strain (reduced RV contractility, increased RV size, flattened or left-shifted septum).

Dramatic *ST segment elevations* may occur during the wash phase (8). These tend to occur with irrigation, correct promptly with cessation, and are not associated with TEE changes or other hemodynamic alterations suggestive of myocardial ischemia. They most likely represent nonischemic electrophysiologic changes related to focal myocardial warming or surface electrolyte changes. No treatment is necessary unless they persist, produce hemodynamic instability, or are confirmed to be associated with wall motion abnormalities by TEE.

Repositioning, Tube Exchange and Emergence

The same principles apply as in standard pneumonectomy (see Chapter 22). The pericardial defect increases the risk of cardiac herniation during repositioning (especially with right EPP). As with standard pneumonectomy, immediate postoperative extubation is the general practice. ICU monitoring post-op is warranted.

Selected References

1. Sugarbaker DJ, Jaklitsch MT, Bueno R, et al. Prevention, early detection, and management of complications after 328 consecutive extrapleural pneumonectomies. J Thorac Cardiovasc Surg. 2004;128:138–46.

2. Chang MY, Sugarbaker DJ. Extrapleural pneumonectomy for diffuse malignant pleural mesothelioma: techniques and complications. Thorac Surg Clin. 2004;14:523–30.

3. Chang MY, Sugarbaker DJ. Innovative therapies: intraoperative intravacitary chemotherapy. Thorac Surg Clin. 2004;14:549–56.

4. Ng JM, Hartigan PM. Anesthetic management of patients undergoing extrapleural pneumonectomy for mesothelioma. Curr Opin Anaesthesiol. 2008;21:21–7.

5. Amar D, Burt ME, Roistacher N, et al. Value of perioperative Doppler echocardiography in patients undergoing major lung resection. Ann Thorac Surg. 1996;61:516–20.

6. Slinger P. Pro: low tidal volume is indicated during one-lung ventilation. Anesth Analg. 2006;103:268–70.

7. Hurford WE, Kolker AC, Strauss HW. The use of ventilation/perfusion lung scans to predict oxygenation during one-lung anesthesia. Anesthesiology. 1987;67:841–4.

8. Brown MJ, Brown DR. Thoracic cavity irrigation: an unusual cause of acute ST segment increase. Anesth Analg. 2002;95:552–4.

Chapter 24
Lung Volume Reduction Surgery

Nelson L. Thaemert

Keywords Lung volume reduction • National Emphysema Treatment Trail • Lung volume reduction surgery • Mechanisms of improvement from LVRS

Introduction

Lung volume reduction surgery (LVRS) is designed to improve respiratory function by resecting the most diseased lung tissue in patients with severe emphysematous COPD. In a selected subset of patients with severe emphysema, LVRS can improve exercise capacity, quality of life, and possibly survival compared to maximum medical therapy. Because it is performed on patients with debilitating pulmonary function and significant comorbidities, it requires proper patient selection and diligent anesthetic planning and implementation.

Successful outcomes require particular attention paid to the following:

- Proper patient selection:
  - Anatomic distribution of disease
  - Functional status
  - Adherence to exclusion criteria

P.M. Hartigan (ed.), *Practical Handbook of Thoracic Anesthesia*,
DOI 10.1007/978-0-387-88493-6_24,

- General anesthetic tailored to early extubation:
  - Optimum lung isolation to allow minimally invasive surgical approach
  - Ventilation strategy appropriate for severe COPD
  - Avoidance of barotrauma and air leaks
  - Excellent narcotic-sparing postoperative pain control

Rationale

Emphysema is characterized as a chronic, slowly progressive disorder of airflow obstruction. It is defined by permanent destruction and enlargement of airways distal to the terminal bronchioles. Characteristic changes in emphysema include loss of normal lung architecture, with loss of elastic recoil of lungs and collapse of small airways. Pure emphysema is unusual: most patients also have variable amounts of secretions and inflammation of small airways. Together, these lead to expiratory flow limitation and hyperinflation of lungs (see Chapter 3).

The resultant enlargement of the thorax (flat diaphragm, hyperexpanded chest wall) disrupts normal respiratory mechanics. Patients with severe COPD, in particular emphysema, are chronically dyspnic and have decreased exercise capacity.

Purported mechanisms of improvement from LVRS include:

- Improved pulmonary mechanics
- Improved diaphragm and chest wall function
- Improved right ventricular cardiac function

Improvement in pulmonary function is achieved by targeting the most emphysematous lung tissue for removal. Resecting these areas allows for improved expansion of less-diseased tissue, with more normal tethering and traction of patent airways and restoration of more uniform lung architecture. Ultimately, this allows for improved elastic recoil and work of breathing, with decreases in both expiratory flow limitation and dynamic hyperinflation.

Diaphragm and chest wall function also benefit, as each resumes a shape more conducive to normal respiration. Stretched muscle fibers of flattened diaphragms and intercostal muscles return to more optimum length at FRC. These mechanical changes lead to improved negative pressure generation from the diaphragm, and improved accessory muscle function during respiration.

Right ventricular cardiac function may also improve by reducing lung hyperinflation (tension physiology) and increasing inspiratory negative-pressure generation, both of which favorably affect venous return to the heart.

Surgical Considerations

Patient Selection

Current selection guidelines (Table 24-1) are drawn from conclusions of the National Emphysema Treatment Trail (NETT), a multicenter, randomized, controlled clinical trial comparing surgery to maximum medical therapy. Two large conclusions were made from the trial.

1. Patients with heterogeneous and predominantly upper lobe disease who underwent LVRS had improvement in exercise capacity and quality of life, compared to those with medical management (1). Moreover, the mortality in the subgroup with low functional capacity and heterogenous, upper lobe disease was reduced compared to medical management alone (controversial – see below).
2. Patients with a high risk of death were ones with (2):
   - $FEV_1 < 20\%$ predicted
   - Homogenous distribution of emphysema
   - DLCO < 20%

The NETT trial results have been widely misunderstood to suggest that LVRS is safer in the subgroup with predominantly upper lobe disease and low functional capacity. In fact, the separation of

Table 24-1 – Selection criteria for LVRS

Typical inclusion criteria for LVRS

- End-stage COPD refractory to medical therapy
- Severe dypsnea
- FEV_1 < 35% predicted
- Hyperinflated lungs by pulmonary function testing and chest X-ray
- Able to participate in pulmonary rehab program

Typical exclusion criteria for LVRS

- Advanced age >75 years
- Failed smoking cessation
- High-dose steroids
- Hypercapnea (controversial)
- Pulmonary hypertension
- DLCO < 30% predicted
- FEV_1 < 20% predicted
- Poor exercise tolerance (shuttle walk <200 m)
- Significant comorbidity

the surgical versus medical survival curves for this subgroup is solely due to the dismal survival of the medical treatment arm rather than from any reduced risk in the surgical arm (Fig 24-1). Patients and surgeons must have a sober understanding of this distinction.

The NETT study and others impacted both selection criteria and reimbursement policy for LVRS. As an aside, LVRS became somewhat of a test case for the perils of prematurely adopting new surgical techniques for desperate patient populations. In addition, the NETT and subsequent trials highlighted the potential, somewhat enduring flow benefits of exercise, and the poor outcomes associated with pulmonary hypertension and small airways disease.

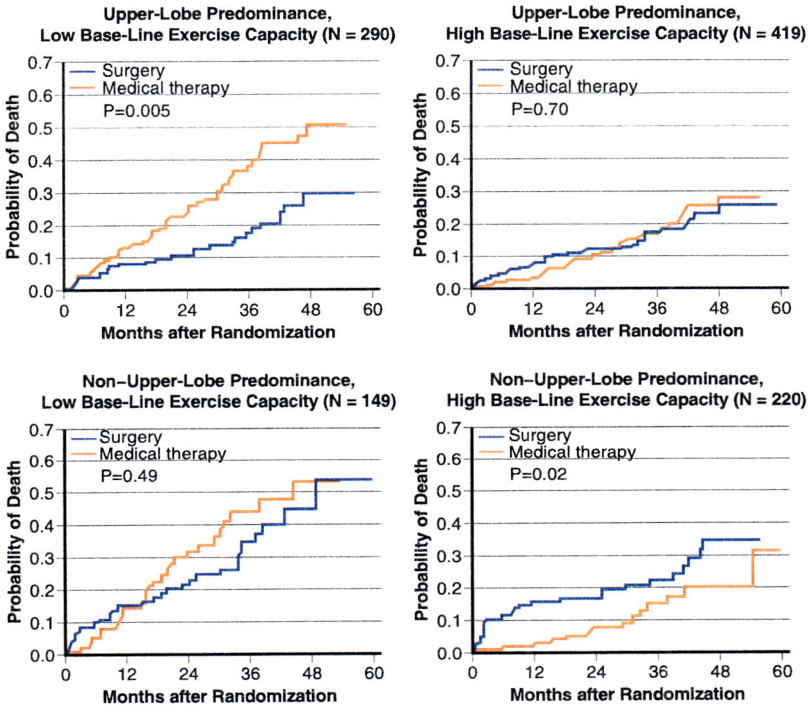

Figure 24-1 – Kaplan–Meyer survival curves from NETT Trial comparing survival following LVRS versus medical therapy for four subgroups of patients as labeled. Adapted with permission from Fishman A, Martinez F, et al. N Engl J Med 2003 (1); see text for explanation

Surgical Technique

Surgical priorities for LVRS include:

- Resection of appropriate amount and regions of lung
- Minimally invasive approach
- Avoidance of air leaks

Identification of the most diseased parts of the lung is based on a preoperative chest CT scan and direct observation. The lung regions slowest to collapse following lung isolation are generally the most emphysematous. The mechanical advantages of resection must not be outweighed by the reduction in parenchyma contributing to gas exchange. As a rough guideline, 20–30% of total lung volume is typically resected.

Maintaining a minimally invasive approach (VATS) has been associated with lower perioperative respiratory failure and mortality (3). Bilateral LVRS provides greater benefit than unilateral surgery, but is better conducted in a staged fashion (4).

Postoperative air leaks are common, owing to the tissue quality at the staple lines. Large, persistent air leaks have major implications, including reintubation, chronic ventilator dependence, and death. Air leak risk factors include pleural adhesions and lower DLCO and FEV_1 (5). Surgical strategies attempting to reduce leaks include buttressing (bovine pericardium, Gore-Tex™, etc.) and plication of staple lines (5). Gentle reinflation and ventilation of the operative lung following resection are believed to be instrumental in minimizing parenchymal stress at staple lines and postoperative air leaks.

Less-invasive alternatives to LVRS, including bronchoscopic LVRS (insertion of one-way valves or bioactive compounds to produce targeted atelectasis) and airway bypass (creation of collateral expiratory conduits), are in development at this writing.

Anesthetic Considerations

From a technical standpoint, LVRS is a comparatively straightforward surgical procedure, but with major anesthetic challenges. Principal among these is tailoring the general anesthetic to immediate postoperative extubation in the setting of lung resection and end-stage pulmonary disease (see Table 24-2). Reintubation or prolonged positive-pressure mechanical ventilation following LVRS increases the risk of volutrauma, major air leak, chronic ventilator dependency, pulmonary infection, aspiration, and other complications of mechanical ventilation. Other challenges include noninjurious ventilation, hemodynamic stability, and aggressive, narcotic-sparing analgesia.

Preoperative Medical Considerations

Patients presenting for LVRS are chronically ill and should be in optimum pulmonary health at the time of surgery. The presence of

Table 24-2 – Causes of respiratory failure following LVRS and strategies for prevention

CAUSES OF FAILED EXTUBATION/REINTUBATION	STRATEGIES TO PREVENT FOLLOWING LVRS
Narcotic-induced respiratory inhibition	Limit/avoid narcotics (except remifentanyl)
	TEA for post-op pain
Residual/trapped inhalational agent	TIVA
Hypercapnea	Judicious ventilation seeking balance between hypercapnea and lung injury
	Limit duration of one-lung phase
	Permissive hypercapnea during OLV
	Correct CO_2 during two-lung vent phase
Pain/splinting	Aggressive narcotic-sparing pain control (TEA, paravertebral, adjuncts, etc.)
Bronchospasm	Bronchodilators. Blunt airway reflexes with remifentanyl during tube exchanges and extubation
Residual muscle weakness	Full paralytic reversal
Mucous plugging	Toilet bronchoscopy at the end of case
	Antisialogogue if profuse
	Mucolytic if viscous
Atelectasis	Gentle recruitment maneuvers following toilet bronch
Unfavorable mechanics	Raise head of bed >45°
Lingering FRC reduction from general anesthetic	May be countered by surgery (unclear how early this effect occurs)

any reversible pulmonary process should be a reason to postpone surgery. In addition, patients should receive maximal medical therapy for end-stage COPD, including long-acting inhaled bronchodilators. A preoperative trial of pulmonary rehab is indicated. Assessment of cardiopulmonary reserve is problematic in severely deconditioned patients.

Patients with a history of heavy cigarette smoking should also be suspected of having indolent underlying coronary artery disease. Performing preoperative stress testing in the absence of other symptoms is controversial, and raises subsequent questions of whether the patient should then proceed to potential coronary intervention for asymptomatic coronary artery disease. Regardless of a workup for coronary artery disease, patients who present for surgery with severe COPD that are taking beta blockers preoperatively should continue them through the perioperative period.

Anesthetic Technique

Premedication

Preoperative sedatives should be used with great caution to avoid somnolence and hypercapnea. A treatment of nebulized bronchodilator may help preempt bronchospasm.

Monitoring

Despite a relatively limited surgical trespass, an arterial line is useful for early recognition of hemodynamic instability and for serial measurements of arterial blood gases. Capnography alone may be misleading, as the large increase in anatomic dead space increases the gradient between end-tidal and arterial pCO_2. Exaggerated postinduction hypotension is common (see below).

Induction and Maintenance

Patients should receive a carefully titrated intravenous induction, with particular attention paid to stable hemodynamics.

Causes and contributing factors to exaggerated hypotension following induction in LVRS patients include:

- Auto-PEEP
- Loss of thoracic pump effect from spontaneous ventilation
- Preexisting volume depletion
- Vasodilation from induction drug
- Test dose of epidural local anesthetic
- Tension pneumothorax
- Myocardial ischemia

Conversion to positive-pressure ventilation in such patients must be mindful of the hazards of air trapping (auto-PEEP), volutrauma, and impaired venous return (see "Ventilation Strategies" below). Should severe hypotension occur, the breathing circuit should be disconnected or opened to atmospheric pressure as the first maneuver. A poor response to vasopressors, inotropes, and fluid administration should prompt consideration of tension pneumothorax, particularly in those with bullous disease.

Maintenance of anesthesia has been described with both inhaled anesthetics and total intravenous anesthetic agents (TIVAs). TIVA consisting of propofol and remifentanyl has advantages: propofol offset is not dependent on pulmonary elimination, and remifentanyl profoundly blunts airway reflexes and reduces propofol requirements with no residual narcotic effect. Conversely, in patients with severe emphysema, emergence from an inhaled anesthetic can be particularly delayed.

Lung Isolation

VATS LVRS depends on excellent atelectasis. Flow limitation, secretions, and poor elastic recoil impair the degree and rate of onset of atelectasis. A DLT is typically preferred over a bronchial blocker because it better enables suctioning of the operative lung and may accomplish faster or more complete collapse. The impact of suctioning with severe flow limitation is likely limited because the airways quickly collapse, but attempts at secretion removal will likely help.

Ventilation

LVRS patients are at high risk of barotrauma, gas trapping, and hypercapnea. Target tidal volumes should roughly comply with lung-protective ventilation recommendations (5–6 ml/kg ideal body weight), particularly during the OLV phase. No conclusive study has demonstrated the superiority of one mode of ventilation over another.

Minimizing dynamic hyperinflation requires both a slow respiratory rate and an *I*:*E* ratio to maximize absolute expiratory time. Use of more advanced anesthesia machines capable of displaying flow versus time curves allows for assessment of whether expiration has concluded prior to delivery of the next inspiratory tidal volume. While complete elimination of auto-PEEP in such patients is not generally possible, attention to tidal volume and expiratory flow minimizes the amount of gas trapped (Fig 24-2).

Permissive hypercapnea may be the inevitable result of a low tidal volume and low-respiratory-rate ventilation strategy, particularly during the OLV phase. This is generally tolerated provided that the patient does not have significant pulmonary hypertension or

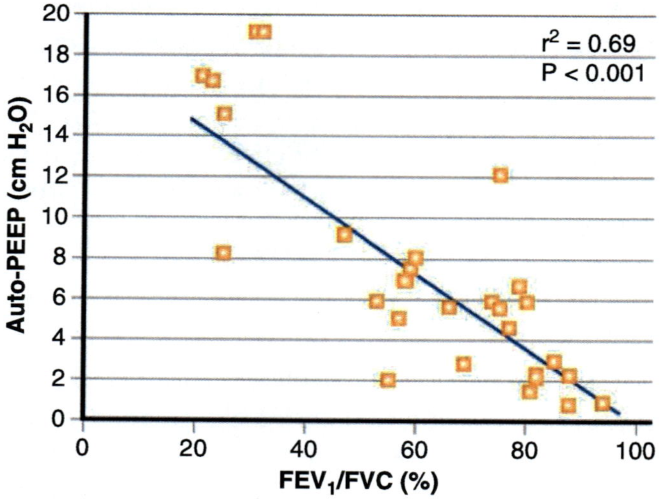

Figure 24-2 – Relationship between the severity of obstructive airways disease (FEV_1/FVC) and auto-PEEP during one-lung ventilation (from Ducros L, Moutafis M, Castelain M, et al. J Cardiothorac Vasc Anesth 1999; 13: 35, with permission)

right heart dysfunction, and is preferable to risking lung injury with more aggressive OLV. If hypercapnea and acidosis become severe, operative lung reinflation may be required for a period of time, necessitating a pause in the surgical procedure. An efficient surgeon helps limit the accumulated CO_2 burden. Obviously, clear communication with the surgeon in these circumstances is important. The limit of tolerable permissive hypercapnea is not defined. However, excessive acidosis can delay emergence by interfering with CNS and diaphragm function. Catch-up ventilation on two lungs following resection must be performed with careful attention to not exacerbate air leaks.

Management of Hypoxia During Lung Isolation

General management principles of hypoxia during OLV are outlined in Chapter 5. Counterintuitively, hypoxia during OLV is unusual during LVRS. This is presumed to be due to the slow or incomplete collapse of the operative lung, short duration of the OLV phase, and the unavoidable auto-PEEP in the dependent lung which prevents dependent lung atelectasis.

Analgesia

Inadequate pain control (splinting) may easily preclude extubation or precipitate reintubation in this fragile population. Excellent postoperative pain control is a critical component of the anesthetic plan for LVRS. Although no single approach is agreed upon, thoracic epidural analgesia (TEA) is most commonly employed as an effective narcotic-sparing technique. Alternatives do exist, including paravertebral blocks, intercostal infusions of local anesthetics, and limited parenteral (PCA) narcotics with adjuncts (NSAIDS, ketamine, etc.) (see Chapter 37). Adjuncts are not infrequently required for referred shoulder pain, even with TEA.

Emergence Strategies and Postoperative Management

Early extubation immediately after surgery is an important goal to limit the risk of air leak, as well as pneumonia and other complications of prolonged mechanical ventilation. A smooth tube exchange for toilet bronchoscopy can be facilitated by a bolus of remifentanyl. Bronchospasm may be preempted with in-line-nebulized bronchodilator treatments. Other impediments to extubation may be addressed as indicated in Table 24-2. Only the FRC effect of general anesthesia is beyond control (Chapter 4), and it is unclear whether the salutary effects of surgery are immediately operative to counter this negative effect. Return of clear sensorium may be slow in many LVRS patients for unclear reasons. Correction of permissive hypercapnea and acidosis can take time depending on the burden accumulated during OLV. As previously mentioned, $ETCO_2$ poorly reflects $PaCO_2$, and an arterial blood gas should be sent when patients are slow to emerge. Patients are impaired in their ability to hyperventilate if extubated with a high $PaCO_2$. Gentle augmentation of spontaneous efforts during emergence is a useful strategy. The many distracting events of this phase make it easy to inadvertently overventilate the patient and exacerbate air leaks. Attention to fine-tuning pain control may be the most important maneuver to prevent reintubation.

Selected References

1. Fishman A, Martinez F, et al. A randomized trial comparing lung-volume reduction surgery with medical therapy for severe emphysema. N Engl J Med. 2003;348(21):2059–73.

2. National Emphysema Trial Treatment Group. Patients at high risk of death after lung-volume reduction surgery. N Engl J Med. 2001;345(15):1075–83.

3. Kotloff RM, Tino G, Bavaria JE, et al. "Bilateral lung volume reduction for advanced emphysema. a comparison of median sternotomy and thoracoscopic approaches." Chest. 1996;100:1399–1406.

4. Brenner M, McKenna RJ, et al. Rate of FEV1 change following lung volume reduction surgery. Chest. 1998;113:652–9.

5. DeCamp MM, Blackstone EH, et al. Patient and surgical factors influencing air leak after lung volume reduction surgery: lessons learned from the national emphysema treatment trial. Ann Thorac Surg. 2006;82(1):197–207.

Suggested Further References

Naunheim KS, Wood DE, et al. Long-term follow-up of patients receiving lung-volume-reduction surgery versus medical therapy for severe emphysema by the National Emphysema Treatment Trial Research Group. Ann Thorac Surg. 2006; 82(2):431–43.

Brister NW, Barnette RE, et al, "Anesthetic considerations in candidates for lung volume reduction surgery". Proc Am Thorac Soc. 2008;1,5(4):432–7. Review.

Hartigan PM, Pedoto A. Anesthetic considerations for lung volume reduction surgery and lung transplantation. Thorac Surg Clin. 2005;15:143–57.

Chapter 25
Plueral Space Procedures

Shannon S. McKenna

Keywords Pleuroscopy • Pleurodesis • Complete or radical pleurectomy • Pleurectomy • Decortication

Introduction

Surgical access to the pleural space allows for observation, drainage, biopsy, mass resection, and debridement/decortication. Common abnormalities that lead to surgical evaluation of the pleural space are listed in Table 25-1.

Pleuroscopy

Pleuroscopy refers to the visual examination of the pleural space using a scope inserted into the chest. The procedure may be performed using either a mediastinoscope or a thoracoscope. Thoracoscopic instruments allow for drainage of fluid, biopsy of tissue, mass resection, stripping of adhesions, and even decortication.

Surgical Considerations for Pleuroscopy

The principal surgical considerations are to enable adequate visualization of the pleural space, fully meet the surgical goals of

P.M. Hartigan (ed.), *Practical Handbook of Thoracic Anesthesia*,
DOI 10.1007/978-0-387-88493-6_25,

Table 25-1 – Pleural space abnormalities

Effusion – benign or malignant
Hemothorax
Infection (empyema)
Tumor/mass
Fibrothorax/adhesions/trapped lung
Pneumothorax

Table 25-2 – Complications of pleuroscopy

Bleeding (port sites, chest wall, lung surface, and tumor at the site of biopsy)
Air leak (parenchymal disruption)
Residual space (failure of lung to completely reexpand)
Pleural effusion
Hemothorax
Empyema
Persistent nonhealing air leak

the procedure (biopsy, drainage, etc.), and to avoid perioperative complications.

Adequate visualization of the pleural space starts with proper patient positioning to allow appropriate port placement. Deflation of the lung on the operative side is needed to create space between the chest wall and lung surface. Adhesions or loculated fluid collections may need to be broken up to allow the lung to fall away from the chest wall. Potential *complications of pleuroscopy* are outlined in Table 25-2.

Anesthetic Considerations for Pleuroscopy

Pleuroscopy is usually performed under *general anesthesia*. It is possible, using adequate local anesthesia and careful sedation, to perform limited pleuroscopy in an awake patient. This approach should be reserved for those patients unable to tolerate general anesthesia, who are motivated to avoid intubation and capable of being still through periods of discomfort. At least a partial pneumothorax occurs in the awake patient with ports open to atmosphere.

Care should be taken in the *preoperative assessment* to identify patients with comorbidities that may affect anesthetic management (see Table 25-3).

Table 25-3 – Concerning comorbidities found in patients having pleuroscopy

COMORBIDITY	POSSIBLE COMPLICATIONS	HELPFUL INTERVENTIONS
Contralateral pleural effusion	Low FRC, hypoxia with induction, hypoxia during OLV, postoperative respiratory failure	Drainage of contralateral effusion prior to procedure; PEEP
Ascites	Low FRC, hypoxia with induction, postoperative respiratory failure	Drainage; reverse Trendelenburg position; PEEP
Pericardial effusion	Hypotension and hypoperfusion	Catheter drainage pre-op
Empyema	Perioperative sepsis, seeding of intravascular and epidural catheters from bacteremia, major bleeding intra-op	Preparation to treat sepsis intraoperatively; consider not placing epidural; preparation for major blood loss
Coagulopathy	Increased bleeding	Reversal prior to surgery; preparation for major blood loss
Parenchymal lung disease	Poor tolerance of OLV, postoperative respiratory failure	Intermittent apnea rather than OLV; PEEP; TIVA and non-narcotic analgesia to facilitate extubation

Positioning: Lateral decubitus or supine depending on where surgeon needs to place ports. If an axillary port is required, arm position must allow full access to axilla.

Lung isolation: OLV with a DLT provides the most flexibility. A bronchial blocker is a viable option, particularly if the lung is already partially deflated secondary to the underlying disease process. If the patient is unable to tolerate OLV, intermittent apnea or continuous ventilation with small tidal volumes often result in tolerable operative conditions. Arterial blood gas monitoring may be of use for more tenuous patients or prolonged procedures.

Hemorrhage: In most cases, bleeding occurs from port sites, chest wall, or surface of the lung. It can be controlled with local compression and directed cautery. Decortication (discussed below) can be associated with substantial blood loss. It is prudent to have adequate IV access and cross-matched blood available.

Air leak: Injury to the lung surface may result in a *persistent air leak*. Difficulty ventilating using an anesthesia ventilator can usually be resolved by turning up the fresh gas flows. It is important to realize that the reported tidal volume on most anesthesia ventilators is the expiratory (returned) tidal volume and not the delivered volume. Excessively large tidal volumes can be delivered if this is not appreciated. Air leaks generally improve with return to supine positioning and resumption of spontaneous ventilation. There are several important anesthetic implications with large air leaks, which are much more common after pleurectomy than pleuroscopy (see below).

Postoperative considerations: Patients with empyema or advanced cancer with pleural spread are often quite sick and may not have the pulmonary reserve to extubate at the end of the procedure. Preoperative evaluation should include an evaluation of the likelihood of extubation. In some cases, modification of the anesthetic technique to employ those techniques used for lung volume reduction surgery (see Chapter 24) may allow for extubation. In contrast, patients who fully reexpand their lungs after the removal of large effusions achieve significant respiratory improvement and readily extubate.

Pleurodesis

Pleurodesis is the obliteration of the pleural cavity. It occurs when the visceral and parietal pleura fuse together. Mechanical or chemical irritation can be used to trigger pleural inflammation. Pleurodesis is used to treat pleural effusions and pneumothorax.

Surgical Considerations for Pleurodesis

The surgical considerations for thoracoscopy, as described above, apply here. In addition, it is critical that complete reexpansion of the lung is achieved. Pleural fusion cannot occur if the visceral pleura does not come into contact with the parietal pleura. When complete lung expansion does not occur, it may be necessary to place a chronic drainage catheter and forego pleurodesis.

Options for pleurodesis are listed in Table 25-4. Talc is the most effective, and thus most commonly used, chemical agent. *Complications* of chemical pleurodesis are described in Table 25-5.

Anesthetic Considerations for Pleurodesis

The anesthetic considerations mirror those for pleuroscopy. In addition, it is important to work with the surgeon to ascertain whether complete lung reexpansion is possible. Brief *selective ventilation of the operative lung* only may allow for full expansion in certain cases. If pleural apposition cannot be achieved, then it is unlikely that pleurodesis will be successful.

Table 25-4 – Agents for pleurodesis

Mechanical irritation
Talc poudrage
Talc slurry
Doxycycline
Bleomycin

Table 25-5 – Complications of pleurodesis

Minor complications
Pain
Fever
Nausea
Major complications (predominately associated with talc)
Respiratory failure/ARDS
Hypotension
Arrhythmias
Empyema

Poudrage, if done using a reservoir attached to air or oxygen to aerosolize the talc, can lead to increased intrathoracic pressure and a *tension pneumothorax*. This is treated by halting aerosolization and allowing the thorax to vent through the port incision. The lung should be deflated during administration of the sclerosing agent to allow free distribution throughout the pleural cavity.

Postoperative *respiratory failure* and *systemic inflammation* can occur within hours of talc administration. Onset may occur in the recovery room. Intubation and mechanical ventilation may be necessary. Pharmacologic support of the blood pressure may also be required. Patients with systemic talc reactions are best cared for in an ICU as they can progress to multiorgan system failure.

Decortication and Pleurectomy

Infections, hemothorax, and chronic noninfectious effusions can all lead to the deposition of fibrous material on the lung and chest wall. The lung can become restricted and entrapped. *Decortication* refers to the stripping of the fibrous layer off the lung and, as needed, the chest wall. Decortication may be done via pleuroscopy, but often requires either mini-thoracotomy with VATS or a full thoracotomy.

Pleurectomy refers to removal of the pleura. Pleurectomy may be partial or complete. A small, partial pleurectomy has surgical and anesthetic considerations that are addressed by the pleuroscopy section. A *complete or radical pleurectomy* implies complete removal of both the visceral and parietal pleura. It is a *major surgical procedure* that has specific anesthesia considerations.

Surgical Considerations for Decortication and Pleurectomy

Adequate visualization may be challenging if the pleural disease is extensive. Significant time may be spent performing lysis of adhesions to free a trapped lung. Once the pleural space is appropriately accessed, the surgeon must strip away all fibrous and diseased tissue. The goal is to allow complete lung expansion. Postoperatively, fusion of the lung to the chest wall obliterates the pleural space and prevents accumulation of fluid, hematoma, or pus.

If *complete pleurectomy* is the goal (e.g., for mesothelioma), the surgeon will dissect down to the parietal pleura and then proceed to strip the pleura off the chest wall. It is generally not possible to fully strip diseased pleura from the pericardium and diaphragm. This can be dealt with surgically by excising the portions of pericardium and diaphragm that are in contact with the pleura and reconstructing these structures with Gore-Tex™ or a similar material. Once the parietal pleura is removed, it may be necessary to partially or completely strip the visceral pleura off of the lung. Complications of decortication and pleurectomy are detailed in Table 25-6.

Anesthesia Considerations for Decortication and Pleurectomy

Decortication and pleurectomy are generally major procedures associated with significant surgical trespass. The anesthesiologist must anticipate a number of intraoperative and postoperative problems. The issues of positioning and lung isolation discussed in the pleuroscopy section apply here. On occasion, the surgeon may opt

Table 25-6 – Complications of decortication and pleurectomy

Bleeding (chest wall, lung surface, major intrathoracic vessels)
Air leak (parenchymal disruption)
Residual space (failure of lung to completely reexpand)
Pleural effusion
Hemothorax
Empyema
Persistent nonhealing air leak
Thoracic duct injury (usually, with right-side surgery)
Recurrent laryngeal nerve injury (usually, with left-side surgery)
Esophageal injury

to perform part of the visceral decortication while the operative lung is being ventilated as this may make it easier to identify the proper tissue planes. It is critical that the anesthesiologist have the ability to smoothly transition back and forth between OLV and two-lung ventilation.

Mucous plugging: Patients with an empyema may have *copious purulent secretions* in the operative lung and even on the non-operative side. Frequent suctioning, often through a bronchoscope, is required to keep the large airways and the double-lumen ETT patent. Visceral decortication causes significant trauma to the lung parenchyma and frequently results in endobronchial hemorrhage. *Blood clots* can obstruct the airways or even the lumen of the endotracheal tube. This can prevent lung reinflation at the end of the case and is best dealt with via bronchoscopic examination and suctioning.

Hemorrhage: Parietal pleurectomy/decortication results in diffuse bleeding from the chest wall. Likewise, visceral decortication can result in diffuse bleeding from the lung surface. Both sites can be controlled to a significant extent with packing, pressure, and cautery. However, *significant occult blood loss* may occur. Bleeding from

Table 25-7 – Vessels vulnerable to injury during pleurectomy

Superior vena cava
Subclavian vessels
Azygous vein (most common)
Internal mammary vessels
Aorta
Bronchial arteries
Pulmonary artery
Pulmonary veins
Intercostal vessels
Coronary artery bypass grafts

these sites may persist for 1–2 days and become a source of ongoing blood loss. It is important to monitor the hemoglobin concentration periodically as blood loss may "hide" in sponges, drapes, and in the thoracic cavity.

Pleural disease may cover and obscure the major intrathoracic and mediastinal vessels. Blind dissection in this setting can result in injury to major blood vessels and *massive blood loss*. Vessels vulnerable to injury are listed in Table 25-7. It is necessary to have IV access sufficient for major resuscitation, blood products readily available, and the ability to warm blood and fluids.

Arrhythmia: Decortication of the mediastinal pleura requires mechanical *manipulation* and *compression* of the *heart and great vessels*. Arrhythmias can occur during this phase. Typically, they are atrial (atrial fibrillation, flutter, or SVT) and short lived. Ventricular tachycardia may also occur. Often, immediate cessation of the surgical manipulation leads to restoration of sinus rhythm. Sometimes, treatment with a nodal blocking agent or antiarrhythmic is needed. If the patient is unstable or adequate rate control cannot be achieved, electrical cardioversion may be needed. ECG leads from the defibrillator should be in place to enable synchronized cardioversion if indicated.

Septic shock: Manipulation of empyema cavities can lead to transient bacteremia and the onset of septic shock. The anesthesiologist should be prepared to treat *intraoperative sepsis* in the setting of decortication for empyema. Fluid resuscitation is first-line treatment for septic shock (along with surgical drainage and appropriate antibiotic therapy); however, if the patient does not respond adequately to fluid, vasoactive therapy should be started. Detailed initial management of sepsis can be found on line at the Surviving Sepsis Campaign Web site.

Hypotension: Intraoperative hypotension is common during pleurectomy and major decortication. Common etiologies are hypovolemia (blood loss), mechanical compression of the heart or great vessels, arrhythmias, and vasodilation from sepsis. Treatment must be directed at the underlying cause. Arterial pressure monitoring is invaluable in these cases. Central venous access and monitoring may also be useful. Hypotension resulting from mechanical compression often responds well to judicious volume loading (±vasopressors) timed to the period of maximal surgical manipulation of the heart and great vessels.

Air leak: Visceral decortication can lead to *massive air leak*. This has important implications for the anesthesiologist, including management of ventilation, fire hazard, choice of anesthetics, safe transport, and postoperative ventilation.

Management of ventilation with large air leak: It may be difficult to ventilate the patient at the time of transition back to two-lung ventilation. Very high fresh gas flows may be needed. Rarely, it is necessary to bleed additional oxygen from a supplemental source into the anesthesia circuit or to transition intraoperatively to an ICU ventilator. Since most anesthesia machines measure tidal volume as the expiratory volume returned to the circuit, the tidal volume is spuriously low with large air leaks. If extra fresh gas flow is bled into the circuit, the expiratory (and delivered) volumes will be significantly larger than the volume set on the ventilator. Volume control ventilation, thus, may result in incessant alarms for incorrect tidal volume delivery. In this regard, pressure control mode may be easier to use.

A distinction should be made between the two purposes served by ventilation in this setting: (1) CO_2 removal and (2) expanding the lungs. Lung expansion is important to recruit lung and bring together lung and chest wall to abate bleeding and air leaks. Gas exchange can be quite satisfactory despite large air leaks and poor expansion. Air that leaks from the lung surface participates in gas exchange and contributes to effective minute ventilation even though it is not accounted by the ventilator. Serial measurement of arterial blood gasses is necessary to assess CO_2 removal.

In the face of a large air leak, there is likely an advantage of pressure control mode compared to volume control due to the different flow versus time profile. Pressure control may achieve lung expansion better in the presence of large air leaks, but also may ventilate excessively. It is important to monitor the inspired tidal volumes (via spirometry) when using pressure control to make sure that excessive volumes are not being administered.

An air leak in excess of the capacity of the chest tubes and pleurovac results in a pneumothorax. Air leaks typically improve when the patient is turned back to the supine position, and improve further with spontaneous ventilation.

Fire hazard: It is important to note that any parenchymal injury allows ventilated gas to escape from the lung surface into the thoracic cavity if that lung is being ventilated. Typically, patients are maintained on high inspired oxygen levels during thoracic surgery. Cavitary oxygen concentrations are a mixture of atmospheric and leaked (delivered) FiO_2, and will likely vary with proximity to the parenchymal defects and respiratory cycle. Use of electrosurgical devices (cautery), argon beam coagulator, or other high-energy potential ignition sources may result in an *intrathoracic fire*. It is prudent to maintain OLV until hemostasis has been achieved and to hold ventilation or resume lung isolation if/when further electrocautery is to be used. Clear communication with surgeons on this matter is obviously important.

Choice of anesthetics with large air leaks: TIVA techniques are preferable to inhalational agents to prevent contamination of the OR and for more predictable delivery.

Transport of patients with large air leaks: Standard regulators often have maximum flows of 25 L/min. Even with the chest drain on water seal for transport to the ICU, this may be inadequate to overcome the leak. Monitoring of adequacy of ventilation during patient transport is limited (often to observation of chest wall rise). Prudence dictates that one should not leave the OR on standard ambu bag ventilation from a standard oxygen tank regulator if ventilation is in doubt. A brief trial followed by a blood gas analysis is one strategy to assure safety. Use of portable ventilators is a better option when transporting patients with large parenchymal air leaks. If a transport ventilator is not available, two oxygen tanks may be Y connected together to increase gas flow. PEEP may aid in limiting air leak during transport. If difficulties occur with oxygenation or ventilation during transport, one should first rule out a kinked chest tube as the most common cause of pneumothorax during transport in this setting.

Postoperative ventilation: Patients with substantial blood loss, major air leaks, or an operative lung that does not expand well at the end of surgery may benefit from postoperative ventilation. Mechanical ventilation for 12–24 h helps to fully expand the lung and promote apposition of the lung to the chest wall. This process minimizes postoperative bleeding and allows for more rapid closure of persistent air leaks. Some clinicians advocate the use of elevated PEEP (8–10 cm H_2O) to help maintain FRC and prevent atelectasis. Large air leaks may require balancing chest tube suction level (versus water seal) with ventilator settings to optimize the distribution of ventilation and lung expansion.

Pain: Substantial pain should be anticipated following decortication or pleurectomy. Thoracic epidural analgesia is the most common strategy employed, when not contraindicated by coagulation status or bacteremia. This and alternative strategies are discussed in Chapter 37.

Suggested Reading

Swanson SJ, Sugarbaker DJ. Surgery of the pleural space: fibrothorax, thoracoscopy, and pleurectomy. In: Baum GL et al. editors. Textbook of pulmonary diseases. 6th ed. Philadelphia: Lippincott-Raven Publishers; 1998.

Heffner JE. Chemical pleurodesis. UpToDate. Version 17.1. 2008. www.uptodate.com.

Dresler CM, et al. Phase III intergroup study of talc poudrage vs. talc slurry sclerosis for malignant pleural effusion. Chest. 2005;127:909–15.

Rusch VW. Pleurectomy/decortication in the setting of multimodality treatment for diffuse malignant pleural mesothelioma. Semin Thorac Cardiovasc Surg. 1997;9:367–72.

Surviving Sepsis Campaign. Guidelines for management of severe sepsis and septic shock. 2008. www.survivingsepsis.org.

Chapter 26
Rigid Bronchoscopy

Eric D. Skolnick

Keywords Apneic oxygenation • Jet ventilation • Rigid bronchoscopy • Anesthetic considerations

Introduction

Rigid bronchoscopy enables a thorough evaluation of the trachea and proximal bronchi. Since indications for this procedure include airway obstruction or bleeding, patients often present with impaired respiratory reserve or significant comorbidities. The procedure is most commonly performed under general anesthesia and, depending on the patient's pathology, may be better suited to either spontaneous or positive pressure ventilation.

Rigid bronchoscopes are long, stainless steel tubes, open at either end, that enable the surgeon to view tracheal (and to some extent bronchial) anatomy (Figs 26-1 and 26-2). Modifications include a side port that adapts to a standard anesthesia circuit, allowing for intermittent positive pressure ventilation (PPV) and a glass cover at the proximal end, offering a view of the surgical field during ventilation. There is no distal cuff, so some air leak is generally present during PPV.

P.M. Hartigan (ed.), *Practical Handbook of Thoracic Anesthesia*,
DOI 10.1007/978-0-387-88493-6_26, © Springer Science+Business Media, LLC 2012

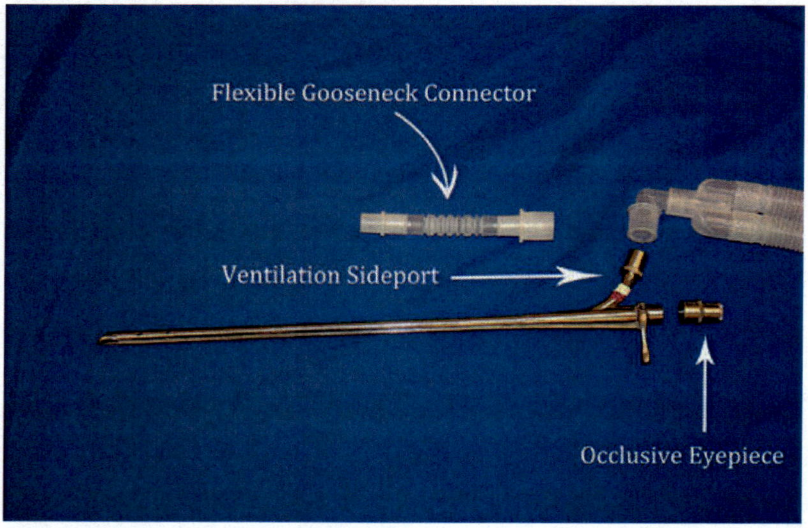

Figure 26-1 – Standard Rigid Bronchoscope. The tip is rounded to minimize trauma, but beveled to facilitate insertion and coring out of lesions. The ventilating side port fits standard 15 mm connectors for anesthesia breathing circuits (small scopes may require an adapter). A flexible gooseneck connector between the breathing circuit and scope facilitates operation. The eyepiece has an occlusive glass window, allowing ventilation and viewing, but is removed for insertion of instruments. Ventilation should be held when the eyepiece is removed.

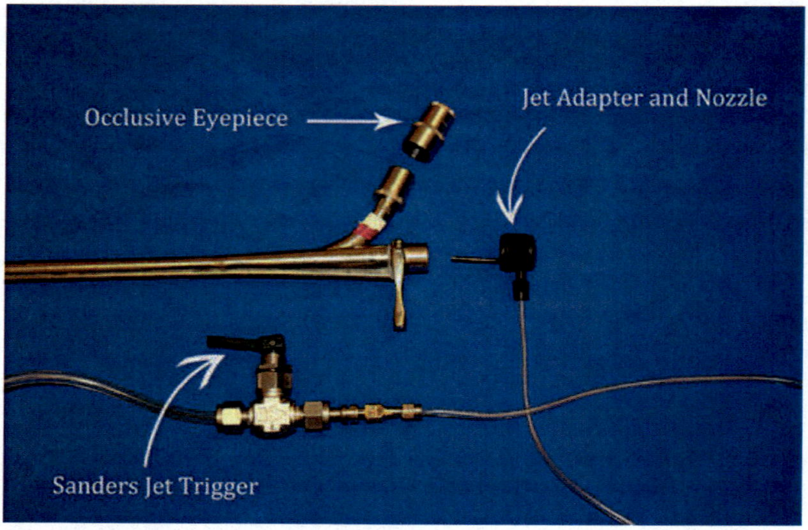

Figure 26-2 – Rigid Bronchoscope with Jet Ventilator. A simple Sanders jet ventilator mounted at the proximal end allows unobstructed view and uninterrupted access for the surgeon. The occlusive eyepiece may be used to cover the ventilating side port if present. Alternatively, the jet could be mounted on the side port.

Surgical Considerations

The *surgical indications* for rigid (Table 26-1) and flexible (Chapter 18) bronchoscopy overlap considerably. In general, rigid bronchoscopy provides more room for direct instrumentation and access, but requires more experience and is more stimulating and potentially traumatic.

Preoperatively, one should be sure that the airway distal to an obstruction can be accessed by the rigid scope. If so, it may be used as a rescue maneuver to stent open and ventilate a collapsed airway. Patient positioning can be critical to surgical success. Often, the operating table is turned 90° after induction and a transverse shoulder roll is placed, hyperextending the neck to facilitate intubation with the rigid scope. The upper teeth are protected with a bite block or moist gauze. The surgeon's thumb, interposed between the teeth and the scope while grasping the maxilla, provides the most important dental protection. The thumb acts as the fulcrum as the scope is advanced under the epiglottis (Fig 26-3).

Surgical complications directly related to rigid bronchoscopy, or to the procedures performed through rigid scopes, are listed in

Table 26-1 – Surgical Indications for Rigid Bronchoscopy

- Massive hemoptysis; Evaluation & treatment
- Foreign body retrieval
- Tracheal/bronchial stenosis; Evaluation and treatment
  - Mechanical core-out
  - Laser therapy
  - Placement or extraction of stents
- Rescue of compressed or obstructed airway
- Evaluation and treatment of fistulae (bronchopleural, tracheoesophageal)

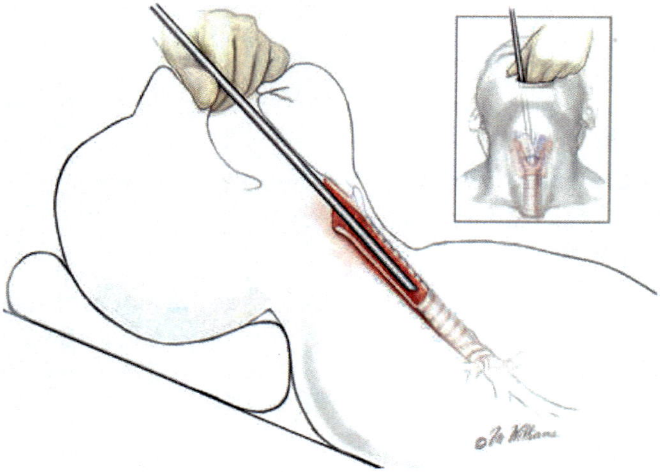

Figure 26-3 – The thumb acts as the fulcrum as the scope is advanced under the epiglottis.

Table 26-2 – Surgical complications of rigid bronchoscopy

- Airway obstruction from manipulation of tumor, foreign body, stent, etc.
- Hemorrhage
- Tracheal/bronchial laceration, dissection, disruption
- Hyperextension injury of cervical neck or spinal cord
- Vocal cord edema/trauma, with post-op stridor
- Atelectasis from excessive suctioning
- Airway fire or other complications of laser (Chapter 27)
- Dental injury

Table 26-2. Other threats to patients during rigid bronchocopy relate to the pathophysiology produced by the lesions (airway obstruction, mediator release from carcinoid tumors, etc.), or to anesthetic management (see below).

Anesthetic Considerations

- *Preoperative:* Assessment of the CT scan, discussion of the surgical plan, and direct patient evaluation are critical to the decisions that follow, and to preempt complications. Specifically, one should seek information on the following:
  - Extent and position of tracheal/bronchial stenosis or lesion
  - Intraluminal vs. extrinsic airway lesion
  - Positional dyspnea/coughing
  - Paraneoplastic symptoms
  - Difficult airway anatomy
  - Cervical (spine) pathology, including stenosis, instability, or limited range of motion
  - Bronchospasm (vs. wheezing from lesion-related obstruction)
  - Extent of hemoptysis, if applicable, and coagulation parameters if biopsy is planned

It is critical to discuss the exact nature and extent of the airway pathology if obstruction is a possibility. Distal tracheal obstructions, which do not allow advancement of the scope beyond to assure rescue ventilation, are the greatest risk. For patients with significant dynamic airway obstruction (e.g., anterior mediastinal mass), the principals of management outlined in Chapter 20 would apply.

- *Positioning*: Approximating the surgical position while the patient is awake allows one to define the extent of tolerable neck extension under anesthesia. This often includes a transverse shoulder roll and soft ring pillow under the head.
- *Induction & Ventilation Decisions*: Fundamental decisions are how to induce, and whether to use spontaneous or positive pressure ventilation (PPV). In patients with a difficult airway, foreign body causing a ball-valve effect, or those in whom successful placement of the endotracheal tube distal to the lesion

may be in question (stenosis, fistula), spontaneous ventilation is preferred until the surgeon secures the airway with the rigid scope. In patients with compressible proximal lesions or known anatomy, one can generally proceed immediately to positive pressure ventilation.

Positive pressure ventilation is hampered by foreword airflow resistance (stenotic lesions) and the inevitable air leak resulting from the lack of a cuff on the rigid scope. Adequate tidal volume delivery requires increased flows and prolonged inspiratory times. Many practitioners find manual ventilation advantageous, since the degree of volume loss can be variable from breath-to-breath, and interruptions are frequent. Caution must be exercised to avoid air trapping distal to stenoses.

Air leak around the bronchoscope can be reduced by packing the hypopharynx with moist gauze, pressing down on the larynx, pinching the lips and nares closed, or by fitting an inflatable cuff around the bronchoscope.

- *Jet Ventilation*: (Sanders or High Frequency Jet Ventilation) is preferred in some centers over side-port PPV for rigid bronchoscopy. Jet ventilation may be delivered through a 16 gauge cannula mounted on the proximal port of the rigid bronchoscope, or its side ventilation port. Alternatively, a catheter may be positioned within or alongside the rigid bronchoscope through which jet ventilation may be delivered. Advocates of jet ventilation cite the advantage that surgical progress can continue uninterrupted. With PPV, the surgery must halt and the viewing port must be occluded when delivering a breath through the ventilation port. Disadvantages of jet ventilation include risk of barotrauma, inability to deliver volatile agents, and inability to regulate FiO_2 or monitor extent of ventilation. In addition, the jet airflow can blow blood and debris distally, potentially affecting gas exchange. Limitations to the amount of airway pressure that jet ventilation delivers may result in inadequate ventilation of patients with reduced airway compliance. Adequacy of ventilation relies on attention to chest rise, intermittent blood gas analysis, or transcutaneous CO_2 monitoring if available. Jet ventilation is discussed more fully in Chapter 11.

- *Apneic oxygenation* is a technique in which 100% oxygen is continuously delivered through a catheter to the airway of an open system such as during rigid bronchoscopy (1). When patients are preoxygenated with 100% oxygen, rigid bronchoscopy with apneic oxygenation can proceed uninterrupted for significant periods of time before desaturation occurs. CO_2 levels continuously rise during the period of apnea. Apneic oxygenation can conveniently be utilized together with intermittent periods of side-port ventilation to provide the surgeon with long stretches of operating time.

- *Choice of Anesthetics*: Rigid bronchoscopy is intensely stimulating. Nonetheless, for emergency relief of central airway obstruction, local anesthesia with sedation may be the safest choice (2). For general anesthesia with spontaneous ventilation, an inhalational approach may be easier to titrate to respiratory drive (compared to intravenous anesthetics). During the surgical portion, the required intermittent apnea causes both oscillating anesthetic depth and exposure of the OR staff to unscavenged volatile agent. This can be avoided by use of total intravenous anesthesia (TIVA) once the airway is secured.

In choosing drugs for a TIVA, keep in mind the intense surgical stimulation with minimal postoperative pain. Short-acting drugs are best, for which infusions of propofol and remifentanil are ideally suited. An antisialagogue such as glycopyrolate can be helpful.

- *Muscle Relaxation*: Paralysis is greatly beneficial (and occasionally critical) to facilitate intubation with the rigid scope. Additionally, it helps to avoid the risk of tracheal laceration or rupture from bucking against the instruments. Consider an infusion of either mivacurium or succinylcholine. Should Sugammadex receive FDA approval in the near future, then bolus doses of steroid based neuromuscular blockers may be an option. If maintaining spontaneous ventilation, insure a profound depth of anesthesia prior to start of laryngoscopy.

- *Monitoring Gas Exchange*: In the paralyzed patient, gas exchange depends upon brief periods of ventilation separated by episodes of apnea. Permissive hypercapnea is to be expected. Brief oxygen desaturation into the low 90s or even upper 80s can be tolerated by the otherwise healthy patient.

As with flexible bronchoscopy, frequent suctioning, air leak, and intermittent periods of apnea render machine readings of FiO_2, $ETCO_2$, ET Agent, tidal volume, and capnogram shape difficult to interpret. Observation of chest rise is helpful to assess ventilation. During prolonged apnea, the rise in $PaCO_2$ may be approximated to increase by 6 mmHg during the first minute, followed by 3 mmHg each subsequent minute (3). Transcutaneous CO_2 monitoring may be useful during prolonged procedures (4).

- *Fire/Burn Hazards*: Laser or electrosurgical device usage via rigid bronchoscopes may result in airway fire when charred tissue or a foreign body acts as fuel and the FiO_2 is high. Reflection of the laser from the rigid scope may injure unintended tissue or cause vocal cord burns by the "hot tube effect." Other hazards of lasers would apply, including eye injuries and OR fires from ignition of the drapes (see Chapter 27). If photodynamic therapy is employed, the patient's skin and eyes must be protected from ambient light, and the pulse oximeter should be periodically rotated to a different site (5) (see Chapter 27)
- *Airway Obstruction Hazard*: Rigid bronchoscopy is often performed to address lesions which threaten total tracheal occlusion. Tight lesions of the distal trachea are the greatest risk. Nearly obstructive situations may become totally obstructive by several mechanisms:
  - Reduced caliber of airways with induction of anesthesia due to reduction in functional residual capacity
  - Conversion of laminar to turbulent airflow
  - Alteration in the position of a foreign body during attempted extraction
  - Folding of airway stent during attempted manipulation
  - Edema of airway tumor due to manipulation, biopsy, etc.
  - Occlusion of stenotic lesion by secretions, blood clots, etc.

When the offending obstruction is a foreign body, the surgeon must promptly remove it or advance it into one mainstem bronchus. When the obstruction is from an intrinsic or extrinsic mass, advancing the rigid bronchoscope or an endotracheal tube beyond the stenosis to stent open the airway is often the rescue maneuver of choice. *It should be evident that loss of the airway due to a distal tracheal stenosis cannot be remedied by a cricoidthyrotomy*.

- *Massive Hemoptysis*: Biopsy of lesions occasionally results in brisk bleeding. Carcinoid tumors are prone to this. Tamponade of the source using an instrument, balloon tipped catheter (e.g., embolectomy catheter, bronchial blocker, etc.), or by advancing the rigid bronchoscope, may abate the bleeding. Temporary apnea would be required for balloon tamponade of tracheal bleeding lesions. Intubation of the trachea such that the endotracheal tube cuff tamponades the bleeding source is an alternative that allows ventilation. Minor bleeding is addressed with electrocautery or by spraying a vasoconstrictor (dilute epinephrine) on the source.
- *Emergence*: During emergence from anesthesia, consider whether to switch directly from the rigid bronchoscope to mask anesthesia or to replace it with an endotracheal tube or LMA. In patients with difficult airway anatomy, bronchospasm, persistent stenosis, prolonged neuromuscular blockade, or impaired oxygenation, intubation prior to emergence is recommended. In either case, recruitment maneuvers are important to counter the inevitable lung volume loss resulting from the air leak, apneic periods, suctioning, and absorption atelectasis. Intubation facilitates such recruitment maneuvers and allows for a final flexible bronchoscopy to assess any previously unrecognized injury or residual tumor. Owing to its angle of takeoff, the left mainstem bronchus has blind spots for rigid bronchoscopes that are better assessed by flexible scopes prior to emergence.
- *Postoperative Considerations*: Many rigid bronchoscopy patients are sent home on the day of surgery. Postoperative considerations consist of a search for and treatment of common complications (Table 26-3). Patients with significant airway obstruction, hemoptysis, or limited reserve may warrant admission and observation.

Table 26-3 – Postoperative considerations following rigid bronchoscopy

- Chest X-ray to rule out pneumothorax
- Beta-agonist for bronchospasm
- Racemic epinephrine and/or steroids for airway edema
- Intravenous or nebulized lidocaine for airway irritation/coughing
- Humidified oxygen

Selected References

1. Furmin MJ, Epstein RM, Cohen G. Apneic oxygenation in man. Anesthesiology. 1959;20:789–93.

2. Conacher ID, Curran E. Local aneaesthesia and sedation for rigid bronchoscopy for emergency relief of central airway obstruction. Anaesthesia. 2004;59(3):290–2.

3. Eger EI, Severinghaus JW. The rate of rise of $PaCO_2$ in the apneic anesthetized man. Anesthesiology. 1961;22:419–22.

4. Simon M, Gottschall R, Gugel M, et al. Comparison of transcutaneous and end-tidal CO2 monitoring for rigid bronchoscopy during high-frequency jet ventilation. Acta Anaesthesiol Scand. 2003;47(7):861–7.

5. Farber NE, McNeely J. Rosner d, Skin burn associated with pulse oximetry during perioperative photodynamic therapy. Anesthesiology. 1996;84(4):983–5.

Further Reading

Mentzer SJ. Bronchoscopy, rigid and flexible. In: Sugarbaker DJ, Bueno R, Krasna M, Mentzer S, Zellos L, editors. Adult Chest Surgery. New York: McGraw Hill Medical; 2009. p. 438–44. Chapter 52.

Wain JC. Rigid bronchoscopy: the value of a venerable procedure. Chest Surg Clin N Am. 2001;11(4):691–9.

Farrell PT. Rigid bronchoscopy for foreign body removal: anesthesia and ventilation. Paediatr Anaesth. 2004;14(1):84–9.

Chapter 27
Laser Surgery of the Airway and Laser Safety

Gyorgy Frendl

Keywords LASER • Endobronchial laser tumor ablation • Potential hazards of lasers • Airway fire • Anesthetic considerations of lasers • Photodynamic therapy

Introduction

Light Amplification by Stimulated Emission of Radiation (LASER), an electromagnetic energy of high intensity, has several applications in thoracic surgery. The focus of this chapter is laser function and safety, mainly in the context of *endobronchial laser tumor ablation*. Anesthetic concerns including the choice of endotracheal tubes, ventilation strategies, and gas medium needed to safely manage laser airway cases are discussed.

Advantages of laser include the ability to:

- Deliver high energy into small, focused areas and therefore improving the precision of tumor treatment.
- Cause less bleeding (heat cauterizes blood vessels), edema, and scarring.
- Be delivered via flexible devices and reach challenging or restricted spaces.

P.M. Hartigan (ed.), *Practical Handbook of Thoracic Anesthesia*,
DOI 10.1007/978-0-387-88493-6_27,

Indications of laser therapy in the context of thoracic surgery are:

- The ablation of endoluminal (endobronchial) tumors or strictures.
- Photodynamic therapy.
- Hemostasis.

During laser therapy, the *goals* are to:

- Maximize the biologic effect (delivering the maximum amount of heat/energy into the target tissue).
- Minimize the damage to surrounding normal tissues.
- Avoid injury to the patient and OR personnel.

When lasers are in use, important considerations include:

- Fire hazard and general laser safety issues.
- Maintaining patency of threatened major airways.
- Shared airway with the surgical team.

The LASER

The high degree of monochromaticity, coherence, and collimation are the important characteristics of laser, which allow for a very concentrated energy delivery. The degree of tissue penetration is principally a function of wavelength. Lasers can operate in either the continuous (constant output when laser is "on") or pulsed wave (rapidly alternating "on" and "off" pulse periods) mode. Pulsed wave laser delivers short bursts of high energy, ideal for tissue ablation (Table 27-1).

Mechanisms of Laser Effects on Tissues

Photothermal effects: Micro to millisecond long pulses cause rapid but selective heating of the target tissue with thermal injury.

Table 27-1 – Commonly used medical lasers

TYPE (WAVELENGTH)	DELIVERY	PROPERTIES	INDICATIONS
Carbon dioxide, CO_2 (10,600 nm)	Transmitted by mirrors through an articulated arm with a hand-held coupler	Completely absorbed by water in the first few layers of cells (shallow penetration)	Upper airway and proximal tracheal lesions
Neodymium-doped: yttrium aluminum garnet, Nd:YAG (1,064 nm)	Transmitted by a quartz monofilament via a flexible endoscope	Penetrates deeper tissues	Superior for tumor debulking, resection of lower tracheal, and bronchial lesions
Potassium titanyl phosphate, KTP-YAG laser (532 nm – green visible spectrum)	Often delivered via a rigid bronchoscope	Allows for slower, more gentle heating, and coagulation of the vessels	Tumor ablation and photocoagulation Ideal for the treatment of highly vascular tumors
Pulsed dye (any chosen wavelength over fraction of visible spectrum)		Highly versatile	Ideal for treating highly vascular tissues
Argon plasma coagulator (blue and green visible spectrum)	Flexible fiberoptic device	Noncontact mode of tissue coagulation. Contraindication is the presence of a pacemaker susceptible to electrical interference	Photocoagulation Bronchoscopic management of central airway obstruction or hemoptysis

Photochemical effects: Laser energy causing chemical changes in tissue. In photodynamic therapy (PDT), laser or narrow-band light energy can trigger a chemical reaction directly by interacting with photosensitizing compounds in cells.

Photomechanical effects: Nanosecond pulses of laser will induce rapid heating and formation of expanding thermal plasma, causing it to collapse and send shock waves, mechanically disrupting the target.

Surgical Considerations

The decision to employ laser, rather than mechanical core-out, or other options (dilation, stenting, radiation seeds, sleeve resection, etc.) is individualized, based on patient, surgical, and situational factors (Fig 27-1). Often, laser ablation is just part of a multimodality approach to treat or palliate malignancies of the central airways.

Laser can be used for airway procedures with either rigid or flexible bronchoscopy. While laser airway procedures are most frequently performed via flexible fiberoptic bronchoscopy, rigid bronchoscopy has the advantages of better visibility, easier removal of larger size tumor debris, decreased risk of airway fire, and easier maintenance of open airway. The Nd-YAG laser is most commonly employed for endobronchial heat ablation of tumors (photothermal effect) because of its high energy level and higher tissue penetration (up to 10 mm) (1).

Complications (perforation, unintended target, etc.) are avoided by tight control of laser direction, timing, and total power of laser delivery. It is best to have a motionless field, to use multiple short bursts, and to limit the total power for the case. A basic rule would be to laser parallel to the airway, and to avoid laser use when the airway distal to the lesion cannot be visualized. Targeting is guided by a pilot light (the Nd:YAG laser beam itself is not visible), which should be confirmed by pretesting, to ensure that it corresponds to

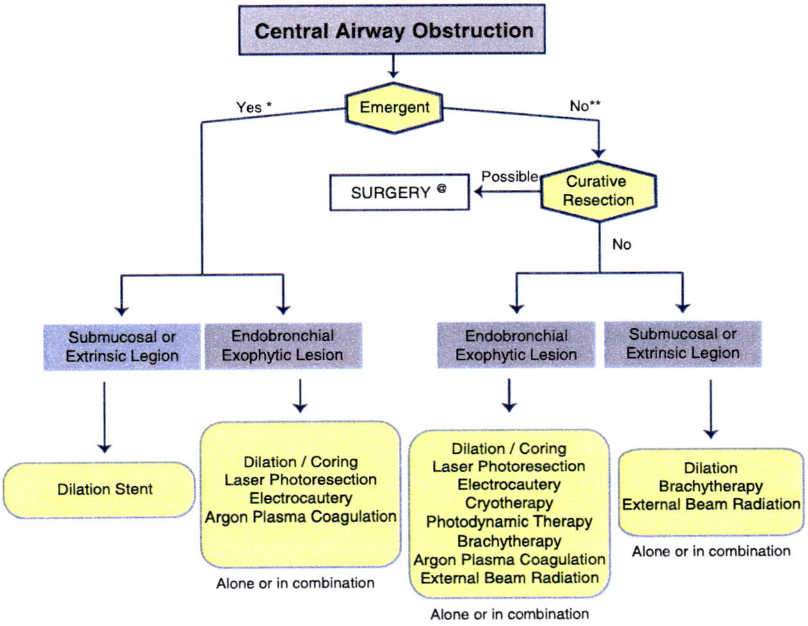

Figure 27-1 – Algorithm for the management of endobronchial tumors. *Awake fiberoptic or rigid bronchoscopic evaluation. **Nonemergent airway evaluation includes CT scan, plus possible flexible bronchoscopy, endobronchial ultrasound, autofluorescence. @Possibly with presurgical intervention. *Adapted with permission from Ernst A, Feller-Kopman D, Becker H, Mehta A. Central airway obstruction. Am J Resp Crit Care Med. 2004;169:1278–97.*

the laser aim. When not firing the laser, it should be on standby mode. Unambiguous, closed loop communication between all team members in the OR is an essential safety measure when the laser is turned on and off.

Caution should be employed with vascular metastatic airway tumors (e.g., renal cell carcinoma and melanoma), as there may be significant bleeding when treated with laser ablation. This bleeding often responds well to cold saline washes and the instillation of dilute epinephrine solutions. Rarely, the bleeding may be significant enough to warrant conversion to rigid bronchoscopy (as laser does not coagulate vessels over 5 mm size very well) or require isolation of the bleeding lung segment with a bronchial blocker.

Laser Safety

Potential Hazards of Lasers

The three major categories are:

- Fire, electric shock, and explosion.
- Damage to the eye, skin, and mucosa.
- Inhalation of noxious fumes.

Fire Hazard in the Operating Room

The greatest concern is the *risk of fire in the OR, particularly an airway fire*. Fire requires the presence of three components: energy (ignition), combustibles (fuel), and oxygen. Fire occurs when these three components are present and enough energy is delivered for the combustible materials to reach their ignition point (temperature). Fires can cause *thermal injury* (direct burn) and/or *inhalational injury* (from toxic fumes derived from burning plastic, synthetic material [CO, CO_2, HCl, cyanide, etc.] or CO poisoning).

Airway Fire

Airway fire is a special risk of airway laser surgery, with high risk of serious morbidity (scarring, stricture, etc.) and mortality. Approximately 650 surgical fires are reported in US hospitals each year, and another three to four times as many are "near misses" or unreported events (2–4). Approximately 20% of those reported fires result in serious patient injury. Endoscopic airway surgery is one of the highest risk operations for OR fire (3–20% of all OR fires, in various reports),

An ignited endotracheal tube becomes a blowtorch if oxygen flow continues (Fig 27-2). Tissue damage is immediate, placing a premium on prevention over treatment (Tables 27-2 and 27-3).

Box 27-1 outlines the recommended interventions should airway fire occur (5). This is the joint responsibility of surgeons, anesthesiologists, and all support personnel in the OR.

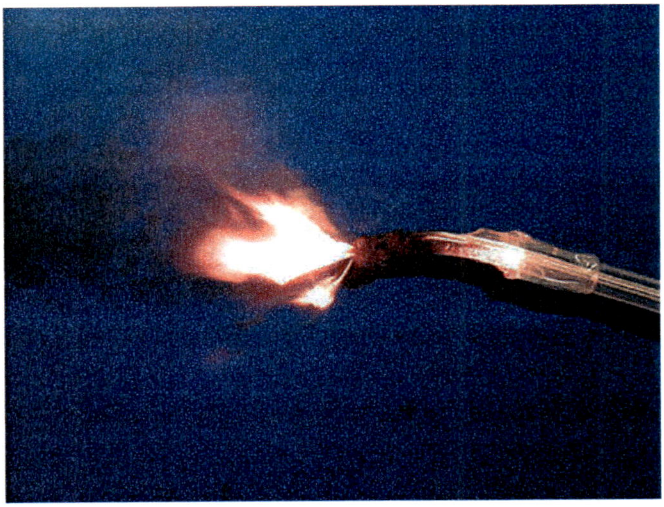

Figure 27-2 – A double-lumen PVC endotracheal tube is ignited with 5 l/min flow of oxygen (100%) demonstrating a dramatic blowtorch effect.

Table 27-2 – Primary prevention of airway fire

OR PERSONNEL (NURSING, SURGICAL, AND ANESTHESIA TEAMS)	
Training and education	Credentialing of surgeons for the operation of laser equipment
	Safety checklist during laser utilization
	Protocols for management of airway fire
Maintenance of standards	Equipment checks
	Quality assurance

The most important maneuvers are to cease oxygen delivery, extinguish the flame, and remove any airway device that might be on fire or sufficiently hot to be damaging. This often requires the reflex disconnect of the circuit while the surgeon squirts a prefilled

Table 27-3 – Secondary prevention of airway fire

	STEPS IN THE PREVENTION OF AIRWAY FIRE
Environment	Warning signs posted at entry points
	Have cold water/saline, and wet sponges immediately available to extinguish fire (prefilled large bulb syringe is best)
Laser equipment	*Test and calibrate laser* prior to use (including true aim)
	Protective eyewear for OR personnel and patient
Surgery	*Clear warning by operator when laser is activated* ("Laser-On" vs. "Standby"), with closed-loop communication
	Avoid laser or electrocautery for hemostasis when O_2 concentration is high (use packing, ties, instillation of epinephrine, etc.)
	Remove charred tissue from the area of laser use (including tip of laser or bronchoscope)
Anesthesia	*Choice of Airway device*:
	▪ LMA (maximizes distance between flammable airway device and laser)
	▪ Rigid bronchoscopy or jet ventilation (avoids tube altogether)
	▪ Laser-resistant tubes (less combustible than PVC)
	FiO_2 should be the minimum tolerated by the patient. (dilute O_2 with helium, N_2, or air)
	Hold ventilation (as tolerated) when laser is fired

large bulb syringe of cold saline down the ETT, followed immediately by removal of the ETT by the anesthesiologist. Whether the airway device should be removed when the airway may be difficult to resecure (or it is felt highly unlikely that the ETT is on fire) is controversial. When in doubt, one should err on the side of removing the device to limit damage.

Box 27-1 – Recommended Interventions When Airway Fire Occurs

(http://www.guideline.gov/summary/summary.aspx?doc_id=12547&nbr=006463&string=laser+and+%22thoracic+surgery%22)

The following steps should be taken once fire in the airway occurs:

- *Remove or minimize the oxygen delivered*: disconnect the patient from the source of oxygen if possible, if this is not possible then lower to 21% FiO_2.
- *Extinguish the fire* with cold saline or cold saline soaked cloth.
- *Assess injuries* with fiberoptic bronchoscopy and direct laryngoscopy and assess if the removal of the damaged endotracheal tube is safe and the airway can be safely secured. *The benefit of removing the damaged endotracheal tube has to be weighed against the risks of potential difficulties of securing the airway*; this has to be judged on a case-by-case bases.
- *Remove all external burning objects* from patient.
- *Resume ventilation and oxygen delivery* as soon as safely possible.
- *Prevent re-ignition*:
  - Continue cooling the area of fire.
  - Resume ventilation with the lowest tolerated FiO_2.
- *Formulate alternate plans*:
  - If the procedure is a tracheostomy, then proceed with tracheostomy expeditiously before removing the burned endotracheal tube if it was on fire.
  - If the initial surgical procedure was not a tracheostomy, after assessing the airway, consider prophylactic tracheostomy.
  - Assess whether the patient needs to be kept intubated after the procedure.
  - Monitor the patient for signs of lung injury.

Risks of Laser Injuries to the Patients and Providers

High energy lasers can cause inadvertent injuries to both the patient (Box 27-2) and health care provider (Box 27-3).

Box 27-2 – Potential Hazards to Patients During Laser-Assisted Surgery

- Fire (airway or operating room fire).
- Severe eye injuries by direct or reflected laser beams.
- Venous gas embolism.
- Bleeding.
- Inadvertent airway perforation (secondary pneumothorax, pneumomediastinum, or perforation-related tracheo-esophageal fistula).
- Respiratory hazards when breathing laser-generated airborne contaminants (LGAC).
- Scarring.
- Skin burn from direct beam when incidentally misdirected.
- Incomplete treatment of the target lesion.
- Pain.

Box 27-3 – Potential Hazards to Health Care Providers due to Laser Exposure

- Severe eye injuries by direct or reflected laser beams.
- Skin burn from direct beam when incidentally misdirected.
- Skin color changes at exposed areas.
- Operating room fire.
- Respiratory hazards when breathing LGAC.

Eye Injuries

Direct or reflected laser beams may cause *impaired vision or blindness*. The extent of eye damage depends on the wavelength of the laser as well as the intensity and duration of exposure.

Carbon dioxide lasers can cause corneal opacification. The energy produced by the Nd:YAG laser are transmitted by the lens to the back of the eye and injure the retina. *Eye protection*: Protective wavelength-specific polycarbonate goggles with side shields are mandatory for all OR personnel and the patient. In addition, many recommend saline soaked gauze eye patches to shield the patient's eyes under the goggles. Warning signs must be posted at entry points, and windows must be shielded by blinds.

Because the infrared wavelength of the carbon dioxide laser is absorbed by almost all surfaces, eye wear of any color, even clear glasses (but not necessarily plastic lenses), will stop the beam and prevent ocular damage.

Skin Injuries

Errant laser strikes to skin or mucous membranes cause injuries ranging from mild erythema to severe burn or perforation. Prevention hinges on tight control of laser direction and timing by the operator, as well as a motionless field. Calibration of the pilot light with the Nd:YAG beam must be confirmed prior to use in the patient (see section on "Surgical Considerations" above).

OR personnel may also incur skin injuries if struck by an errant laser on exposed skin. Nylon, synthetic fiber, or plastic-based clothing should be avoided. Cotton/rayon will fare better as less toxic (carcinogenic) fumes will be generated if a fire occurs.

Federal regulations classify lasers primarily by their ability to cause damage to the eye and skin (Class I [no hazard] to Class IV [serious hazard]). Most lasers used for surgical procedures belong to the Class IV safety class. The regulatory agency websites (5, 6) detail mandated safety requirements.

Respiratory Hazards

Vaporized tissues produce smoke (plume), which may be mutagenic or infectious. LGAC are a minimal but potentially important risk of the use of laser. When infrared lasers are used, toxic fumes must be evacuated by suction of smoke and carbonaceous debris away from the operative site. N95 respirators are recommended when the plume is hazardous.

Tracheo-Bronchial Wall Injury

Excessive or misdirected laser in the airway may result in a mucosal, or transmural injury (air leak, pneumothorax, tracheo-esophageal fistula, bleeding, etc.). As above, control of laser direction and power, and a motionless field help prevent this. The depth of penetration with Nd:YAG lasers is not easily apparent to the operator, and must be continually reassessed. Lasering off-parallel to the bronchial lumen should be avoided.

Anesthetic Considerations

Apart from the laser hazards discussed earlier, the main anesthesia concerns include the method used to secure the airway, ventilation strategies, and postoperative challenges.

Choice of Airway Devices

Supraglottic Devices

Laryngeal mask airways (LMA) or similar supraglottic devices are advantageous because they maximize the distance between the laser beam and the device (potential fuel). In addition, the vocal cords and entire trachea can be viewed and evaluated. With a bronchoscope inserted through an LMA, airflow resistance is less than it otherwise would be through a large ETT (8). The disadvantage is that it is a less secure airway, vulnerable to laryngospasm, aspiration, and air leak during positive pressure ventilation.

Rigid Bronchoscope

For cases of high-grade airway obstruction (particularly for proximal tumor or stenosis), rigid bronchoscopy is commonly used as the airway device and conduit for flexible bronchoscopy and delivery of laser. Advantages of this approach include:

- Ability to advance the rigid scope as a stent to maintain airway patency.
- Convenient conduit to mainstem bronchus, through which flexible scope may be advanced to distal targets.
- Metal, fire-resistant material.
- Direct visual field, and conduit for forceps, suction, etc.

Rigid bronchoscopy typically requires general anesthesia. Implications for the mode of ventilation (periodic positive pressure ventilation via side-port, jet ventilation, or high frequency jet ventilation) are discussed in Chapter 26. If positive pressure ventilation is employed, periodic interruptions are necessary, and attention to avoid hypercarbia is important. Due to the inevitable air leak, TIVA is most often employed over inhalation-based anesthetics, and muscle paralysis is useful to aid insertion of the bronchoscope.

"Laser-Resistant" Endotracheal Tubes

No tube is completely laser-safe, and many fires have been reported with laser-resistant tubes (9). Various tubes are available with a variety of features designed to reduce the risk. However, these features principally reduce risk from laser strikes to the external midshaft or cuff (i.e., appropriate for laser surgery of the larynx or pharynx). With endobronchial laser procedures, the bronchoscope/laser is passed through the tube lumen, extending beyond the tip. Inadvertent laser strikes to the tube exterior midshaft are unlikely. The distal tip of the tube, which is closest to the laser beam, is the most susceptible to ignition, and is unprotected in currently available laser-resistant tubes.

Two general strategies have been pursued in designs of laser-resistant tubes: (1) metal tubes, and (2) wrapped tubes. *It is emphasized that unless the distal tip is metal or wrapped with fire-resistant material, these tubes offer limited protection from fire during endobronchial laser surgery.*

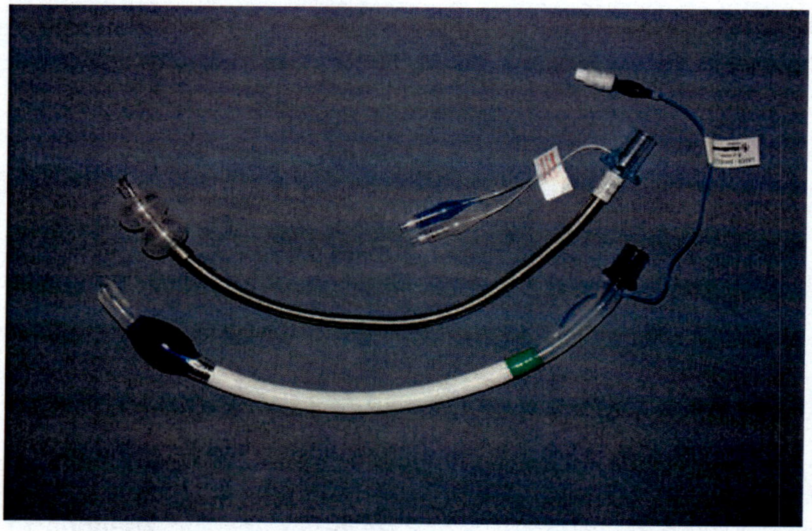

Figure 27-3 – Laser-resistant tubes. Examples of metal (Laser-Flex [Mallincrodt, Inc., St Louis, MO]), and wrapped "laser-resistant" endotracheal tubes (Laser-Shield II [Medtronic Xomed, Inc. Jacksonville, FL]). See text for discussion of features.

Metal tubes (e.g., Laser-Flex, Mallincrodt, Inc., St Louis, MO) (Fig 27-3) have a very high ignition temperature, but still may burn in high oxygen environments. When struck by lasers they may also deflect energy to unintended targets, become incandescent, and burn the airway or vocal cords by a "hot tube effect." A matte finish reduces risk by defocusing reflected laser beams. Although mostly metal, they have cuffs and pilot balloons/cannulae which may burn or melt. Double cuffs are designed to be filled with saline so that a laser strike to the proximal one will be extinguished, and the distal cuff will prevent backflow of oxygen. Metal tubes have unfavorable internal-to-external diameter ratios and are relatively rough and traumatic. The distal tip is PVC to reduce trauma, but becomes a potential fuel source. At this writing, no metal tube is approved by the FDA for Nd:YAG laser use.

The alternative strategy is to wrap tubes with reflective and/or absorptive material. Examples include Laser-Shield II (Medtronic Xomed, Inc., Jacksonville, FL) (Fig 27-3), Lasertubus (Teleflex Medical, Rusch, Inc., Duluth, GA), and Fome-Cuff (Bivona® Smiths Medical,

St Paul, MN). Alternatively, silver, aluminum, or copper foil adhesive strips (3M No. 425, or Venture Copper) can be wrapped in overlapping fashion over standard PVC tubes, but it is difficult/impossible to adequately protect the cuff, distal end, or internal tube.

Induction Strategies (Avoiding Airway Obstruction)

Patients with high-grade tracheal obstruction warrant induction techniques that preserve spontaneous ventilation (either awake fiberoptic intubation or inhalational induction). When in doubt, an awake fiberoptic exam is the safest approach. Depending on the lesion, the obstruction may be fixed, variable, or most commonly a combination of the two (see Chapters 20 and 30). Lesions that are predominantly fixed (e.g., tracheal scar from intubation injury) are lower risk of collapse with induction. Back-up plans for a lost airway include advancing a small ETT across the stenosis, rigid bronchoscopy, and rapid return to upright, awake, spontaneously breathing state. Bronchial lesions are also lower risk, as long as the patient can tolerate contralateral single-lung ventilation. Standard induction techniques are generally safe for endobronchial lesions which do not extend above the carina.

Ventilation Strategies

If spontaneous ventilation is required to maintain airway patency, care must be taken to assure sufficient depth for a motionless field during use of the laser. Controlled ventilation is more common and convenient, when feasible, and may be delivered through an LMA, ETT, or the side port of a rigid bronchoscope. Alternatives, include jet ventilation and high frequency jet ventilation (see Chapter 11). Disadvantages of jet ventilation are that it can result in gastric dilatation, cause barotrauma, pneumothorax, pneumomediastinum, or subcutaneous emphysema, and can lead to aspiration of surgical debris, and of secretions. All open techniques require TIVA. Additionally, the supraglottic air/O_2 insufflation technique can be used with either spontaneous breathing as a form of shorter term, continuous flow, apneic oxygenation.

Gas Medium

It is recommended that the FiO_2 be maintained below *0.4* during the use of laser, although ignition is still possible below this level. Nitrogen, air, or helium can be used in the inhaled gas mixture to reduce the level of oxygen. *Heliox* (79% helium; 21% oxygen) has the additional advantage of lower resistance to air flow through a stenosis due to its lower density (Chapter 30). Nitrous oxide should not be used as it supports combustion.

Emergence and Extubation

The anesthetic plan should be tailored to rapid emergence with sufficient respiratory strength and efforts to assure successful extubation. This is best accomplished with short acting medications of IV anesthetics and muscle relaxants. Remifentanil facilitates a smooth emergence, reduces the risk of long lasting narcosis, and suppresses coughing from airway irritation. Spraying local anesthetic on the mucosal site of laser surgery may also reduce coughing. Table 27-4 summarizes the postoperative challenges and their management.

Photodynamic Therapy

PDT is a palliative procedure for patients with central airway tumors not amenable to other treatments and less than 1 cm in diameter. PDT employs the use of a photosensitizer called porfimer sodium (injected intravenously and absorbed by all cells but enriched in tumor cells).

During an incubation period, the cells produce a photosensitizer, typically a porphyrin, which in the presence of molecular oxygen will generate cytotoxic singlet oxygen, and target cell death. The energy required for this is delivered by a laser beam (630 nm for porfimer; photochemical effect) targeted onto the tissue (generally by a cable passed through a fiberoptic bronchoscope).

Table 27-4 – Challenges encountered postoperatively

CHALLENGES	ETIOLOGY	MANAGEMENT
Vocal cord edema (Dyspnea, stridor)	▪ Rigid bronchoscopy (trauma) ▪ Repeated airway instrumentation	Nebulized racemic epinephrine Corticosteroids (controversial) Elevate the head of the bed Close monitoring for trend, and need for reintubation
Coughing spells (common) (may exacerbate bleeding or displace stents)	▪ Blood, debris in airway ▪ Bronchospasm ▪ Mucosal injury or trauma	Antitussives (judicious narcotics) Humidified oxygen Close monitoring Repeat bronchoscopy
Respiratory failure (uncommon)	Severe preexisting respiratory disease, not immediately relieved by the laser surgery	Delayed extubation

Anesthetic Considerations for PDT

The laser utilized in PDT is a KTP laser of wavelength in the UV range. Cell kill is accomplished by photochemical, rather than thermal means. Fire risk is therefore minimal compared to Nd:YAG. Patient stimulation is limited to the presence of the fiberoptic scope. PDT is thus amenable to awake, sedated techniques (with topical anesthesia), or light general anesthetics (LMA). Cell kill takes days, so obstructive symptoms from the tumor will not be immediately relieved. Because all cells are photosensitized to some extent, patients' skin should be protected from UV range light, including ambient. They should wear dark glasses pre- and postoperatively, and should have skin surfaces covered. During laser activation, wavelength specific goggles must be worn by patient and personnel, and other laser safety protocols must be followed. The pulse oximeter may cause skin burns or fingernail damage, and should be rotated to different sites if the procedure becomes prolonged.

Selected References

1. Ernst A, Feller-Kopman D, Becker H, Mehta A. State of the art: central airway obstruction. Am J Respir Crit Care Med. 2004;169:1278–97.

2. Prasad R, Quezado Z, St Andre A, et al. Fires in the operating room and intensive care unit: awareness is the key to prevention. Anesth Analg. 2006;102(1):172–4.

3. Ehrenwerth J, Seifert HA. Fire safety in the operating room. ASA Refresher Courses in Anesthesiology. Am Soc Anesthesiol. 2003;31:25–33.

4. ECRI. The patient is on fire! A surgical fires primer (Guidance article). Health Devices. 1992;21(1):19–34.

5. Practice advisory for the prevention and management of operating room fires. (http://www.guideline.gov/content.aspx?id=12547&search=laser+safety).

6. US government guidelines for the risk classification of laser medical instruments and the use of medical lasers. (http://webstore.ansi.org/FindStandards.aspx?Action=displaydept&DeptID=310&Acro=ISO%20&DpName=ISO%20ICS%2031%20Electronics%20%28Laser%20Equipment,%20etc.%29).

7. Standards and safety supplies for medical laser use. (http://webstore.ansi.org/FindStandards.aspx?Action=displaydept&DeptID=310&Acro=ISO%20&DpName=ISO%20ICS%2031%20Electronics%20%28Laser%20Equipment,%20etc.%29).

8. Slinger P, Robinson R, Shennib H, Benumof J, Eisenkraft J. Alternative technique for laser resection of a carinal obstruction. J Cardiothorac Vasc Anesth. 1992;6(6):749–55.

9. Sesterhenn AM, Dünne A-A, Braulke D, Lippert BM, Folz BJ, Werner JA. Value of endotracheal tube safety in laryngeal laser surgery. Lasers Surg Med. 2003; 32(5):384–90.

Further Suggested Reading

Cerfolio RJ. Laser Bronchoscopy. In: Franco KL, Putnam JB, editors. Advanced therapy in thoracic surgery. Hamilton: BC Decker; 2005.

Sugarbaker DJ, Bueno R, Krasna M, Mentzer S, Zellos L, editors. Adult chest surgery. New York: McGraw-Hill; 2009.

Kaplan JA, Slinger PD, editors. Thoracic Anesthesia. Churchill Livingstone: Elsevier; 2003.

Chapter 28
Tracheal Stent Placement

David A. Silver

Keywords Airway stenting • Airway stenosis • Tube stents • Mesh stents • Stenotic lesion • Spirometry • Subglottic • Proximal tracheal lesions • Distal tracheal and carinal lesions • Endobronchial lesions

Introduction

Patients presenting for stenting of central airways typically have symptomatic, subcritical stenosis. The central concern is to provide safe anesthesia and surgical conditions without loss of the airway. Anesthetic strategy depends on the patient's condition, the location, severity and nature of the lesion, and the choice and deployment technique of the stent. A basic understanding of surgical techniques and stent types helps inform the anesthetic strategy. Not infrequently, the surgical plan unfolds based on the initial bronchoscopic exam, emphasizing the value of broad preparation and a flexible approach to these potentially high-risk cases.

Surgical Considerations

Indications for Airway Stenting

A number of options are available to treat airway stenosis of various causes (Box 28-1) (see also algorithm; Chapter 27).

P.M. Hartigan (ed.), *Practical Handbook of Thoracic Anesthesia*,
DOI 10.1007/978-0-387-88493-6_28, © Springer Science+Business Media, LLC 2012

Box 28-1 – Therapeutic Options for Central Airway Stenosis

- Balloon dilation
- Photodynamic therapy
- Cryotherapy
- Brachytherapy
- External beam radiation
- Core-out (mechanical or laser)
- Chemotherapy
- Tracheal resection/reconstruction
- Temporary or permanent stent

Box 28-2 – Potential Complications of Airway Stenting

- Airway obstruction
- Airway rupture/perforation/erosion
- Stent migration/misplacement/folding/fracture
- Fistula formation
- Impaired clearance of secretions
- Stent occlusion
- Infection
- Granuloma formation (especially at ends of bare metal stents)
- Halitosis

While stenting often provides immediate and dramatic relief of symptoms, it is fraught with important potential complications (Box 28-2), and so is commonly reserved for palliative or rescue situations (1). Airway stents require close management, including periodic bronchoscopic exams and intermittent adjustment,

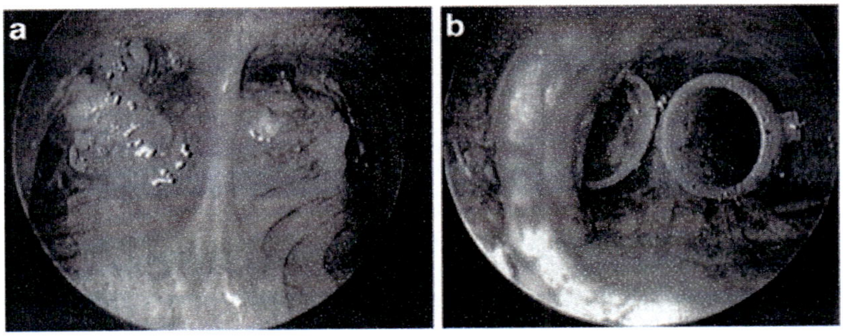

Figure 28-1 – Severe bilateral mainstem bronchial occlusion by locally advanced nonsmall cell lung cancer before (**A**) and after (**B**) stenting using two silicone tube stents. From Wood DE, Liu YH, Vallieres E et al. Airway stenting for malignant and benign tracheobronchial stenosis. Ann Thorac Surg. 2003;76:167–74.

maintenance, or replacement. The surgical decision to employ an airway stent is impacted by the patient's situation and prognosis, as well as the location and nature of the lesion.

Malignancy. In the setting of malignancy (Fig 28-1), airway stenting is primarily a palliative maneuver in patients who are not candidates for surgical resection, either due to extent of disease or prohibitive comorbidies. Stenting may be used in end-of-life palliation, or to temporize while adjuvant chemotherapy or external beam radiation takes effect to shrink tumor mass (2). Not infrequently, stenting of a malignant airway stenosis is the final step of a multimodality approach.

Anastomotic strictures. Post-lung transplant bronchial anastamotic complications occur in over 10% of recipients. While dilation and laser debridement are preferred initially in the management of these strictures, the use of airway stents provides rapid relief of dyspnea and is largely safe (3). Stent dislodgment (Fig 28-2), inspissation of secretions, and development of granulation tissue within stents are all common reasons for repeated bronchoscopy and intervention in the transplant population (3, 4). Strictures following sleeve resection or bronchoplasty may also rarely require stents.

Other indications. Other lesions which may require stenting include postintubation or posttracheotomy scar tissue, airway burn injuries, congenital or acquired tracheomalacia (rare), and

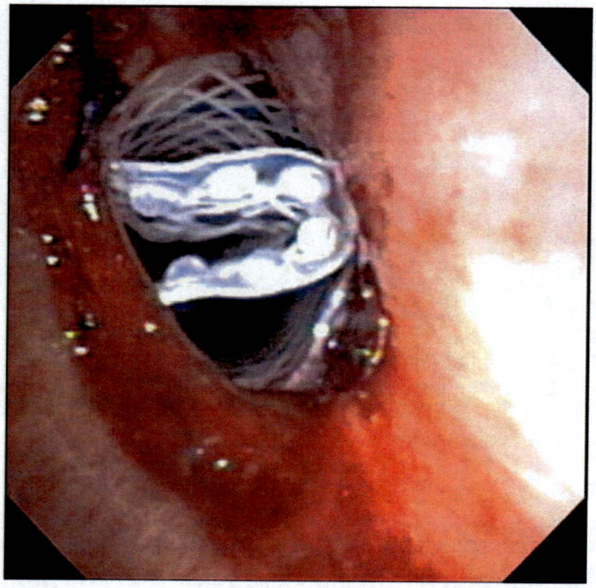

Figure 28-2 – Self-expanding stent at bronchial anastomotic stricture folding upon itself with partial bronchial occlusion.

inflammatory diseases (amyloidosis, relapsing polychondritis, amyloidosis, tuberculosis). Further nonmalignant indications for stenting include extraluminal compression due to aortic aneurysm, and laryngeal injury or stricture, in which tracheal stenting may be combined with tracheotomy. In recent years, the development of an array of stents designed for endovascular use has led to the application of these devices in small airways as well. Because patients with nonmalignant airway strictures generally have a longer life expectancy than those with cancer, they are more likely to need future interventions for airway maintenance, including cleanout, restenting, and eventual stent removal. Covered stents may also be employed for temporary or terminal occlusion of airway fistulae. In the case of tracheoesophageal fistula (TEF), an esophageal stent is generally preferred over a stent on the tracheal side. Use of adjacent stents (trachea and esophagus) is discouraged due to the risk of friction erosion of intervening tissue.

Surgical Approach

Airway stenting may involve a combination of suspension laryngoscopy, rigid bronchoscopy, or flexible fiberoptic bronchoscopy via LMA or ETT. In addition to surgical preference, the approach depends on the location of the stricture to be treated (from the subglottis to lobar airways), adjunctive therapies planned, and the type of stent to be employed. Increasingly, airway stent procedures are performed by interventional pulmonologists in endoscopy suite settings.

Stent Selection

Various types of stents are available for use (Fig 28-3 and Table 28-1). Compared to carinal and more distal lesions, a larger variety of stents are available for the trachea. Stents may also be custom manufactured.

Stents may be categorized by design (tube versus mesh) or by material (silicone versus metal). *Tube stents,* largely descendents of the Montgomery T-tube, are usually composed of silicone, are of fixed shape and diameter, radiolucent, and generally placed via rigid bronchoscopy. *Mesh stents* can be introduced in nonexpanded form over a guidewire, utilizing a flexible bronchoscope to position the guidewire and fluoroscopy to position the stent itself, and may be balloon-expanded or self-expanding (Fig 28-3) (4). Balloon-expandable stents should generally not be used in the central airways, as they are more likely to deform and migrate or dislodge with coughing. Bare metal stents have been associated with a disproportionate number of serious complications, including bronchial wall perforation, blood vessel laceration, stent dislodgment and fracture, and granuloma formation (5–7). All of the above, and patient intolerance, may be seen to some degree with any airway stent, but bare metal stents should generally be avoided in benign airway strictures as the risk of complications (including esophageal erosion) likely outweighs potential benefits (7).

Table 28-1 – Types of airway stents

STENT TYPE/ EXAMPLES	ADVANTAGES	DISADVANTAGES/RISKS
Silicone (Tube)		
Dumon, Endoxan (*Novatech, Abayone, France*) Dynamic Y, Freitag (*Rusch, Kernan, Germany*)	▪ Time-tested ▪ Easy to remove ▪ Resistant to tumor growth ▪ Resistant to granulation tissue	▪ Require rigid bronchoscope for placement ▪ High incidence of migration ▪ Eliminate mucociliary clearance ▪ Retained secretions ▪ Thick wall, low internal to external diameter ratio
Mesh (Metallic)		
Ultraflex (nitinol) Wallstent (elgiloy) (*Boston Scientific, Natick, MA*)	▪ With or without polyurethane coating ▪ Deploy with small sheaths or flexible bronchoscopy ▪ Reduced disruption of mucociliary clearance (uncovered stent) ▪ Less prone to migration ▪ Preserved airflow in subsegmental airways (uncovered stent) ▪ Less tumor ingrowth (covered stent)	▪ Granulation tissue buildup, especially at bare metal edges, leading to restenosis ▪ Significant shrinking and elongating with respiration/ coughing (Wallstent) irritates mucosa, elicit granulation response ▪ Incorporation into mucosa, difficult to remove ▪ Airway laceration, damage to adjacent (vascular) structures

After Walser EM, Stent placement for tracheobronchial disease. Eur J Radiology. 2005;55:321–30.

Anesthetic Considerations

Placement, deployment, or manipulation of an airway stent can be performed with sedation (dexmedetomidine, ketamine, etc.), but is often sufficiently stimulating to warrant general anesthesia.

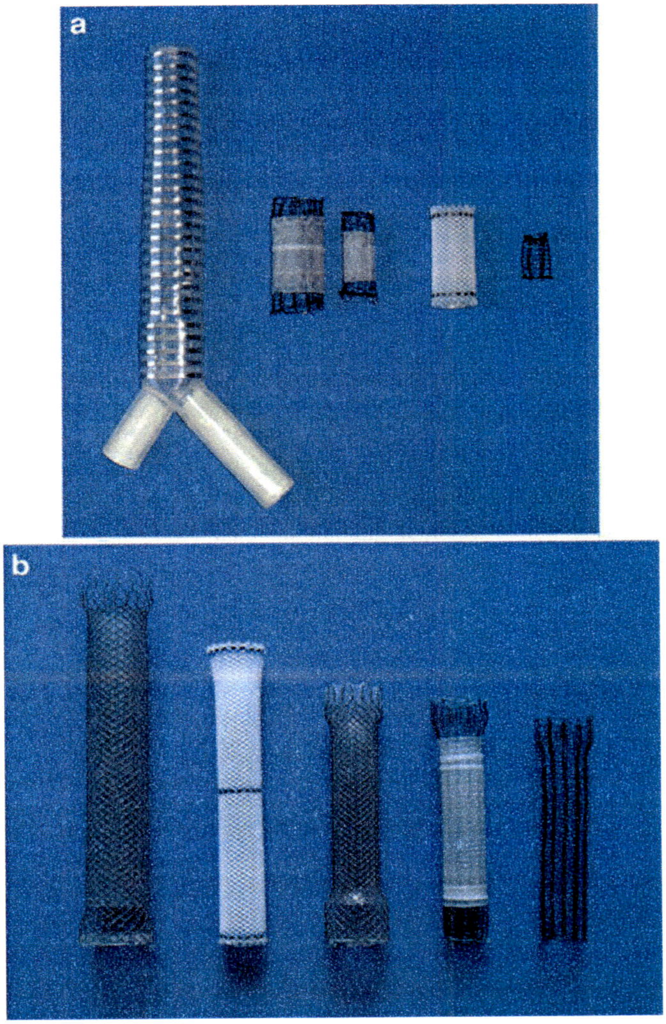

Figure 28-3 – Examples of various modern (**A**) tracheal/bronchial stents and (**B**) esophageal stents.

When airway patency is threatened by the lesion, defense of airway patency is the principal anesthetic concern. An overview strategy for anesthetic management is presented in Box 28-3, though variation may be dictated by the lesion (location, nature, and degree of stenosis), and the surgical approach (rigid vs. flexible bronchoscopy).

Box 28-3 – Overview: Anesthetic Management for Airway Stents for Tracheal Stenosis

- Initial flexible bronchoscopy:
  - Awake/sedated/topicalized vs. general anesthetic.
  - Direct vs. via conduit (LMA, ETT, etc.).
- Induction tailored to perceived threat to airway patency (based on imaging, symptoms, bronchoscopy, and known features of lesion) (see below).
- Establish ventilation. Reevaluate airway patency and security.
- Maintenance, tailored to extubation:
  - TIVA advantageous for intermittent apneic periods (especially if rigid bronchoscopy anticipated).
  - Judicious paralysis with attention to evolving surgical plan/duration.
- Provision for significant airway stimulation (remifentanil).
- Provision for potential intermittent inability to ventilate:
  - Hyperventilate prior to apneic periods when possible.
  - Monitor $PaCO_2$ rise "by-the-clock" (6 mmHg first minute, 3 mmHg/min thereafter).
  - Prepare to intervene with air insufflation, jet ventilation, intubation/LMA, or side-port ventilation via rigid scope.
- Back-up plans for lost airway:
  - Intubate beyond stenosis.
  - Ventilate via rigid bronchoscope passed beyond stenosis.
  - Temporize with insufflation or jet ventilation via catheter or flexible scope passed beyond stenosis.
  - Return to spontaneous ventilation or reposition if variable obstruction.
  - Emergent removal of folded stent or mass via rigid bronchoscope.
  - Dislodgement and temporary advancement of obstructing mass into mainstem bronchus, allowing OLV if removal is not immediately possible.

(continued)

Box 28-3 – (continued)

- Surgical airway access, including mediastinal tracheotomy via sternotomy for proximal tracheal obstructions (extremis).
- Contingency planning for emergent use of cardiopulmonary bypass or ECMO, where appropriate (controversial).

- Mitigation of coughing on emergence:
  - Remifentanil emergence.
  - Judicious longer acting narcotics.
  - Diligent toilet bronchoscopy prior to emergence.
  - Local anesthetic via bronchoscope to mucosal surfaces (limited efficacy and duration).
- Preparation for specific lesion-associated complications:
  - Spillage of postobstructive contents to "clean" areas of lung:
    - Toilet bronchoscopy.
    - Contaminated area in dependent position.
  - Massive hemoptysis:
    - Isolation of nonbleeding lung via selective endobronchial intubation.
    - Compression with ETT cuff or rigid bronchoscope (often double-lumen tube is most convenient).
    - Electrocautery (Fire hazard; must reduce FiO_2).
    - Angiographic embolization.
    - Convert to open surgical exploration.
  - Carcinoid crisis:
    - Octreotide (initial bolus for adults = 50 mcg).
    - Avoid Beta-adrenergic agonists.
  - Damage to aortic aneurysm:
    - Potential for endovascular stenting.
    - Emergent open repair.

Assessment of the Stenotic Lesion

Lesion assessment is based on history, imaging, spirometry (if available), and most importantly, an initial awake bronchoscopy when concern is significant.

History: Patients presenting for stents will generally have been previously assessed (including bronchoscopy). If available, pictures, video, or report from prior bronchoscopy is invaluable. Often the nature of the lesion is known (e.g., fixed stricture, dynamic extrinsic compression, tracheomalacia, etc.) as well as the extent of stenosis. A history of new or increased symptoms (wheezing, stridor, dyspnea, reduced exercise tolerance) suggests progression of stenosis, and the need for extra caution. Any positional preference should be sought and respected, and may indicate a variable component to the obstruction. Other historical data with management implications include:

- Hemoptysis (risk of hemorrhage with manipulation).
- Purulent expectoration or symptoms of infection (postobstructive pneumonia with potential for cross-contamination when obstruction is relieved).
- Symptoms of carcinoid syndrome.

Spirometry

Peak expiratory flow rate relates to the severity of obstruction (flow limitation). Flow-volume loops may distinguish between a fixed vs. variable obstructive lesion, but are effort dependent. Classically, fixed intrathoracic tracheal obstructions result in truncation of both expiratory and inspiratory limbs, while variable obstructions limit expiratory flow more than inspiratory flow. This distinction is germane because, in theory, variable obstructions are exacerbated by induction of general anesthesia while fixed obstructions are not (see Chapter 30). Often this is assumed from the nature of the lesion, but many lesions exhibit mixed features, with some variable component, and compromise of both inspiratory and expiratory airflow. *In general, patients who are symptomatic at rest should receive an awake bronchoscopic evaluation prior to induction* even if spirometry suggests a fixed obstruction.

Imaging

High-resolution CT scans are typically used to assess location and extent of stenosis. An "airway CT" is preferred, as it provides thinner cuts than a standard chest CT. 3D reconstructions (Fig 28-4) can provide details of a complex lesion and virtual bronchoscopic images. The position (proximal/distal), length, and tortuosity of the stenotic portion influence the anticipated ease of negotiating a tube or rigid bronchoscope beyond the lesion. For technical reasons, CT imaging may overestimate the degree of stenosis, reemphasizing the value of bronchoscopy.

There is no consensus as to the acceptable degree of radiographic stenosis for safe induction. Normal adult tracheal diameters range from 18 to 25 mm. Symptoms at rest occur when the tracheal lumen is reduced to approximately 5 mm. In children, a 50% reduction in tracheal cross-sectional area has been safely employed as the threshold beyond which airway stenosis from an anterior mediastinal mass should be treated more conservatively (8). Clearly other

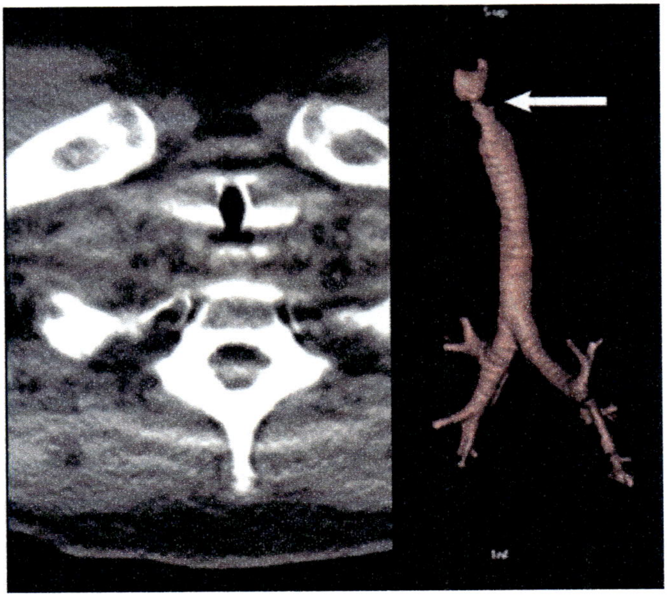

Figure 28-4 – Subglottic tracheal stenosis (*arrow*) due to Wegener's granulomatosis by CT scan and 3D reconstruction.

factors influence the approach to induction. Imaging can only help with what is ultimately a judgment: whether airway patency will be threatened by induction, and whether it can be rescued by intubating beyond the stenosis.

Imaging also provides information regarding related mass effects in the case of extrinsic compression (see Chapter 20). Contrast enhancement may reveal vascularity of the lesion, and risk of hemorrhage. Postobstructive pneumonia will also be evident on CT scan as well as CXR.

Location of Lesion

Subglottic, proximal tracheal lesions (e.g., stricture from a cuff injury) generally present a lower risk for loss of airway than distal obstructions. However, one needs to rule out serial lesions (such as with burn injury) which extend distally. This is best done by CT scan. Generally, high discrete stenotic lesions are fixed in nature. If variable (e.g., extrinsic compression by a mass) they can generally be easily rescued by advancing an ETT (or rigid scope in more dire circumstances). Exceptions include extremely tight or tortuous lesions, or certain inflammatory lesions (such as polychondritis) which may rapidly become edematous and completely obstructive when instrumented. The surgical approach for proximal tracheal lesions may be suspension laryngoscopy, or rigid or flexible bronchoscopy.

The risk of airway loss is higher with *distal tracheal and carinal lesions*. Because it is more difficult to negotiate a tube or rigid bronchoscope beyond the carina as a rescue maneuver, such lesions warrant a more conservative approach. Awake bronchoscopy is indicated prior to induction for patients with tight lesions who are symptomatic at rest, even if the obstruction is primarily fixed.

Endobronchial lesions pose limited risk, and induction of general anesthesia is generally safe if the contralateral lung is open and functional. If the contralateral lung is also compromised, however (Fig 28-1A), the airway should be approached with the caution accorded a distal tracheal lesion.

Induction

While the foregoing data helps assess risk, defense of airway patency with induction is never guaranteed, and backup plans and equipment must be available (Box 28-3). Strategies for safe induction with extrinsic variable tracheal obstruction are discussed in Chapter 20, while issues with fixed stenotic lesions are discussed further in Chapter 30. There is little to be lost by an awake, topicalized bronchoscopic exam prior to induction for worrisome cases. Once it is established that the stenosis can be negotiated with a scope or tube, induction can proceed.

Ventilation Issues

Following induction, some time should be spent reassessing the security of the airway, and hyperventilating in anticipation of interruptions in ventilation. Tight lesions may be completely obstructed by the presence of a bronchoscope or stent deployment device. Intermittent apnea is often required, and constant attention must be paid to the field, as events which may threaten ventilation (bleeding, edema, displacement or folding of stent, eruption of pus from postobstructive pneumonia, etc.) must be immediately recognized. When a stent is malpositioned and obstructive, the surgeon should immediately remove it via a rigid or flexible scope using forceps. If the latter is employed, extubation may be required to remove the stent (forceps, stent, and ETT removed together), followed by prompt reestablishment of an airway. Silicone "Y" stents for carinal placement (Fig 28-5) can be particularly difficult to pass through the glottis and often require multiple attempts, long periods of apnea, and can easily obstruct the airway if not seated properly. Alternatives for ventilation and other back-up plans for lost airway are listed in Box 28-3. Forethought and preparation are necessary to rapidly respond to the lost airway situation during stent procedures (Box 28-4).

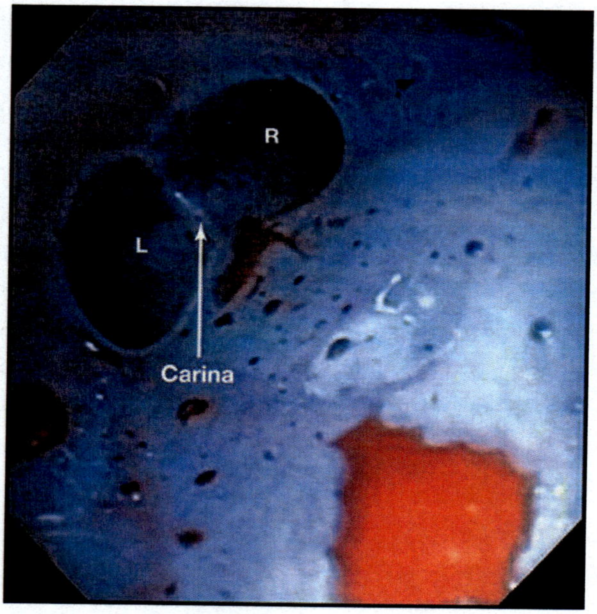

Figure 28-5 – Bronchoscopic view of silicone Y-stent in place at carina. The patient presented with distal tracheomalacia. R: right mainstem bronchus; L: left mainstem bronchus.

Box 28-4 – Recommended Equipment for Anesthesia for Tracheal Stenting

- Rigid bronchoscopes of various sizes, with long handled forceps.
- Appropriately sized LMAs with aperture bars\removed to facilitate bronchoscopy.
- ETTs of various sizes, including very small (5.0, 5.5, 6.0) in case of need to advance tube past lesion.
- Jet ventilator (Sanders or high frequency) with appropriate attachment for rigid bronchoscope and catheters for use in the airway.
- Magill forceps.
- Tracheostomy kit (if very proximal tracheal stenosis).

Emergence Strategies

Violent coughing can displace stents. Various strategies work to effect a smooth emergence, including remifentanil-based deep narcotic emergence, deep extubation, dexmedetomidine-based gradual emergence, aggressive use of local anesthetics to the airway, or combinations of the above. Narcotics are more important for their antitussive properties than their analgesic effects, since postprocedure pain is generally limited. Bronchoscopy is typically performed prior to emergence to assess stent position and patency, as well as to clear the airway of debris.

Other Stent-Related Procedures

Stenting is rarely performed for emergent relief of critical stenosis. This usually involves self-expanding metal stents, deployed via flexible scopes under topical local anesthesia and judicious sedation. More often, balloon dilation is the first maneuver to stabilize the patient and stenting is performed only after a more complete evaluation. In contrast to patients who undergo dilation or stenting, those who are merely being evaluated for planning (e.g., for creation of a custom stent) will not have immediate relief postoperatively, and may require ICU observation and management, including Heliox, depending on symptoms and the stability of the airway.

The patient with a *central airway fistula* may have a covered stent placed to control air leak [or lung soilage in the case of TEF]. Pinhole fistulas are straightforward because air leak is minimal. A large fistula is best approached with maintenance of spontaneous ventilation (asleep or awake), or better by immediate isolation of the fistula by contralateral endobronchial intubation. A double-lumen tube or endobronchial tube should be advanced under bronchoscopic guidance to prevent further disruption of the airway at the fistula site.

References

1. Wood DE, Liu YH, Vallieres E, et al. Airway stenting for malignant and benign tracheobronchial stenosis. Ann Thorac Surg. 2003;76:167–74.

2. Witt C, Dinges S, Schmidt B, et al. Temporary tracheobronchial stenting in malignant stenoses. Eur J Cancer. 1997;33(2):204–8.

3. Sonnett JR, Keenan RJ, Ferson PF, et al. Endobronchial management of benign, malignant and lung transplantation airway stenoses. Ann Thorac Surg. 1995;59:1417–22.

4. Rafanan AL, Mehta AC. Stenting of the tracheobronchial tree. Radiol Clin North Am. 2000;38(2):395–408.

5. Puma F, Farabi R, Urbani M, et al. Long-term safety and tolerance of silicone and self-expandable airway stents: an experimental study. Ann Thorac Surg. 2000;69:1030–4.

6. Zakaluzny SA, Lane JD, Mair EA. Complications of tracheobronchial airway stents. Otolaryngol Head Neck Surg. 2003;128:478–88.

7. Gaissert HA, Grillo HC, Wright CD, et al. Complication of benign tracheobronchial strictures by self-expanding metal stents. J Thorac Cardiovasc Surg. 2003;126:744–7.

8. Shamberger RC, Holzman RS, Griscom NT, Tarbell NJ, Weinstein HJ, Wohl ME. Prospective evaluation by computed tomography and pulmonary function tests of children with mediastinal masses. Surgery. 1995;118:468–71.

Further Suggested Reading

Carre P, Rousseau H, Lombart L, et al. Balloon dilatation and self-expanding metal Wallstent insertion for management of bronchostenosis following lung transplantation. Chest. 1994;105:343–8.

Conacher ID. Anaesthesia and tracheobronchial stenting for central airway obstruction in adults. Br J Anaesth. 2003;90:367–74.

Daumerie G, Su S, Ochroch EA. Anesthesia for the patient with tracheal stenosis. Anesthesiol Clin. 2010;28:157–74.

Korpela A, Aarnio P, Sariola H, et al. Bioabsorbable, self-reinforced poly-L-lactide, metallic, and silicone stents in the management of experimental tracheal stenosis. Chest. 1999;115:490–5.

Martinez-Ballarin JI, Diaz-Jimenez JP, Castro MJ, Moya JA. Silicone stents in the management of benign tracheobronchial stenoses: tolerance and early results in 63 patients. Chest. 1996;109:626–9.

Noppen M, Schlesser M, Meysman M, et al. Bronchoscopic balloon dilatation in the combined management of postintubation stenosis of the trachea in adults. Chest. 1997;112:1136–40.

Puma F, Farabi R, Urbani M, et al. Long-term safety and tolerance of silicone and self-expandable airway stents: an experimental study. Ann Thorac Surg. 2000;69:1030–4.

Strachan LM, Patey RE, Casson WR. Anesthesia and tracheobronchial stenting for central airway obstruction in adults (letter to the editor). Br J Anaesth. 2003;91(3):450.

Sonnett JR, Keenan RJ, Ferson PF, et al. Endobronchial management of benign, malignant and lung transplantation airway stenoses. Ann Thorac Surg. 1995;59:1417–22.

Walser EM. Stent placement for tracheobronchial disease. Eur J Radiol. 2005;55:321–30.

Zakaluzny SA, Lane JD, Mair EA. Complications of tracheobronchial airway stents. Otolaryngol Head Neck Surg. 2003;128:478–88.

Chapter 29
Anesthesia for Tracheotomy

David A. Silver

Keywords Tracheotomy • Tracheostomy • Risks/benefits of tracheotomy

Introduction

Tracheotomy, either percutaneous or open, is a procedure frequently performed by thoracic surgeons. Patients in need of tracheotomy are often critically ill, with an anticipated ongoing requirement for mechanical ventilation (MV). The principal anesthetic concern is *loss of the airway*. Other potential hazards include those associated with patient transport, airway fire, bleeding, and aspiration.

Tracheotomy and tracheostomy are often used interchangeably; the former refers to the operation, the latter refers to the opening created in the trachea. Tracheotomies may be emergent or elective, open or percutaneous, awake (local) or asleep, and in intubated or unintubated patients. The most common scenario is open, under general anesthesia in a chronically intubated patient from an ICU.

Surgical Considerations

Surgeons share the airway, as well as the principal concern (loss of airway), with their anesthesia team. Coordination of the tube exchange (endotracheal tube-for-tracheostomy cannula) as

P.M. Hartigan (ed.), *Practical Handbook of Thoracic Anesthesia*,
DOI 10.1007/978-0-387-88493-6_29,

described under section "Anesthetic Considerations" below is critical. Other surgical concerns may be summarized as follows:

Location of Procedure: Tracheotomy in the OR vs. ICU is both a logistical and clinical decision. The logistics of a bedside percutaneous tracheotomy are relatively simple, but anesthesia personnel and a bronchoscope should be on hand, and the patient's anatomy should be appropriate. Bedside open tracheotomy may increase the risk of infection, and of dealing with a lost airway. Equipment issues, lighting, and the width of ICU beds make bedside tracheotomies more challenging for the surgeon. But patients too unstable to transport may be better served by this option. The patient with a very difficult airway is better off in the OR, whereas those with cumbersome equipment (ventricular assist devices, renal replacement therapy, etc.) may be so challenging to move that it is better to bring the OR to the patient.

Proper Site: Generally, the level of tracheal rings 2–4 is chosen (Fig 29-1). More cephalad risks injury to the cricoid cartilage, and

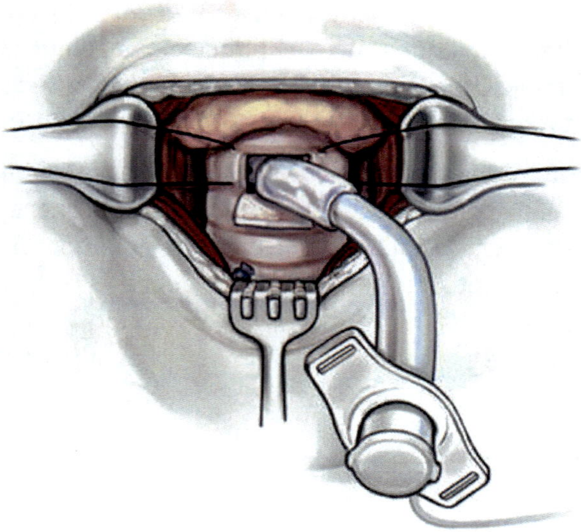

Figure 29-1 – Open surgical tracheostomy. A flap is created at the third tracheal cartilage and held open with hooks or stay sutures to admit an appropriately sized tracheostomy tube, which is advanced into the trachea with respect to its curvature. Just prior to this, the endotracheal tube was withdrawn just far enough to admit the tracheostomy tube. *(Reproduced with permission from Sugarbaker DJ, et al. editors. Adult chest surgery. New York: McGraw-Hill; 2009. Artwork copyright of Marcia Williams).*

subsequent subglottic stenosis. Too low may cause the cannula to abut the carina. The angle of the tracheostomy tube is designed for 2–4 cartilaginous rings. Pressure from a low tracheostomy tube or cuff on the innominate artery may result in erosion, fistula formation, and innominate bleeding (Fig 29-2).

Hemostasis: Electrocautery use after the trachea is open may result in fire (see below). Significant bleeding sources include the thyroid vessels and innominate artery. Bleeding from minor vessels may be problematic due to movement and rubbing of the cannula against the wound. An end-inspiratory hold maneuver (valsalva) may be useful at the end of the procedure to help identify small venous bleeding sources.

Choice of Cannula: Appropriate length, caliber, and curvature must be considered to prevent dislodgement with patient movement. Examples are depicted in Fig 29-3. Depth (skin-to-trachea distance) is most critical, as a cannula that is too short may retract into the wound. Fenestrated ("talking" trachs) or uncuffed tracheostomy

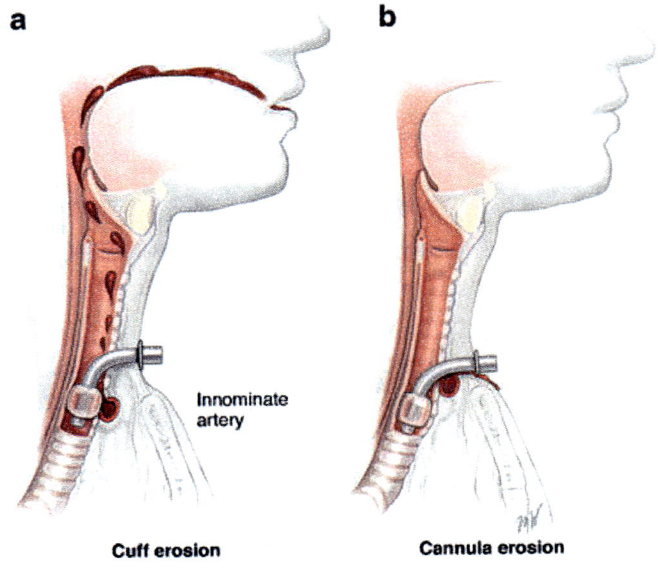

Figure 29-2 – Tracheo-innominate artery fistula may occur as a result of pressure from the cuff (**A**), or from a low lying tracheostomy cannula (**B**). *(Reproduced with permission from Sugarbaker DJ, et al. editors. Adult chest surgery. New York: McGraw-Hill; 2009. Artwork copyright of Marcia Williams).*

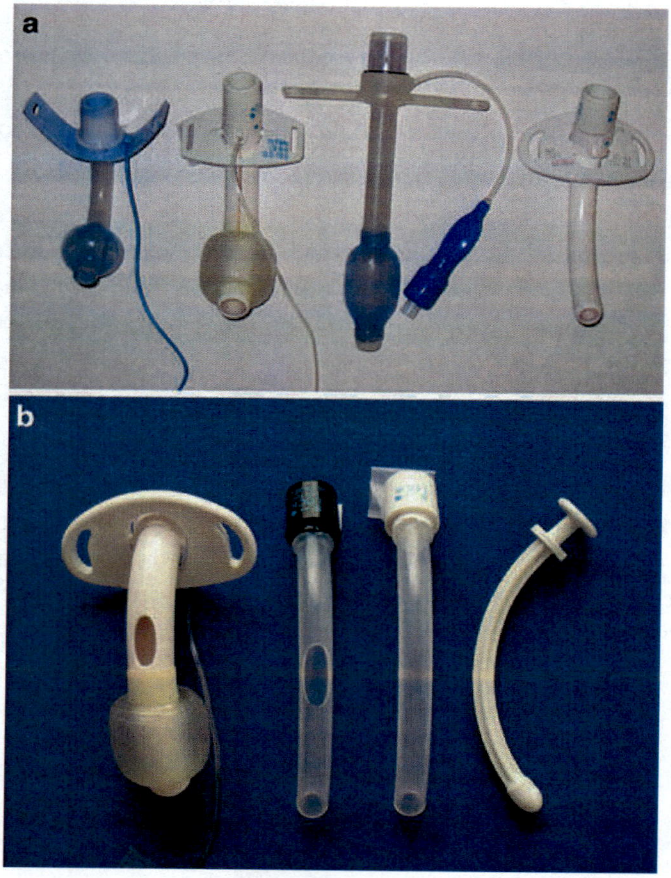

Figure 29-3 – (**A**) Examples of Tracheostomy Cannulae. (**B**) A fenestrated trach can accommodate either a fenestrated or a nonfenestrated disposable inner cannula. On the right is an obturator, used only in initial placement of the tracheotomy tube.

tubes are not generally employed at the time of initial surgical tracheotomy.

Safe Cannulation: This critical juncture is aided by use of tracheal hooks or stay sutures to maintain control of the trachea, and lift it anteriorly as the cannula is inserted. The cannula and tracheostomy must be appropriately sized, and *the existing ETT should not be withdrawn beyond the glottis until the tracheostomy cannula position is confirmed* (see section "Anesthetic Considerations," below).

Confirmation of Cannulation: Bronchoscopy is recommended to definitively rule out a partial false lumen (flap) which might provide end-tidal CO_2 return, but which is at risk for dissection or misplacement with transport or neck movement. Bronchoscopy also confirms proper depth and hemostasis, and allows removal of blood and secretions.

Percutaneous Tracheostomy: Kits are available which utilize the principles of the Seldinger Technique to advance a tracheostomy cannula into the trachea. Online instructional videos are available at http://www.cookmedical.com/cc/educationResource.do?id=Educational_Video.

Anesthetic Considerations

Timing/Location Decisions

Risks/benefits of tracheotomy are generally most favorable for the patient with chronic respiratory insufficiency (Table 29-1). Tracheotomy is generally ill-advised for patients in severe acute

Table 29-1 – Benefits of tracheostomy

- Increased patient comfort (decreased sedation/analgesia requirements)
- Decreased airway resistance, dead space, and work of breathing
- Ventilator-free intervals (facilitates separation from/return to mechanical ventilation)
- Decreased risk of aspiration
- More secure airway (less likely to dislodge)
- Enhanced patient mobility
- Potential to speak (e.g., Passy-Muir™-style one-way valve)
- Conduit for improved toilette bronchoscopy and suctioning
- Decreased risk of subglottic stenosis or vocal cord injury
- Decreased rate of sinusitis

Table 29-2 – Limitations of tracheostomy

▪ Loss of ability to cough
▪ Upper respiratory colonization
▪ Potential for cuff injury, stricture, or granulation tissue
▪ Impaired humidification (thicker, dryer secretions)

respiratory failure (excluding emergent), or those with high oxygen or PEEP requirements. Such patients may be at excessive risk for hypoxemia due to the low FiO_2 and interrupted or limited ventilation required during the open trachea phase. Patients with severe restrictive physiology and high PEEP requirements may suffer hypoxemia and derecruitment. ARDS patients may desaturate with manipulation, suctioning, or other minor perterbations. Transport of such patients may present risks that exceed benefits. Thresholds for cancellation (vs. bedside open, or percutaneous tracheotomy) require judgment, consideration of patient and surgeon factors, and dialogue with ICU and surgical staff. Postponement is worth considering if it is anticipated to reduce requirements for oxygen, PEEP, suctioning of copious secretions, hemodynamic support, etc. But this must be balanced against postponing the benefits of a tracheostomy (Table 29-2).

Other Preoperative Considerations

Factors relevant to reintubation should be assessed due to the risk of lost airway. These include physical exam, intubation records, and available imaging. Insights to surgical difficulties may also be appreciated, related to anatomy, obesity, anasarca, etc. Standard fasting guidelines apply; postpyloric (duodenal or jejunal) feeding tube nutrition need not be withheld, but gastric tube feedings should be held for 4–6 h. Coagulation parameters should be normal.

The extent of, and stability of ventilatory and hemodynamic support must be carefully considered.

Safe Transport

Before leaving the ICU, a period of ventilatory and hemodynamic stability should be demonstrated. If ambu bag ventilation is poorly tolerated, a portable ventilator may be employed, or the wisdom of transport should be reevaluated.

Patient Position

A transverse shoulder roll helps extend the neck, helps lifts the thyroid isthmus above the third tracheal ring, moves the chin out of the way, and delivers the trachea to a more anterior position. Self-evident considerations would apply for patients with unstable or fused cervical spines, or excessive adipose tissue about the neck. Rarely, the severe kyphotic which precludes a standard approach may require a mediastinal tracheotomy.

Anesthetic Choices

TIVA during the open trachea phase prevents gas exposure by personnel, but often this phase is so brief that TIVA is unnecessary. When performed in the ICU, TIVA is the most practical. Sufficient depth and/or paralysis are required to prevent movement with tracheal manipulation.

Entering the Trachea

With the strap muscles retracted, the thyroid isthmus divided or retracted, the pretracheal fascia incised, and hemostasis achieved, the trachea is entered with a knife (*not electrocautery*) at the third tracheal cartilage, and a flap is created (Fig 29-1). Two hazards must be avoided at this point:

1. Airway fire.
2. Ruptured ETT cuff by the surgical blade.

Airway Fire

Airway Fire is prevented by minimizing FiO_2 and eliminating use of electrocautery after entering the trachea. $FiO_2 < 0.4$ is desirable if electrocautery must be used. It takes time for the surgical environment's ambient oxygen levels to drop after turning down the FiO_2, since exhaled oxygen tension may still be high for a number of breaths. Apnea may be safer at this time. Saline to flood the field should be immediately available. Should a fire occur, the following steps must take place as concurrently and quickly as possible:

- Eliminate oxygen delivery.
- Flood field with saline.
- Remove ETT (and tracheostomy tube if in place).

After extinguishing the fire, the airway should be resecured by whatever means, and bronchoscopy should be performed to assess airway damage.

Ruptured ETT Cuff

Ruptured ETT Cuff is prevented by several strategies. One is to briefly deflate the cuff completely at the time the knife enters the trachea. A second strategy is to advance the ETT, positioning the cuff distal to the knife entry point. With the latter strategy, the cuff can remain inflated, preventing backflow of oxygen from the lungs. It also allows continued ventilation and use of higher FiO_2 for patients who do not tolerate low FiO_2 or apnea.

Cannulation

After creating and dilating the tracheostomy hole, the surgeon will be ready to insert the pretested tracheotomy device. He/she will request that the ETT be withdrawn slowly, until the tip is just above the tracheostomy opening. Three points deserve emphasis;

1. *Take care not to withdraw the ETT too far*. The surgeon will announce when to stop. If there is difficulty with cannulation, one would like the option of readvancing the ETT. If it

comes out beyond the glottis, this rescue maneuver is lost. Withdrawing the ETT over a bronchoscope or stylet in high risk airways may provide extra safety. Care should be exercised to avoid obstructing cannulation by "playing it safe."

2. *Suction secretions from the posterior pharynx prior to deflating the ETT cuff to prevent aspiration.* This is a simple point, but often forgotten, with potentially serious consequences.

3. *After cannulation (and cuff inflation), immediately pass the breathing circuit over the drapes to connect to the tracheostomy tube, ventilate, and observe for $ETCO_2$ and chest rise.*

With percutaneous tracheotomy, the presence of *a FOB in the airway* can ensure that the introducer needle, wire, and dilator are all appropriately placed, and can detect damage to the membranous trachea.

Confirmation

End-tidal CO_2, and surgical bronchoscopy are the most important confirmatory tests. As noted above, bronchoscopy via the tracheostomy rules out partial false lumen or flap, which might provide $ETCO_2$, but predispose to dissection or displacement. Bronchoscopy via the existing (partially withdrawn) ETT can help guide and confirm placement. This may be particularly valuable to surgeons during a difficult percutaneous tracheostomy (Fig 29-4).

Failure to Cannulate

If cannulation fails and the surgeon needs time to adjust his approach, the best option is to re-advance the oral (or nasal) ETT such that the cuff occludes, or is distal to the tracheostomy. This may be performed blindly, or over a stylet or bronchoscope. Alternatively, a small (sterile) ETT (e.g., 6.0 O.D.) may be placed through the tracheostomy by the surgeon, and connected to the circuit over the field. Endobronchial intubation is difficult to avoid with this technique. A sterile cannula connected to a jet ventilator would also work. A third (desperate) option, if the oral ETT is not able to be

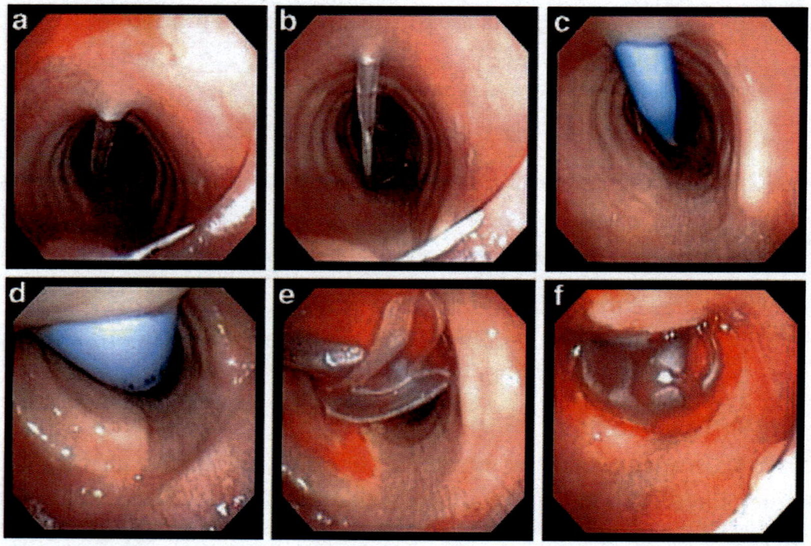

Figure 29-4 – A bronchoscope passed through an existing (partially withdrawn) endotracheal tube can help guide and confirm surgical efforts during a percutaneous tracheostomy. Photos confirm midline tracheal impalement and proper finder needle depth (**A**), guidewire advancement (**B**), dilation steps (**C, D**), cannula advancement with cuff deflated (**E**) and final position with cuff inflated (**F**).

advanced, is to ventilate by facemask, LMA, or jet, with the surgeon occluding the tracheostomy hole with his thumb. These latter are obviously temporizing maneuvers, and will not be adequate for patients with high PEEP requirements. Some surgeons elect to tie silk sutures through the ETT Murphy eye as a means to retrieve the ETT should it be dislodged above the glottis.

Transport

Flexible gooseneck connectors between the tracheostomy and ambu connector help prevent traction of the cannula against the wound. As with initial transport, patients with special ventilatory requirements (high PEEP, high flows, etc.) should undergo a trial with the ambu bag before leaving the operating room. If a fresh tracheotomy becomes decannulated, it is generally better to intubate orally than attempt to recannulate through the fresh wound.

Chapter 30
Tracheal Resection and Reconstruction

David A. Silver and Philip M. Hartigan

Keywords Tracheal surgery • Tracheal resection reconstruction • Induction considerations • Ventilation strategies • Orotracheal/endobronchial intubation for TRR • Intubating over the field

Introduction

Tracheal surgery requires close teamwork between the anesthesia and surgical teams in both planning and execution, with ongoing communication throughout, as they "share the airway." Critical aspects of anesthetic management particular to tracheal resection/reconstruction (TRR) are *(1) preservation of a patent airway with induction* and *(2) safe ventilation while the airway is divided.*

Carinal pneumonectomy is considered here as well, as the concerns of airway manipulation and instrumentation are similar to those of tracheal resection. More distal resections involving an airway anastomosis, such as subcarinal sleeve resection, are covered elsewhere in this text (Chapter 21).

P.M. Hartigan (ed.), *Practical Handbook of Thoracic Anesthesia*,
DOI 10.1007/978-0-387-88493-6_30, © Springer Science+Business Media, LLC 2012

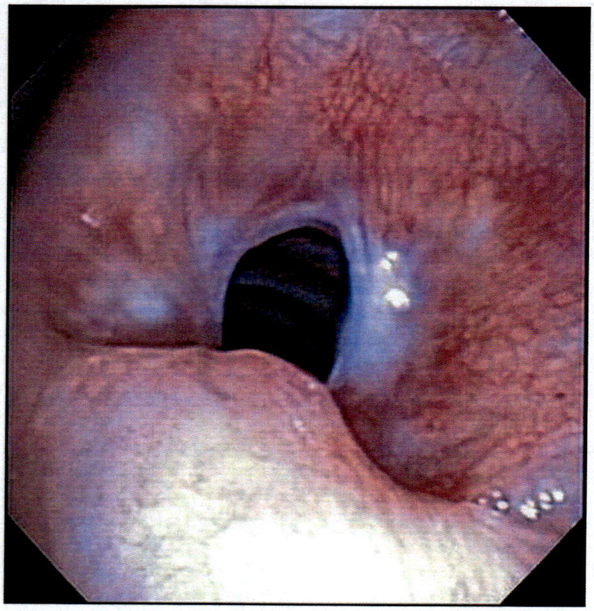

Figure 30-1 – Tracheal stenosis from scarring, following cuff injury.

Lesions treated with tracheal resection include "benign" *strictures* (such as those resulting from prolonged intubation or tracheotomy) (Fig 30-1), *tracheomalacia* (Fig 30-2), and tracheal *neoplasms* (Fig 30-3). Patients with tracheal lesions may present with associated wheezing or stridor (at airway diameters of <5–6 mm), hemoptysis, SVC syndrome, and chronic bronchitis, depending on the etiology of the lesion, and are occasionally misdiagnosed with asthma.

Surgical Considerations

The principal surgical considerations are to accomplish the appropriate resection and create an anastomosis that heals. Surgical decisions include the trade-off between optimal oncologic margins and a tension-free anastomosis. Excessive tension, disruption of circulation, infection, and prolonged positive pressure ventilation

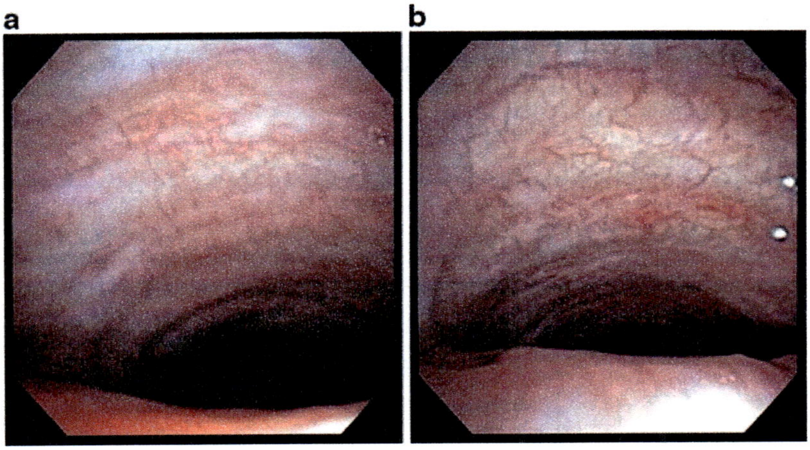

Figure 30-2 – Tracheomalacia is defined as weakening of the cartilaginous walls of the trachea. This figure depicts the trachea of a 64-year-old male with severe dyspnea on exertion due to tracheomalacia from recurrent infections. Note that at end inspiration (**A**), the airway is patent, but seen at the same level at end expiration (**B**), the coronal dimensions of the trachea broaden allowing membranous impingement on the lumen, and the anterior–posterior dimensions become stenotic resulting in expiratory obstruction (photos courtesy of Armin Ernst, M.D.).

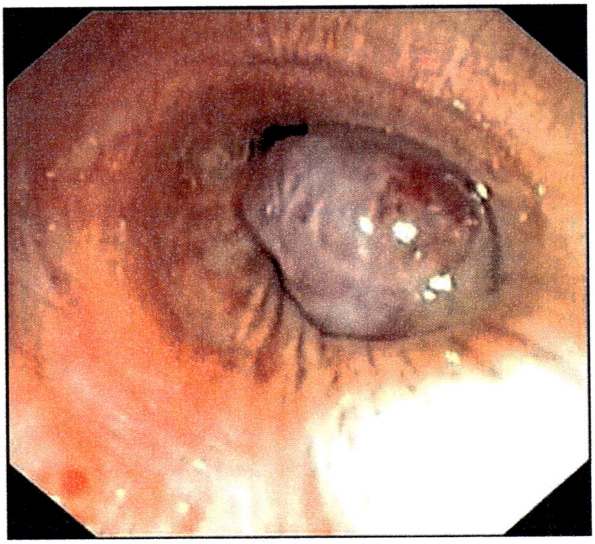

Figure 30-3 – Endoluminal carcinoid tumor.

Table 30-1 – Surgical strategies to prevent tracheal anastomotic failure (note that some depend on anesthetic management)

▪ Limit resection to < 6 cm. More than 6 cm is considered an "extended" tracheal resection
▪ Minimize steroids
▪ Avoid extensive lymph node dissection or skeletonization (devascularization) of tracheal ends
▪ Mobilize trachea by division of inferior pulmonary ligament and/or suprahyoid laryngeal release (principally, for extended resections only)
▪ Attention to suture tension (approximate to prevent air leak, but not strangulate tissue at anastomosis)
▪ Reinforce anastomosis with circumferential vascular tissue flap (intercostal muscle, pericardium, omentum, etc.)
▪ Minimize edema
▪ Maintain neck flexion during emergence and post-op with "guardian" suture between chin and chest
▪ Prevent post-op retching, coughing, agitation, etc.
▪ Minimize positive pressure ventilation to the anastomosis

are considered threats to healing (Table 30-1). Early resection on a virgin trachea fares better than a more extensive resection following repeated palliative procedures (stents, core-outs, etc.). At this writing, no suitable prosthetic tracheal device is available, but tissue-engineered tracheal prostheses and tracheal allotransplantation hold promise (1).

Immediate postoperative extubation is a strong preference of most surgeons to avoid potential disruption of the anastomosis by direct tube trauma or neck hyperxtension from a thrashing patient. Positive pressure ventilation exerts pressure against the anastomosis, but the impact of this is controversial. Higher pressures are typically generated by coughing. ICU monitoring postoperatively is generally indicated.

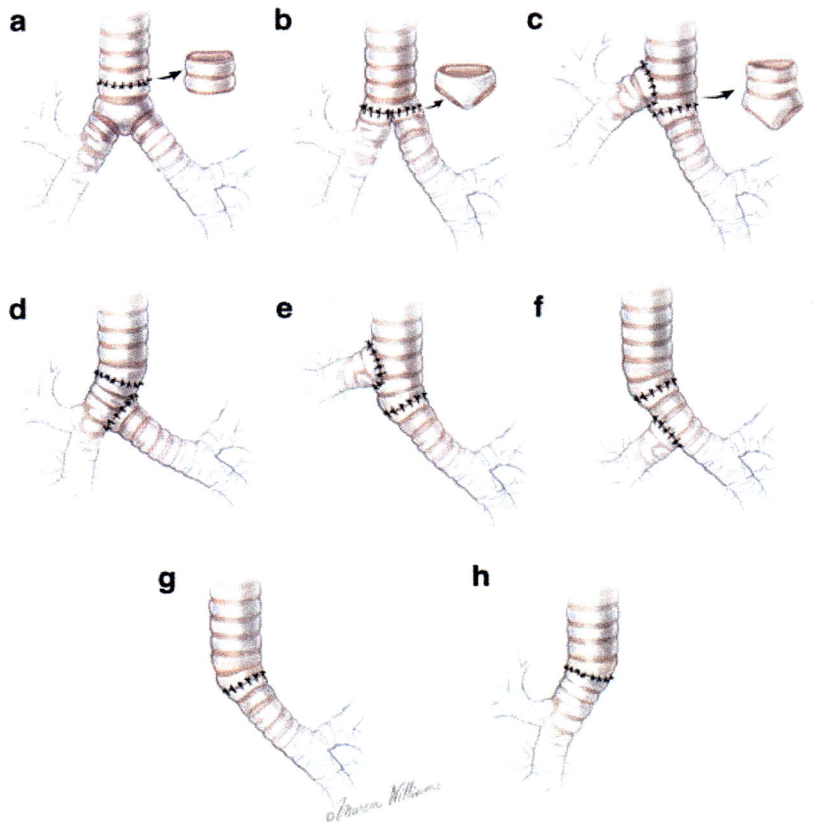

Figure 30-4 – Examples of various options for tracheal/carinal resection/ reconstruction. (**A**) Simple sleeve resection of trachea. (**B–F**) Carinal resections with end-to-end and end-to-side anastomoses. (**G** and **H**) Carinal pneumonectomy. *Adapted with permission from Sugarbaker DJ. Adult Thoracic Surgery. Copyright Marcia Williams 2009.*

The surgical plan is dictated by the location of the lesion. For distal tracheal/carinal lesions, many options exist (Fig 30-4), generally approached by right thoracotomy, median sternotomy, or clamshell incision. High tracheal lesions are approached by neck incision or sternotomy. The surgical anastomosis strategy impacts anesthetic plans for ventilation during the period of open airway.

Early complications of TRR include air leak or frank dehiscence, pneumonia, aspiration, and atrial arrhythmias. Later complications include stenosis or excessive granulation tissue at the anastomosis. Emergent reintubation is to be assiduously avoided due to the danger of mechanical disruption of the repair. Precipitators include subcutaneous emphysema from coughing, failure to clear thick secretions, aspiration of blood or gastric contents, glottic edema following subglottic TRR, and oversedation. When concern is high, some surgeons perform a prophylactic tracheostomy.

Anesthetic Considerations

The principal anesthetic considerations for TRR may be organized as follows, and are elaborated upon below:

- Preoperative assessment of risk of airway obstruction with anesthesia
- Induction considerations
- Safe ventilation during open airway phase
- Early extubation
- Mitigation of stress to anastomosis

Preoperative Assessment of Risk of Airway Obstruction

Induction of general anesthesia may potentially convert subcritical airway obstruction to critical. Assessment of this risk is ultimately a judgment, based on history, physical examination, and available radiolologic and spirometric data. As with any tight airway, an awake, bronchoscopic exam should be performed prior to induction when there is significant concern or doubt about the ability to defend a patent airway with induction.

Radiologic data should be reviewed with particular attention to the following.

Lesion location (upper, mid, or lower trachea or carina). *Proximal lesions* are of lower risk when there is room beyond the lesion to position an endotracheal tube (ETT) to stent open the airway.

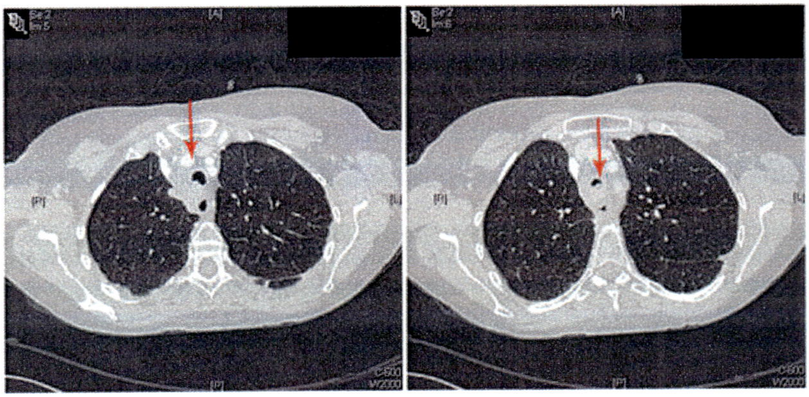

Figure 30-5 – Tracheal obstruction (*red arrows*) on sequential slices of high-resolution chest CT demonstrate a tortuous stenotic lumen.

Lower tracheal and *carinal lesions* are of higher risk because it is more difficult to negotiate an endobronchial tube or rigid bronchoscope into a mainstem bronchus as a rescue maneuver.

Caliber and position of airway lumen. There is increased risk when lumen is small, displaced, or tortuous (Fig 30-5) (see also Chapter 20). One should bear in mind that images are generally obtained during deep inspiratory hold.

Length of stenotic portion. Long or multiple stenotic regions pose higher risk.

Tracheomalacia. The presence or extent of malacia may be evident from CT, but often requires bronchoscopy.

Vascularity of lesion (contrast-enhanced CT). High vascularity or a history of hemoptysis obviously implies greater risk of bleeding and may predict a friable lesion which is easily disrupted by intubation.

Timing of the radiographic study. An airway lesion may have progressed since imaging was obtained.

History and physical examination should seek to delineate respiratory reserve. Surprisingly tight airway lesions may be asymptomatic at rest, but unmasked by exertion. In general, symptoms become evident in adults when tracheal diameter is <6 mm. Increased respiratory demand and airflow velocity may lead to increased turbulence of airflow, dyspnea, wheezing (intrathoracic obstruction), and work of breathing in patients with minimal symptoms at rest. A positional nature of symptoms would be important to note, particularly if the supine position elicits dyspnea or coughing. Disproportionate respiratory distress may be reported during upper respiratory infections as small changes in the diameter (due to secretions or edema) have dramatic effects on airflow in already stenotic airways.

Functional status assessment includes careful questioning of the patient regarding *orthopnea*, as well as both objective and subjective *limitations to inspiratory and expiratory flow (supine vs. upright, rest vs. exertional)*, in an attempt to predict the patient's respiratory reserve, tolerance for the supine position, and induction of anesthesia.

Fixed vs. Variable Obstructive Lesions

Fixed obstruction: A purely fixed tracheal stenosis is unaffected by the respiratory cycle or induction of anesthesia. Lesions such as circumferential anastomotic scars or endotracheal intubation-related stenoses, are examples. Flow limitation and symptoms (stridor) are evident with both inspiration and expiration.

Variable obstruction: Most lesions have a variable component such that the degree of obstruction is exacerbated by position, respiratory cycle, thoracic volume, or in some cases by a ball valve effect. The FRC reduction associated with anesthesia tends to worsen variable tracheal obstructive lesions. The classic scenario of an anterior mediastinal mass is such an example (Chapter 20), but intraluminal tumors may behave as variable obstructions as the membranous trachea bows further anterior with the FRC effect of anesthetic induction.

In theory, fixed tracheal stenoses are not exacerbated by induction. In practice, most lesions have some dynamic component and deserve respect if tight or symptomatic. Even fixed stenoses may become more obstructive with manipulation, mucosal edema, hematoma, displacement of existing stents, or other intraoperative events.

Flow-volume loops are not essential, but if available can help distinguish fixed from variable obstructions (and may be useful as a baseline for follow-up). Classically, with variable intrathoracic obstruction, expiratory flow is compromised more than inspiratory flow, whereas a fixed obstruction limits both inspiratory and expiratory flow equally (Fig 30-6).

With mild/moderate stenosis, flow is relatively laminar and governed roughly by the Poiseuille relationship in which resistance is inversely proportional to the radius raised to the fourth power. With more severe stenosis (or at branch points, such as the carina), flow becomes increasingly turbulent, and density and flow rate become more prominent determinants of the pressure difference (proximal vs. distal to the obstruction) (2). (See Appendix below.) Lower velocity air flow or lower density gas mixtures (heliox) may restore more laminar flow.

Induction Considerations

If there is concern about airway patency following induction, several questions should be addressed.

- *Can this patient be ventilated* by mask or laryngeal mask airway (LMA)?
- *Can this patient be intubated*?
- *Is intubation beyond the lesion a viable rescue maneuver for this patient*?
- Is *rigid bronchoscopy* a viable option in case of difficulty with oxygenation or ventilation, or if significant bleeding develops?
- What is the likelihood of provoking *significant airway hemorrhage*?

If the answer to any of these is unclear, caution dictates an initial *awake fiber optic examination* of the trachea. Awake placement of an LMA with topical anesthesia can provide a convenient conduit for bronchoscopy with delivery of high FiO_2. *If there is concern that airway patency will be worsened or lost by induction* (e.g., variable or

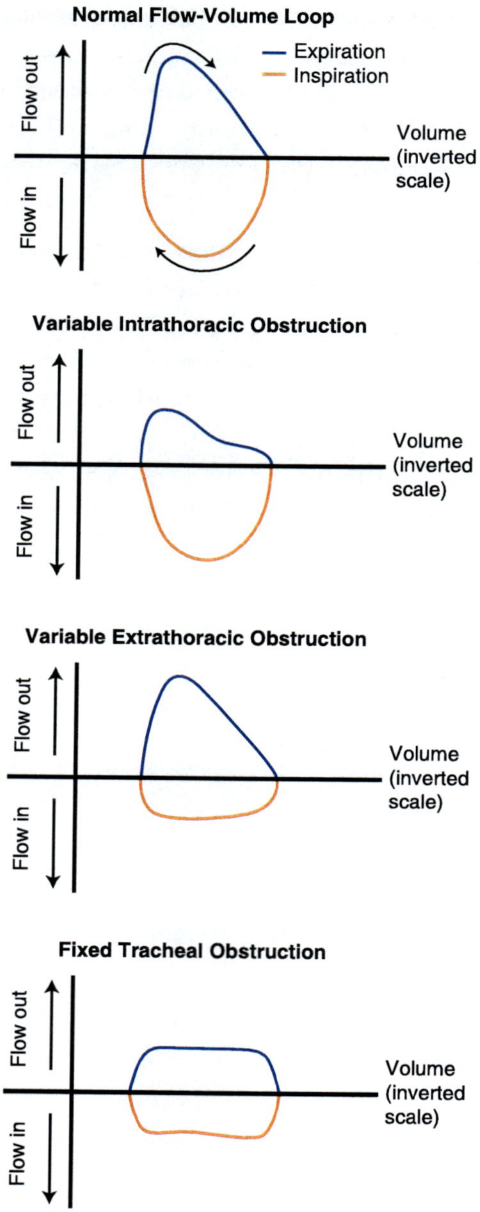

Figure 30-6 – Flow-volume loops for fixed and variable obstructions are contrasted with normal. Figures are idealized. In actual spirometry, volumes would be reduced for all forms of obstruction and the effect on flow would rarely be confined to just the inspiratory or expiratory limb. However, intrathoracic obstructions predominately reduce expiratory flow and produce a "scooping" shape while extrathoracic obstructions affect inspiratory flow more than expiratory. Fixed tracheal obstructions affect both inspiration and expiration relatively equivalently.

extremely tight fixed obstruction) and the awake bronchoscopy is nonreassuring, one should:

- *Maintain patient-preferred position* (usually, sitting up)
- *Maintain spontaneous ventilation* (inhalation induction, no neuromuscular blockade)
- *Stent open stenotic portion with small ETT if possible prior to induction* (unless tissue is particularly friable or hemorrhagic)
- *Have a backup plan available* (rigid bronchoscopy, rapid return to awake, etc.)
- *Consider Heliox*
- *Prepare for emergent extracorporeal support* (ECMO, cardiopulmonary bypass) (controversial)

Many of the guidelines outlined for anterior mediastinal masses (Chapter 20) also apply here, except that gravitational (positional) effects are less important.

Other Anesthetic Choices

- Spontaneously breathing inhalational induction may be preferred (controversial).
- General anesthetic tailored to immediate extubation at conclusion of surgery.
- Total intravenous anesthesia (TIVA) during open airway phase.
- Relative narcotic-sparing techniques to minimize reintubation risk.
- Thoracic epidural to optimize analgesia for thoracotomy or clamshell approaches.

Ventilation Strategies During Open Airway

Aside from accomplishing safe induction, this is the most critical set of decisions for anesthetic management of TRR. The options fall into several categories (Table 30-2). The prudent anesthesiologist is

Table 30-2 – Options for ventilation during open airway

- Orotracheal intubation:
  - Via standard ETT for discrete proximal lesions (Fig 30-7 and 30-10A)
  - Via a long endotracheal or endobronchial tube for more distal lesions. Options include:
    - Double-lumen tube with distal tracheal lumen cut away (Fig 30-8)
    - Straightened nasal Rae tube (passed orally)
    - "Extended" ETT made by connecting two standard endotracheal tubes (Fig 30-9)
    - Specialty endobronchial tube (limited availability in the USA)
- Intubation from the surgical field
  - Into open trachea or mainstem bronchus via an ETT and sterile circuit passed over the drapes (Fig 30-10)
- Jet ventilation
  - May be delivered via orotracheal route or via the surgical field directly into the airway (Fig 30-10)
- Combined ventilatory techniques
  - In distal tracheal/carinal resections, one lung may be selectively intubated either from the trachea or via the surgical field, and the other may be oxygenated via apneic oxygenation, insufflation, CPAP, jet ventilation, or positive pressure ventilation via a second tube and separate ventilator (Fig 30-10)

prepared for all eventualities because the surgical plan may change Box 30-1. Generally, the choice is dictated by the lesion position and the surgical plan.

Proximal tracheal lesions and limited mid-tracheal lesions which permit distal passage of an ETT are relatively simple. They may require a customized elongated tube or endobronchial intubation. Surgeons can often work around a small ETT. One must be prepared for accidental rupture of the ETT cuff by surgical knife or needle. Replacement of the tube may require the use of a fiber optic bronchoscope or tube exchange catheter. Alternatively, the surgeon can

Box 30-1 – Specialized Equipment for TRR Ventilation

- Sterilized anesthesia machine circuit and $ETCO_2$ sampling line.
- Standard ETT.
- Sterile 10-mL syringe for ETT cuff on field.
- Extra-long ETTs (straightened nasal rae, connected standard tubes, or modified double-lumen tubes).
- Tube exchange catheter.
- Various sizes armored ETTs, in sterile packaging.
- Jet ventilator with associated sterile catheters.
- If two lungs are to be ventilated separately, means for ventilation of each (mechanical ventilator, bag-valve device, jet ventilator, CPAP attachment) available.

tie a heavy suture to the distal end of the first ETT, which can then be swapped to the distal end of the new ETT after extubation and used to guide (pull) the new tube into position. Some situations require backing the tube out for brief periods and re-advancing it. When withdrawn, if the airway is open distally, positive-pressure ventilation must be suspended. If apnea is prolonged, ventilation can resume by intubating distally over the field, by jet ventilation, or by re-advancing the original ETT intermittently. The surgeon relies on the anesthesiologist to inform him when ventilation is necessary. Tracking $PaCO_2$ by the relatively predictable rate of rise over time (6 mmHg the first minute followed by 3 mmHg/min thereafter) can be useful.

Distal tracheal and carinal lesions generally require significant periods of apnea and intubation of at least one mainstem bronchus over the field.

Technical Aspects of Orotracheal/Endobronchial Intubation for TRR

Surgeons can often perform much of their work around a small ETT which has been advanced (via oral route) beyond the distal divi-

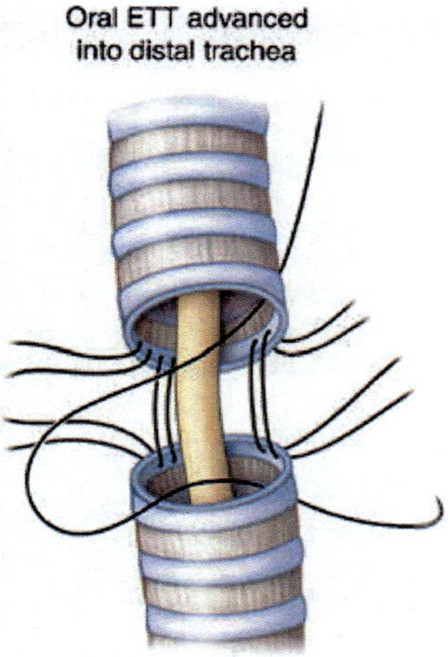

Figure 30-7 – A simple high-sleeve tracheal resection may be performed largely or entirely around a small endotracheal tube.

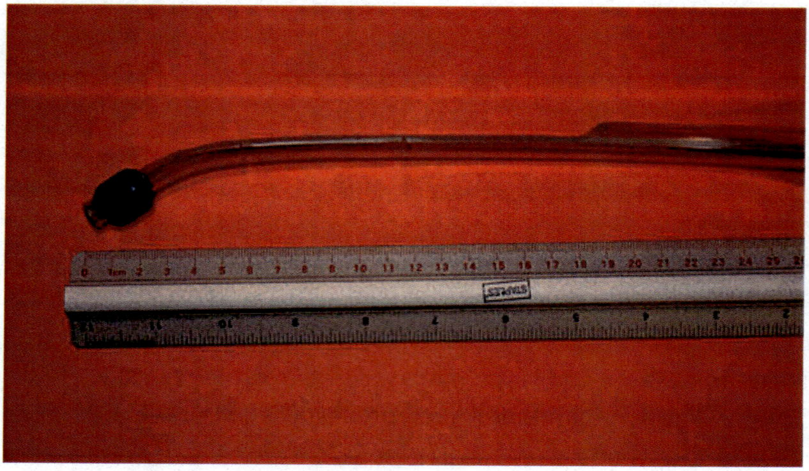

Figure 30-8 – A modified double-lumen endotracheal tube created by cutting off the distal portion of the tracheal lumen, along with the tracheal cuff. Special care must be exercised to smooth out sharp edges (personal communication courtesy of Paul Alfille, M.D.).

sion of the airway (Fig 30-7). The cuffed tip may be in the distal trachea for very high lesions or more commonly in a mainstem bronchus (one-lung ventilation). The ideal tube for this should be extra long, and have a short distance from the top of the cuff to the tip of the tube. This cuff-to-tip distance varies with tube type, size, and

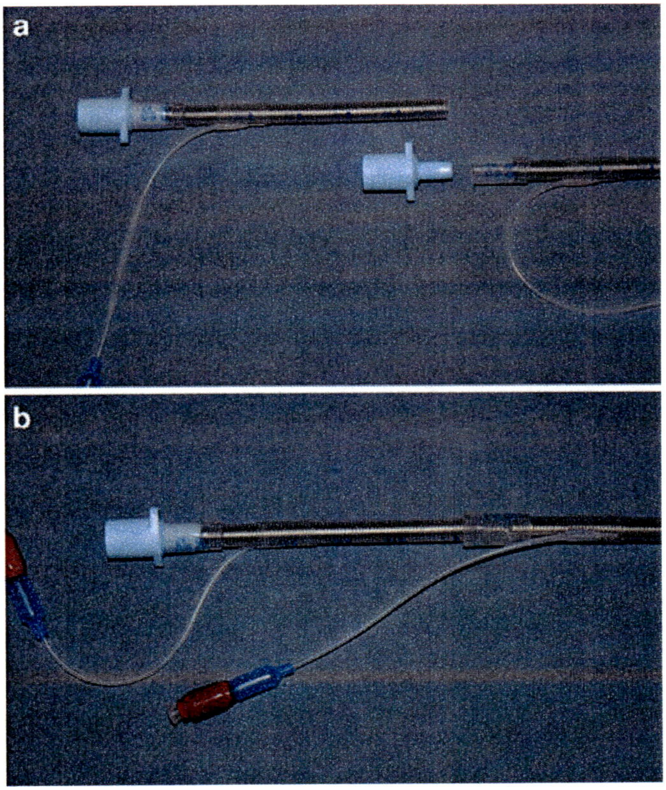

Figure 30-9 – Extended tubes may be created by removing the 15-mm connector and inserting the distal (cut) end of a second tube. A sleeve of PVC makes an effective friction seal to prevent detachment. The tube(s) pictured (Phycon, Fuji Systems Corp, Fukushima-Ken, Japan) are wire reinforced, have relatively short cuff-to-tip distance, and come with a PVC sleeve in place (personal communication courtesy of Paul Alfille, M.D.).

manufacturer. Simply trimming the distal tip of an ETT typically renders the cuff incompetent. Endobronchial tubes especially designed for this are not available in the USA at this writing, but are available in Europe. Certain laser-resistant tubes (e.g., Laser-Flex, Mallinckrodt Inc. St Louis, MO) have double-cuff systems, and if only the distal cuff is utilized, the cuff-to-tip distance is short. Other creative alternatives include options listed in Table 30-2. The bronchial cuffs of double-lumen tubes are favorably designed for TRR. One alternative is to "trim" the distal portion of the tracheal lumen from a standard double-lumen tube (including removing the tracheal cuff), yielding what is effectively a single-lumen endobronchial tube with a very short, distal cuff-to-tip distance (3) (Fig 30-8). The remnant of the tracheal lumen continues to offer access to the upper airway for suctioning, bronchoscopy, jet ventilator tubing, etc.

Adequate length is also an important feature for endobronchial tubes. Nasal Rae tubes have sufficient length when straightened out and passed orally. Tubes can also be extended by end-to-end connections using PVC tubing with tight friction fitting (Fig 30-9).

When utilizing an orotracheal/endobronchial tube strategy, one must be prepared for cuff rupture by the surgeons or requests to withdraw or advance the tube. If one-lung ventilation is not tolerated, one must be prepared to convert to other techniques, including combined ventilatory techniques (see below).

Technical Aspects of Intubating Over the Field for TRR

One should always be prepared to ventilate "over the field" during TRR, whether as the planned ventilation strategy or as a rescue maneuver. It is imperative to have a sterile breathing circuit, sterile CO_2 sampling tubing, and an array of tubes available. The surgeon intubates the divided trachea or bronchus, inflates the cuff, attaches the circuit to the ETT, and hands the proximal limbs of the circuit (with CO_2 sample line) over the drapes to be attached to the ventilator. As noted above, a short cuff-to-tip distance is desirable for the ETT to avoid intubating too deeply. The tube is often intermittently removed to provide surgical access, requiring coordinated efforts to ensure safe gas exchange. At times, it may be secured in place with a tight curvature. Wire-reinforced tubes are advantageous for this as

Figure 30-10 – Various options for ventilation during distal tracheal resection/reconstruction. (**A**) For high discrete tracheal resections, surgeons can sometimes work around a small single-lumen tube. The tube can be also transiently withdrawn above the lesion with a period of apnea if necessary. (**B**) Distal tracheal or carinal resections often can be managed with a single-wire-reinforced endobronchial tube placed "over the field" and withdrawn as the last few anterior sutures are placed. (**C**) When oxygenation is unsatisfactory with single-lung ventilation, it may be supplemented by various combinations of one-lung ventilation with air insufflation, CPAP, jet ventilation, or separate, independent, two-lung ventilation using a second tube passed via the trachea or over the field or a small gage catheter passed via the ETT or over the field. Modified from Sugarbaker DJ, et al. Adult Chest Surgery. McGraw-Hill, 2009. Illustration by Marcia Williams MSMI.

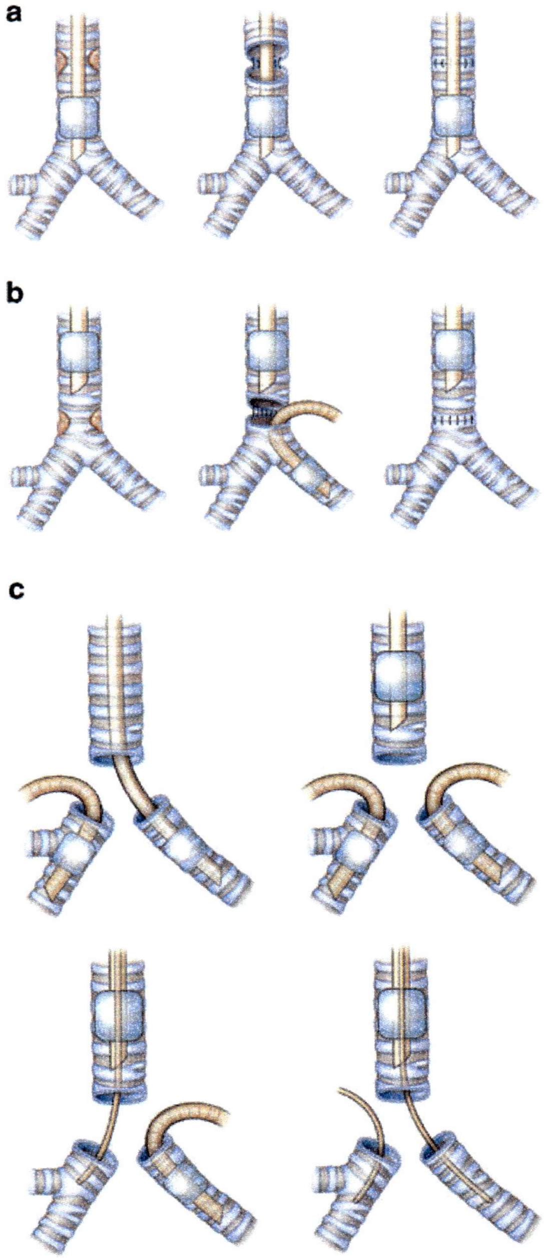
a
b
c

they are flexible and resist kinking (Fig 30-11). Laser-Flex[R], laser-resistant metal tubes (Mallinckrodt, Inc, St Louis, MO), also resist kinking and have a short cuff-to-tip distance when just the distal cuff is inflated. If the right bronchus requires intubation, often right upper lobe ventilation must be sacrificed and the tube is secured in the bronchus intermedius.

Combined Ventilatory Techniques

Under some circumstances, especially during carinal reconstruction, there may be a need to ventilate each lung separately. If this is anticipated, potential strategies include:

- A single endotracheal or over-the-field endobronchial tube intermittently repositioned by bronchoscope or surgical manipulation
- One ETT directed to a mainstem bronchus, and another positioned over the field into the opposite bronchus
- A jet ventilator catheter positioned either endotracheally or over the surgical field into the bronchus opposite a tube
- Two small ETTs, both through the vocal cords, one into each mainstem bronchus

If separate, simultaneous (non-jet) ventilation of both lungs is desired, a second anesthesia or portable/transport ventilator may be employed or a manual (Ambu™ style) bag may be used. Often, very slow respiratory rates and small tidal volumes suffice. Alternatively, a continuous positive airway pressure (CPAP) attachment may be used, unilateral jet ventilation may be employed, or the lungs may be ventilated on an alternating basis.

Technical Aspects of Jet Ventilation for TRR

Jet ventilators deliver pulses of oxygen from a high-pressure source (20–50 psi) via a narrow-orifice attachment or catheter placed

Box 30.2 – Potential Disadvantages of Jet Ventilation

- Risk of barotrauma and volutrauma.
- FiO^2 cannot be readily measured.
- Tidal volume cannot be readily measured.
- $ETCO_2$ cannot be easily monitored to assess adequacy of ventilation.
- Dry (nonhumidified) gas may cause inspissated secretions and pulmonary dehydration; adequate humidification is difficult to provide.
- Volatile anesthetic cannot be easily delivered via this route.
- Blood and secretions from the airways become aerosolized in the atmosphere.
- Spray from the jet may interfere with surgery or contaminate the field.
- The small catheter is easily dislodged from the airways and must be frequently repositioned.

either through the vocal cords and within the trachea or over the drapes into the trachea or bronchus. If a catheter is used, it should be relatively stiff and well-secured at the distal tip to prevent recoil movement. Jet ventilation eliminates the physical interference and fire hazard of an ETT. Ambient air is entrained at the mouth of the jet (Bernoulli's principle), increasing Vt and decreasing FiO_2 by unpredictable amounts. These and other disadvantages are discussed in Chapter 11 and listed in Box 30.2. Jet ventilators are most often used during tracheal resections as a temporary means to intermittently augment oxygenation in one lung when the contralateral lung is intubated and ventilated.

Fire hazard (high FiO_2 and open airway) – Though electrocautery tends to be used sparingly, one must be aware of this risk, especially during the open airway phase.

Emergence Strategies

- Goals:
  - Provide conduit for surgeons to perform final bronchoscopy (ETT/LMA)
  - Immediate postoperative extubation avoids pressure of ETT cuff on anastomosis as well as avoids positive-pressure ventilation to the site
  - Avoid coughing, retching, head extension
  - Assure that reintubation is not needed
- Final surgical bronchoscopy can be performed through an LMA to view entire trachea and facilitate smooth emergence.
- Remifentanil provides depth and suppression of cough/airway reflexes for bronchoscopy, with rapid decay profile for early extubation.
- Secretions and blood should be evacuated during bronchoscopy, and local anesthetic may be sprayed on anastomosis to minimize coughing on emergence.
- Chin-to-chest suture makes mask ventilation and reintubation problematic, but LMA can generally be placed.

Postoperative Management

- ICU-level care.
- Maintain neck flexion for at least several days.
- Relative narcotic-sparing pain control to prevent delirium and respiratory depression.
- Aggressive pulmonary toilet, frequently including awake bronchoscopy, with the critical goals of preventing reintubation as well as aspiration pneumonia.
  - Frequent damage to recurrent laryngeal nerve may compromise vocal cord function.

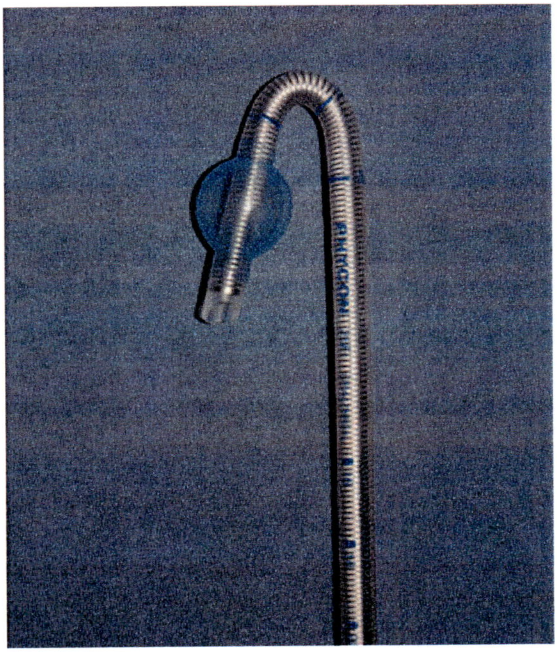

Figure 30-11 – Wire-reinforced endotracheal tubes resist kinking with tight curvatures as often required when intubating "over the field."

- Difficulty expectorating with neck flexion.
- Impaired mucociliary clearance due to surgery.
  - Some surgeons place a "mini-tracheotomy" at the conclusion of surgery to facilitate postoperative subglottic suctioning.
- Antisialagogues, antiemetics.

- LMA at bedside (may be placed with neck flexed if needed).
- Scissors at bedside to cut chin–chest suture if necessary for emergent reintubation.
- Antitussives, nebulized local anesthetics, and humidified respiratory gases for patient comfort.

Post-TRR Anesthesia

If the tracheal resection patient requires anesthesia for future surgeries, the suggested approach may include:

- Avoidance of intubation (regional techniques, LMA) if possible
- Bronchoscopic evaluation of airway prior to ETT placement
- Avoiding placing of ETT cuff within repaired segment (via bronchoscopic guidance)
- Awareness that a surgically shortened trachea increases the risk of inadvertent endobronchial intubation

Appendix

The Hagen–Poiseuille equation (30.1) describes the pressure change occurring with fluid flow through a tube (2). Assumptions include tubular geometry, and that flow is laminar with a parabolic profile. Radius has a profound effect on pressure change, and viscosity is the dominant fluid characteristic. Turbulent flow (30.2) alters this relationship such that radius has an even more profound effect (pressure change is inversely related to radius – raised to the fifth power) and density becomes the dominant fluid characteristic. Note also the increased impact of flow rate and friction factor with turbulent flow.

Laminar Flow
$$\mathbf{P} = \frac{8L\mu\dot{V}}{\pi r^4} \tag{30.1}$$

Turbulent Flow
$$\mathbf{P} = \frac{fLp\dot{V}^2}{4\pi^2 r^5} \tag{30.2}$$

$\mathbf{P}$ = Pressure change, L = Length of tube, μ = Fluid viscosity, $\dot{V}$ = Flow rate, r = Radius, f = Friction factor, p = Density of fluid

Selected References

1. Delaere P, Vranckx J, Verleden G, et al. Tracheal allotransplantation after withdrawal of immunosuppressive therapy. N Engl J Med. 2010;362(2):138–45.

2. Topulos GP, Butler JP. Correction of a recurrent error. Anesthesiology. 1985;63: 563–4.

3. Alfille PH. Anesthesia for tracheal surgery. Chapter 18 in Grillo H. Surgery of the Trachea and Bronchi. Becker, London, 2004.

Suggested Reading

Berry M, Friedberg J. Techniques of tracheal resection. Chapter 54 in Sugarbaker DJ (editor). Adult Chest Surgery. McGraw Hill, New York, 2009; pp458-64.

Lorenz R, Strome M. Subglottic resection of the airway. Chapter 55 in Sugarbaker DJ (editor). Adult Chest Surgery. McGraw Hill, New York, 2009; pp465-72.

Ashiku S, DeCamp M. Resection of the carina. Chapter 56 in Sugarbaker DJ (Editor). Adult Chest Surgery. McGraw Hill, New York, 2009; pp 473-83.

Sandberg W. Anesthesia and airway management for tracheal resection and reconstruction. Int Anesthesiol Clin. 2000;38(1):55–75.

Pinsonneault C, Fortier J, Donati F. Tracheal resection and reconstruction. Can J Anaesth. 1999;46(5 Pt 1):439–55.

Young-Beyer P, Wilson RS. Anesthetic management for tracheal resection and reconstruction. J Cardiothorac Anesth. 1988;2(6):821–35.

Chapter 31
Bronchopleural Fistula

Ju-Mei Ng

Keywords Bronchopleural fistula • Subcutaneous emphysema • Chest drain • Stump dehiscence • Flexible bronchoscopy • Lung isolation • Ventilation • Clagett procedure • Open drainage procedures • High-frequency jet ventilation

Introduction

A bronchopleural fistula (BPF) is a persistent pathological communication between the central airways and the pleural cavity (excluding small peripheral air leaks for the purposes of this discussion). The incidence varies from 4.5 to 20% following pneumonectomy or 0.5% following lobectomy with a high mortality of between 18 and 50% (1). Causes and predisposing factors are listed in Tables 31-1 and 31-2 (1, 2). Most commonly, technical surgical issues or local ischemia are the principal causes of postpneumonectomy BPF.

Symptoms can be variable and subtle. They include dyspnea, productive cough with frothy rust-colored sputum (early presentation, implies contralateral infiltrate), or purulent sputum if presenting late following pulmonary resection. Fever tends to be intermittent. Patients may initially present without fever or leukocytosis.

Signs include subcutaneous emphysema, or if a chest tube is still present, then an intermittent (small BPF) or persistent (large BPF) air leak, and potentially a purulent discharge from the chest tube. If delayed and no chest tube is present, then new air fluid levels

P.M. Hartigan (ed.), *Practical Handbook of Thoracic Anesthesia*,
DOI 10.1007/978-0-387-88493-6_31, © Springer Science+Business Media, LLC 2012

Table 31-1 – Causes of bronchopleural fistula

Breakdown of suture/staple line after pulmonary resection
Spontaneous rupture of a lung abscess, bulla, or cyst
Erosion of bronchial wall by carcinoma, foreign body, chronic inflammatory disease, or infection
Penetrating trauma
Pulmonary infarction
Iatrogenic – Barotrauma from mechanical ventilation, thoracentesis, transbronchial biopsy, traumatic airway manipulation

Table 31-2 – Predisposing factors for BPF

Preoperative radiation therapy
Infection
Right-sided pneumonectomy > left
Residual neoplasm at the bronchial stump
Long bronchial stump without coverage
Prolonged mechanical ventilation

may be seen on chest X-ray. Classically, the air fluid level defines the level of the fistula. It is important to note that symptoms can be surprisingly mild even with relatively large BPFs.

Surgical Considerations

The presentation and treatment of postsurgical BPFs depend on the size of the air leak, the type of resection (pneumonectomy vs. lesser resection), and the time of presentation. While the surgical management of postsurgical air leaks is not standardized, certain principles (Table 31-3) are generally agreed upon.

Table 31-3 – General principles for surgical management of bronchopleural fistulae

Prompt drainage of pleural space
Protect against soilage of remaining lung tissue
Appropriate antibiotics
Respiratory support
Early diagnostic bronchoscopy
Early reclosure for large, central stump dehiscences that occur in the early postoperative period
Address infections before attempting reclosure
Reinforce stumps with vascular tissue flap
Obliteration of residual pleural space
Minimize tension on and airflow through the fistula

From Hartigan PM, Body SC, Sugarbaker DJ. Pulmonary resection. In Kaplan JA, Singer PD, eds. Thoracic Anesthesia, Philadelphia PA, Elsevier Science 2003, with permission

- Small (<3–5 mm), early air leaks following pulmonary resection may be approached more conservatively, with a trial of drainage, antibiotics, serial bronchoscopic evaluations, and possibly the bronchoscopic application of a sealant material.
- Acute major stump dehiscence calls for early reclosure.
- Delayed postpneumonectomy BPFs are almost invariably associated with an infected pleural space (empyema). Empyema must be addressed with closed and/or open drainage procedures, systemic and cavitary antibiotics, nutritional support, debridements, and repeated dressing changes and packing of the cavity with antibiotic-soaked packing material. Closure with obliteration of the pleural space should take place after the infection is well-controlled.

Acute Management

Chest Drain

The goal is to drain the pleural space and, in the case of lobectomy BPF, to promote the reexpansion of remaining ipsilateral lung (if present).

A balance must be struck between adequate drainage and excessive suction.

- Suction is contraindicated in early postpnemonectomy patients since it could result in mediastinal shift, hemodynamic compromise, or even cardiac herniation (following right pneumonectomy with pericardial defect).
- In the case of a BPF following lobectomy, insufficient suction or a chest tube that is too small for the fistula air flow leads to expansion of the air space, failure to fully reexpand remaining ipsilateral lung, and risk of tension pneumothorax (if ventilated).
- Excessive chest tube suction in mechanically ventilated patients with postlobectomy BPF could increase fistula airflow and "steal" tidal volume from remaining lung units (ipsilateral or contralateral) or trigger an inspiration-cycled ventilator.

Stump Dehiscence

Acute postsurgical breakdown of all or part of a stump requires a prompt response with the following guidelines.

- Patient positioning: Elevating the head of the bed and tilting the patient "fistula side down" decrease the probability of further soiling of the contralateral lung.
- Respiratory support: Depending on the size of the leak, respiratory support could require just supplemental oxygen or intubation of the contralateral bronchus with a DLT (or endobronchial tube) followed by single-lung, positive-pressure ventilation. If the fistula is not excluded with lung isolation, positive-pressure ventilation will be ineffective and potentially fatal in the presence of a large BPF. If possible, drainage of the infected space prior to intubation is preferred.
- Diagnostics: CT scan and/or bronchoscopic assessment of stump.
- Establish effective drainage.
- Surgical closure: Barring infection or residual tumor at the stump, early reoperation, and closure of the stump are indicated.

Anesthetic Considerations

Depending on the timing and manner of presentation, size of the BPF, and the surgical therapy planned, the anesthetic issues vary. Different settings are presented individually, including relevant points in the surgical procedure. This chapter discusses only the specific issues of induction and method of lung isolation and ventilation. General principles of thoracic anesthesia regarding monitoring and anesthetic technique (including pain management) may be found in other chapters.

Management goals remain similar regardless of presentation and surgery planned.

- To protect the healthy lung regions from soiling by extrapleural fluid from the affected hemithorax.
- To utilize a ventilation technique which avoids development of a tension pneumothorax in the affected hemithorax or further disrupts the defect.
- Adequate alveolar gas exchange in the presence of a low-resistance air leak.

Flexible Bronchoscopy

This is usually the first step in surgical management and may be therapeutic via the delivery of glue or a sclerosing agent (see Fig 31-1). A chest drain should be in place and the size of the BPF determined. If air bubbles intermittently through the water seal chamber of the chest tube drainage system and occurs only with deep breathing or coughing, then it is likely that the fistula is small. A persistent leak (large leak) indicates involvement of a larger bronchus, and is continuous even with just quiet breathing. Small BPFs can be very difficult to see: one trick is to place fluid on the stump and observe for the disappearance of bubbles with tidal breathing.

Reoperation for Early Closure

Immediate closure with vascular tissue coverage and postoperative irrigation have been successful in patients who are diagnosed

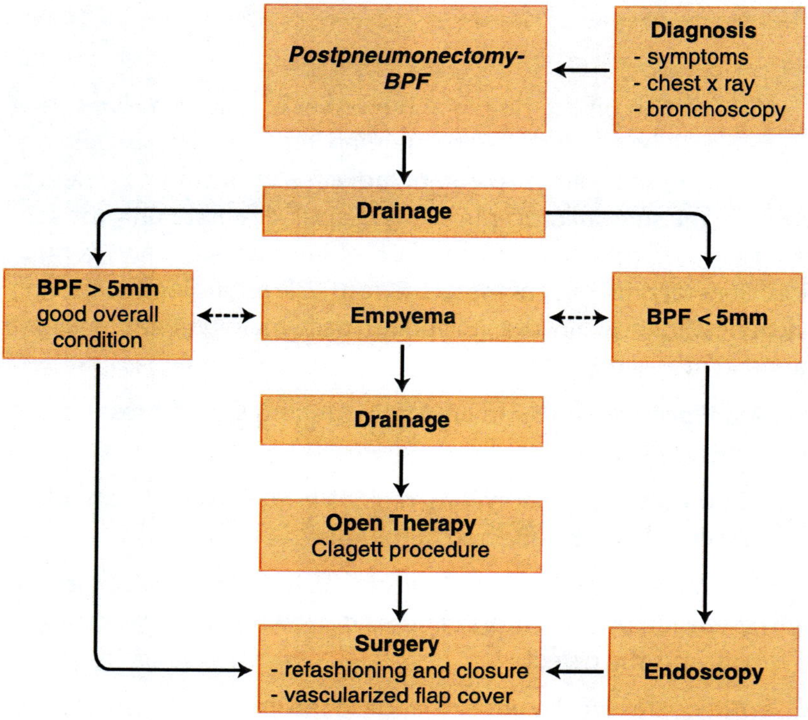

Figure 31-1 – Algorithm for surgical management of bronchopleural fistula following pneumonectomy. (*Modified from in Sirbu H, Busch T, Aleksic I, et al. Ann Thorac Cardiovasc Surg 2001; 7: 330–336, with permission*).

early, have reasonable function in the remaining lung, and do not have infection of the pleural space. Surgical revision is generally reserved for the immediately recognized large BPF, possibly resulting from technical failure of the stump or mechanical disruption.

Flexible Bronchoscopy

Bronchoscopic assessment of the stump is an essential early intervention (see Table 31-4). It serves to clean out and assess soilage of the remaining lung, as well as to observe the size of the fistula directly and assess the stability of the remainder of the stump closure. Depending on the scenario, bronchoscopy may be performed awake or anesthetized.

Table 31-4 – Anesthetic strategies depending on fistula size

FISTULA SIZE	STRATEGIES	NOTES
Small	Intravenous induction with conventional two-lung, positive-pressure ventilation through a single-lumen tube	Utilize normal or small tidal volumes Assess the degree of air leak Chest drain to suction or water seal to prevent a tension pneumothorax Fistula airflow resistance is high (limited lost ventilation)
Moderate to large	Maintenance of spontaneous respiration ± use of a laryngeal mask airway ▪ Awake with airway topicalization + sedation ▪ Inhalational induction ▪ Total intravenous anesthesia ▪ Combination of the above	Spontaneous negative-pressure breathing enables adequate expansion of remaining lung Avoids the risk of a tension pneumothorax Risk of contralateral contamination Meticulous preoxygenation usually enables quick bronchoscopy to be performed before desaturation occurs
	Intravenous induction, intubation with a single-lumen endotracheal tube, and bronchoscopic examination during the period of apnea Establish lung isolation with an appropriate DLT (*positioned under direct fiber-optic guidance*) and bronchoscopy performed via the tracheal lumen with a pediatric bronchoscope	The DLT may be inserted with the patient breathing spontaneously (awake with topicalization ± sedation or anesthetized) or paralyzed with a short-acting relaxant (like succinylcholine). Positive-pressure, one-lung ventilation commenced only after lung isolation secured

Lung Isolation

The most frequently used method to establish lung isolation is intubating the unaffected bronchus with a DLT or endobronchial tube. As previously mentioned, positive-pressure ventilation will be ineffective and potentially fatal in the presence of a large BPF if the fistula is not excluded by lung isolation. The DLT should be placed under direct fiber-optic guidance to ensure rapid, accurate placement and to prevent further disruption of the bronchial stump. Lung isolation protects against soilage of the remaining lung as well as allows effective positive-pressure ventilation. Placement of a protective DLT can be performed in an awake patient with sedation and topical anesthesia or in an anesthetized, spontaneously breathing patient (see Table 31-4). Distal tracheal and carinal topical anesthesia can be applied in a "spray-as-you-go" fashion through the working port of the bronchoscope. If the BPF is sufficiently distal to the carina to permit a bronchial blocker, this option may be preferable.

Ventilation

Lung-protective single (contralateral)-lung ventilation is recommended because that lung is at risk for aspiration and acute lung injury. Inadequate single-lung oxygenation in nonpneumonectomy patients may require alternative support (see below). The goal should generally be to extubate these patients at the end of surgery to avoid positive pressure on the stump.

Open Drainage Therapy (Clagett Procedure)

Pleural space infection following pneumonectomy typically requires creation of a large, open-window thoracostomy (Clagett procedure, Fig 31.2) (3) to facilitate debridement and cleansing of the empyema space and return of healthy granulation tissue covering the walls of the cavity. Intravenous antibiotics are administered and the space is repeatedly irrigated with antibiotic solution and packed with antibiotic-soaked dressings for several days or weeks. Finally, the thoracostomy space is closed after filling the cavity with antibiotic solution.

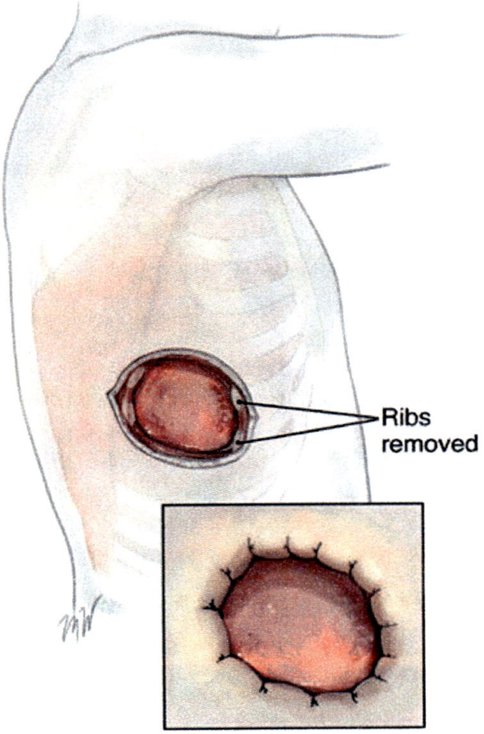

Figure 31.2 – Surgical thoracostomy by means of a Clagett Window. The pleura is joined to the skin to marsupialize the pleural space. The thoracostomy is positioned in the most dependent part of the thorax and two ribs are typically resected. (*From Adult Chest Surgery, Sugarbaker DJ, et al., New York, McGraw-Hill, with permission. Copyright, Marcia Williams, 2009*).

Anesthetic Issues for Open Drainage Procedures

The principal anesthetic issue for patients with an empyema is to prevent the contamination of uninfected lung (see above discussion). Other issues include the following.

- Preoperative effective drainage, antibiotic therapy, intravenous hydration.
- Nutritional and metabolic support, and degree of debilitation by chronic infection.
- Thoracic epidural analgesia has the risk of hematogenous seeding of the catheter from bacteremia.

- Lung isolation is best achieved with a DLT positioned under fiber-optic observation.
- Frequent suctioning of the infected material from the tracheal lumen:
  - Often necessary during the case
  - Should be performed prior to deflating the bronchial cuff at the end of the case

Definitive Fistula Closure with Muscle-Flap Obliteration of Cavity

Obliteration of the pleural cavity can be accomplished by transposition of extrathoracic muscle flaps (latissimus dorsi, serratus anterior, pectoralis major), omentum, or limited thoracoplasty (rare). Reclosure and obliteration of the space may be performed as single- or multistage procedures. The anesthetic considerations are similar to that for open drainage therapy, except that the infection and cross-contamination issues should no longer be a concern.

Ventilation Strategies

Nonpneumonectomy patients with a large BPF and inadequate single-lung oxygenation might require alternative support in the operating room or in the ICU for a period of time until the fistula closes. The options include conventional two-lung ventilation or unconventional two-lung ventilation (high-frequency or independent-lung ventilation). The aim is to minimize airflow across the fistula while maintaining adequate gas exchange. Ventilation strategies should be coordinated with chest tube suction strategies to optimize ventilation and minimize fistula airflow (Table 31-5).

High-Frequency Jet Ventilation

HFJV is the most commonly employed alternative technique for patients with a BPF (see Chapter 11). It has the potential to achieve comparable (or improved) gas exchange at lower peak and mean

Table 31-5 – Ventilation strategies in BPF

	APPROACH	ADVANTAGES	DISADVANTAGES
Conventional two-lung ventilation	Reduce mean airway pressure – Small tidal volumes – Rapid respiratory rates	Simple and familiar One-way valve may be used in chest tube apparatus timed to occlude during inspiration	Conventional extrinsic PEEP not practical Danger of valve malfunction or asynchronous timing Danger of stolen ventilation by excessive fistula airflow
Independent-lung ventilation (ILV) (4, 5)	Unaffected lung ventilated conventionally Lung on the fistula side ventilated at different settings, synchronously or asynchronously, usually with a separate ventilator (Obviously requires DLT and does not apply for pneumonectomy patients)	Optimizes lung recruitment and gas exchange in two lungs of differing compliance Single ventilator with variable-resistance valve on fistula side May be combined with CPAP or high-frequency ventilation to the fistula side	DLT required Management of two ventilators is complex and labor intensive

(continued)

Table 31-5 – (continued)

	APPROACH	ADVANTAGES	DISADVANTAGES
High-frequency ventilation (HFV) (6)	Spectrum of ventilation techniques characterized by respiratory rates in excess of 60 breaths per minute	Adequate gas exchange at lower peak and mean airway pressures May improve recruitment and expansion of residual lung	Lack of standardization Unfamiliar equipment Inability to monitor distal airway pressure or end-tidal CO_2 Risk of barotrauma

airway pressures and may improve recruitment and expansion of residual lung. Despite the theoretical advantages and multiple reports of the successful application of HFJV in patients with BPF, it has not proved universally advantageous in terms of gas exchange, fistula flow, and airway pressures (6–8).

The question of whether HFJV is superior to conventional ventilation for such patients is complicated by the broad diversity of HFJV techniques and settings, the lack of adequately controlled prospective trials, and the variability of the mechanical properties of BPFs (and lungs) between patients and within a given patient over time.

Nevertheless, HFJV should be considered for patients with bilateral or large BPF air leaks who are difficult to manage by conventional ventilatory techniques and in patients with normal lung parenchyma and proximal BPF, (8) provided that adequate technical expertise with the equipment is available.

Selected References

1. Cerfolio RJ. The incidence, etiology, and prevention of postresectional bronchopleural fistula. Semin Thorac Cardiovasc Surg. 2001;13:3–7.

2. Haraguchi S, Koizumi K, Hioki M, et al. Analysis of risk factors for postpneumonectomy bronchopleural fistulas in patients with lung cancer. J Nippon Med Sch. 2006;73:314–9.

3. Clagett O, Geraci J. A procedure for the management of postpneumonectomy empyema. J Thorac Cardiovasc Surg. 1963;45:141–5.

4. Benjaminsson E, Klain M. Intraoperative dual-mode independent lung ventilation of a patient with bronchopleural fistula. Anesth Analg. 1981;60:118–9.

5. Carvalho P, Thompson WH, Riggs R, et al. Management of bronchopleural fistula with a variable-resistance valve and a single ventilator. Chest. 1997;111: 1452–4.

6. Ihra G, Gockner G, Kashanipour A, et al. High-frequency jet ventilation in European and North American institutions, developments and clinical practice. Eur J Anaesthesiol. 2000;17:418–30.

7. Bishop MJ, Benson MD, Sato P, et al. Comparison of high-frequency jet ventilation with conventional mechanical ventilation from bronchopleural fistula. Anesth Analg. 1987;66:833–88.

8. Baumann MH, Sahn SA. Medical management and therapy of bronchopleural fistulas in the mechanically ventilated patient. Chest. 1990;97:721–8.

Chapter 32
Esophagectomy

Ju-Mei Ng

Keywords Minimally invasive esophagectomy • Esophageal resection • Esophagectomy

Introduction

Although perioperative mortality and morbidity from esophagectomy has declined over the past 30 years, overall mortality is still relatively high at 8.8% (1). Outcomes are closely related to the number of esophageal resections performed by individual surgeons and medical centers (2, 3). Mortality at major centers is 2–3%, suggesting the presence of modifiable factors and an impact from perioperative care. Other factors that may predict mortality include advanced age, performance status, pulmonary complications, and need for transfusion. Anesthesia plays an important role in the multimodal approach and/or standardized perioperative clinical care pathways that may help improve the infrastructure for the management of these patients in high-volume centers and improve outcome (4).

Surgical Considerations for Esophagectomy

Esophageal resection and replacement are performed by different surgical approaches, depending on the location and size of the

P.M. Hartigan (ed.), *Practical Handbook of Thoracic Anesthesia*,
DOI 10.1007/978-0-387-88493-6_32,

tumor, the potential for adherence of the esophagus or tumor to mediastinal structures, and the preference of the surgeon (Table 32-1). The healthy stomach is generally the preferred conduit for esophageal replacement, although the colon or jejunum may be utilized.

Minimally invasive esophagectomy (MIE) is emerging in prominence, but should not be thought of as a separate technique. Instead, MIE employs laparoscopic or thoracoscopic techniques to varying degrees to address the surgical objectives of one or another of the techniques in Table 32-1 via more limited incisions. Outcome impacts are likely more closely related to the choice of anastomosis and conduit than to the size of the incisions. Nonetheless, MIE has certain considerations (pneumoperitoneum) and may prove to improve outcome in time.

Anesthetic Considerations for Esophagectomy

Preoperative Patient Considerations

This involves careful evaluation and optimization of the several important conditions, where present:

- Acid gastroesophageal reflux (GER)
- Possible respiratory compromise from chronic tracheal aspiration
- Airway involvement by tumor (potential to be obstructive or to complicate intubation)
- Effects of chemotherapy
- Comorbidities, e.g., coronary artery disease
- Poor nutritional status with hypoalbuminemia, malnutrition, hypochlorhydria, and low hemoglobin

Lines and Monitors

The magnitude of surgery (involving both the thoracic and abdominal cavities) usually calls for *invasive monitoring* and *generous intravenous access*. Continuous intraarterial blood pressure

Table 32-1 – Surgical approaches for esophageal resection

SURGERY	APPROACH	ANESTHETIC CONSIDERATIONS
"Ivor Lewis" 2-stage	1. Upper midline abdominal incision for gastric mobilization 2. Right thoracotomy and tumor resection 3. Stomach anastomosed to proximal esophagus in the chest	OLV (Rt lung deflated) Repositioning supine to lateral
Transhiatal	1. Upper midline abdominal incision for gastric mobilization 2. Blunt intrathoracic dissection 3. Left neck anastomosis	Blunt intrathoracic dissection may cause hemodynamic instability from cardiac compression and there is the possibility of occult perforation of tracheobronchial tree Avoid vascular access in the left neck
Left *thoracoab-dominal*	1. Left anterolateral thoracotomy for esophageal dissection 2. Incision extended to left upper abdomen 3. Anastomosis in the chest	OLV (left lung deflated)
The Brigham tri-incisional or *"Three hole"*	1. Right thoracotomy for esophageal dissection 2. Laparotomy 3. Left neck incision for pull-through and anastomosis	OLV (Rt lung deflated) Repositioning lateral to supine Avoid vascular access in the left neck
Minimally invasive (thoracocscopy, laparoscopy, or laparoscopic assisted)	One or two incisions, plus video port access May involve laparoscopy and neck incision or laparoscopy with thoracoscopy and chest anastomosis	OLV (Rt lung deflated) Potentially prolonged surgery

From Eisendraft JB, Neustein SM. Anesthesia for esophageal and mediastinal surgery. In Kaplan JA, Singer PD, eds. Thoracic Anesthesia. Third edition. Philadelphia PA: Elsevier Science; 2003, with permission monitoring is valuable during mediastinal manipulation in transhiatal esophagectomy and central venous access for prompt delivery of medications and to guide fluid therapy (see "Fluid management").

Thoracic epidural analgesia (TEA) is frequently employed and plays a central role in a multimodal approach or standardized perioperative clinical pathway, which has shown improved outcomes (4). Benefits have been shown in pain relief (particularly dynamic analgesia), reduction in respiratory complications, facilitating immediate or early postoperative tracheal extubation, reducing the length of intensive care stay, and possibly cost reduction (5, 6). A plain local anesthetic solution may be more practical as it permits the concomitant use of patient-controlled analgesia with intravenous opioids to supplement postoperative pain beyond the extent of TEA (see also Chapter 37).

Prevention of Tracheal Aspiration

Most would advocate prophylactic pharmacological management of GER, rapid sequence induction, and securing the airway with a cuffed endotracheal tube. *Gel lubrication* on the tracheal cuff of the single- or double-lumen tube has been shown to reduce pulmonary aspiration in anesthetized patients (7) and should be considered. Simple maneuvers like *proper and repeated suction* of the nasogastric tube and oropharynx prior to and after extubation are fundamental, as is the application of *continuous low-grade suction* to the nasogastric tube.

Surgical Bronchoscopy and EGD

Initial intubation should be with a large (≥8.0 O.D.), single-lumen ETT to allow formal surgical bronchoscopy to rule out invasion of the membranous trachea by tumor. As always, anomalous anatomy germane to the lung isolation plan should be noted at this time. A surgical esophagoscopy is also generally performed at this time. Following this (or after tube exchange), a nasogastric tube should be placed and its position confirmed. Often, this is left in place postoperatively bridging the anastomosis and decompressing the stomach remnant. Some surgical variations may apply.

Lung Isolation and One-Lung Ventilation

An appropriately sized *left-sided double-lumen endotracheal tube (DLT)* may be ideal when lung isolation is required (see Chapter 9). A *bronchial blocker* may be useful in patients with difficult airway anatomy to avoid reinstrumentation of the airway intra- and postoperatively. However, there may be an increased risk of dislodgement when used on the right side. Bronchial blockers are an excellent option when a left thoracoabdominal approach is used.

Lung-protective ventilation strategies during one-lung ventilation (OLV) are currently widely recommended (8). Robust inflammatory responses accompany esophagectomy, and may potentially be related to the development of acute lung injury (ALI). As such, logic suggests that if tolerated, lung-protective ventilatory strategies should be employed. Evidence is lacking as to whether or not this is outcome relevant to esophagectomy patients. Lung-protective ventilation is discussed in Chapter 6, and summarized here:

- 5–6 ml/kg tidal volume
- Optimizing PEEP (setting the PEEP above the lower inflection point of the compliance curve)
- Limiting plateau and peak inspiratory pressures to <25 cm H_2O and <35 cm H_2O, respectively

Fluid Management

There is a delicate balance between the maintenance of perfusion pressure and oxygen delivery to vital organs and the gut mucosa, and the prevention of pulmonary and peripheral edema (9). Hypovolemia and inadequate tissue perfusion may lead to gut hypoperfusion with increased morbidity due to gastric conduit ischemia and duration of hospital stay (10). However, excessive perioperative fluid administration may delay recovery of gastrointestinal function, impair wound/anastomotic healing and coagulation, and impair cardiac and respiratory function (9). Instead of adopting either a "restricted" or "liberal" approach, the amount of fluid should be *individually titrated* to dynamic changes in monitors (urine output, respiratory variation on arterial line, visual assessments blood loss, etc.) recognizing the imperfect nature of all such indicators. TEE is not an option in this surgery, and CVP is not reliable due to surgery-related pressure changes within the chest.

Vasoactive Agents

Caution should be exercised in the use of vasopressors or inotropes with predominantly alpha-adrenergic activity because of the theoretical potential to impair perfusion of the conduit and anastomosis. Hypotension is most commonly due to blood and third space losses, which is better treated with fluid, blood products (when indicated), and mixed alpha–beta adrenergic agonists if necessary. Impediments to venous return (retractor, surgical manipulation, etc.) are also a common cause of transient hypotension.

Tube Exchange

The fluid shifts of this operation can result in significant *airway edema*. For approaches in which the chest dissection precedes the abdominal, the DLT is best exchanged back to an SLT after turning supine, rather than waiting until the end of the case when edema will likely be more extensive. Whichever approach is employed, conservative techniques (tube exchange catheter, FOB, CMac, etc.) should be used when in doubt so as to avoid inadvertent esophageal intubation. Following reintubation with a large SLT, many surgeons want to repeat the bronchoscopy to *examine the membranous trachea for injury* from the dissection phase. This may require partial withdrawal of the ETT to provide an adequate view. The *recurrent laryngeal nerve* is also at risk, and examination of the vocal cords may be performed either during the tube exchange or during extubation.

Timing of Extubation

There is no consensus regarding optimal time of extubation for esophagectomy patients. *Early extubation* has been reported to be safe, not associated with increased respiratory morbidity, and also may reduce the length of ICU stay, potentially reducing costs (4). It also avoids the potential complications associated with mechanical ventilation (including barotrauma, nosocomial pneumonia) and side effects of sedation. Although early extubation does not independently reduce morbidity, when part of a multipronged management plan, it assists in decreasing the number of ventilator days and the duration of ICU stay and contributes to improved outcome as demonstrated in several series.

The counterargument is that pulmonary edema may lead to delayed respiratory failure (exhaustion from increased work of breathing) requiring semiemergent reintubation (late at night), potentially resulting in an esophageal intubation with disruption of the anastomosis. In addition, airway edema may result in upper airway obstruction, further complicating reintubation. Extubation timing decisions need to be individualized to the patient's preexisting comorbidities, intraoperative events, and the postoperative level of care available.

Selected References

1. Jamieson GG, Mathew G, Ludemann R, et al. Postoperative mortality following oesophagectomy and problems in reporting its rate. Br J Surg. 2004;91:943–7.

2. Birkmeyer JD, Stukel TA, Siewers AE, et al. Surgeon volume and operative mortality in the United States. N Engl J Med. 2003;349:2117–27.

3. Ferguson MK, Martin TR, Reeder LB, et al. Mortality after esophagectomy: risk factor analysis. World J Surg. 1997;21:599–604.

4. Brodner G, Pogatzki E, Van Aken H, et al. A multimodal approach to control postoperative pathophysiology and rehabilitation in patients undergoing abdominothoracic esophagectomy. Anesth Analg. 1998;86:228–34.

5. Chandrashekar MV, Irving M, Wayman J, et al. Immediate extubation and epidural analgesia allow safe management in a high-dependency unit after two-state oesophagectomy. Results of eight years of experience in a specialized upper gastrointestinal unit in a district general hospital. Br J Anaesth. 2003;90: 474–9.

6. Cense HA, Lagarde SM, de Jong K, et al. Association of no epidural analgesia with postoperative morbidity and mortality after transthoracic esophageal cancer resection. J Am Coll Surg. 2006;202:395–400.

7. Sanjay PS, Miller SA, Corry PR, et al. The effect of gel lubrication on cuff leakage of double lumen tubes during thoracic surgery. Anaesthesia. 2006;61:133–7.

8. Slinger P. Pro: Low tidal volume is indicated during one-lung ventilation. Anesth Analg. 2006;103:268–70.

9. Holte K, Sharrock NE, Kehlet H. Pathophysiology and clinical implications of perioperative fluid excess. Br J Anaesth. 2002;89:622–32.

10. Mythen MG, Webb AR. Intra-operative gut mucosal hypoperfusion is associated with increased post-operative complications and cost. Intensive Care Med. 1994;20:99–104.

Chapter 33
Esophageal Perforation

Ju-Mei Ng

Keywords Esophageal perforation • Mortality rate • Esophagectomy • Esophagogastroduodenoscopy • Iatrogenic perforations • Hemodynamic management

Introduction

Esophageal perforation is a life-threatening condition whose diagnosis is challenging and management controversial, despite decades of clinical experience and innovation in surgical technique. The mortality rate for esophageal perforation is 19.7% (range 3–67%), and the most important predictor of survival is the interval between injury and initiation of treatment (1). Accurate diagnosis and early treatment are essential to the successful management of patients (Table 33-1).

Surgical Considerations

Principles of Management

The *choice of treatment* is dependent on the cause and location of the perforation (Table 33-2), the presence of underlying esophageal disease, the interval between injury and initiation of treatment,

P.M. Hartigan (ed.), *Practical Handbook of Thoracic Anesthesia*,
DOI 10.1007/978-0-387-88493-6_33, © Springer Science+Business Media, LLC 2012

Table 33-1 – Causes of esophageal perforations

Iatrogenic (>50%)	Endoscopy (most common cause)
	Stricture dilation
	Operative injury (surgery on or in vicinity of esophagus)
	Nasogastic or endotracheal tube. TEE probe
Traumatic	Blunt, penetrating, or ingestion of caustic substance
Barogenic (spontaneous)	Postemetic (Boerhaave's Syndrome)
	Straining (weightlifting, bowel movement, childbirth)
Foreign bodies	
Carcinoma	
Infection	

and the age and general status of the patient (2). Although many treatment options have been used to date, the optimal treatment is still controversial for some scenarios. Treatment options include:

- Nonoperative treatment (antibiotics, non-oral nutrition, observation)
- Drainage
- Fibrin glue, adhesives (for small perforations)
- Primary repair
- Resection (esophagectomy)
- Exclusion
- Stent

Objectives of treatment include prevention of further contamination from the perforation, control of infection, restoration of the integrity of the gastrointestinal tract, and establishment of nutritional support (3). Treatment options diminish with time, and

Table 33-2 – Common operative approaches and implications

LOCATION OF PERFORATION	SURGICAL APPROACH	ANESTHETIC IMPLICATIONS
Cervical	Primary repair or drainage	Cervical incision (commonly left neck) Subcutaneous emphysema Sepsis uncommon (unless >24 h)
Intrathoracic	Primary repair Controlled fistula drainage Resection (transhiatal or transthoracic)	Pneumothorax, pneumomediastinum Pleural effusion Respiratory compromise Sepsis and shock Thoracotomy and OLV
Intraabdominal	Endoscopic treatment (fibrin glue, stent)	Pneumoperitoneum Respiratory compromise Sepsis and shock Upper abdominal incision

esophageal perforation should be treated as a legitimate surgical emergency. Gaining control of the mediastinitis is the first imperative. Twenty-four hours is the typical window for repair. If repair is impossible, exclusion and drainage are performed. Figure 33-1 shows an algorithm for management strategies of esophageal perforation.

Anesthetic Considerations

Esophageal perforation requires a prompt, but flexible and well-prepared, anesthetic response. Communication with the surgeon regarding the anticipated surgical procedure and approach

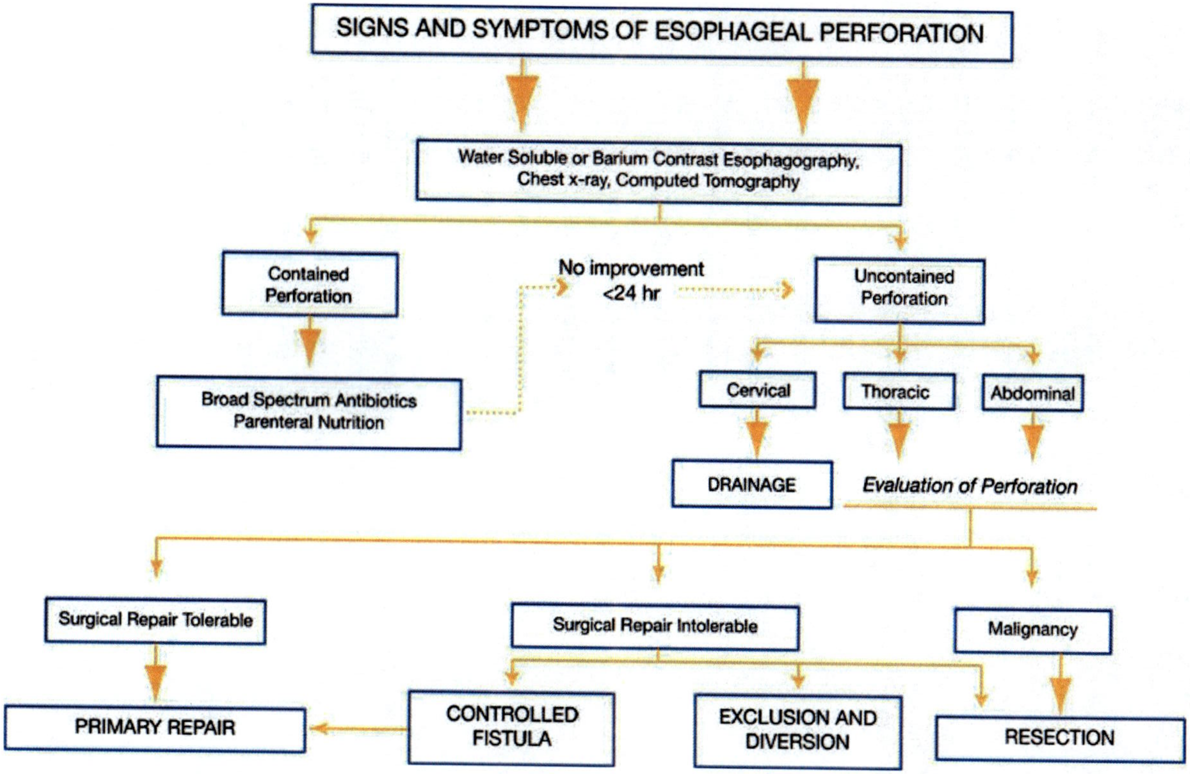

Figure 33-1 – Algorithm for management of esophageal perforation (4), with permission.

is paramount. Flexible esophagogastroduodenoscopy (EGD) is commonly performed initially to localize the rupture or perforation or assess the extent of pathology. Anticipate changes in the surgical plan or anesthetic requirements depending on EGD and intraoperative findings. Anesthetic equipment should be available for all options, including lung isolation and invasive monitoring.

Preoperative Patient Preparation

Patients may present for surgery either early (<24 h) or delayed and in varying degrees of sepsis and/or respiratory compromise. In general, patients with iatrogenic perforations are less ill because they would have been fasted prior to the procedure which led to the perforation. This is in contrast to other causes of perforation, where partially digested food may be found in the thorax or abdomen.

Assessment and considerations include:

- The risk of *aspiration* and need for pharmacological prophylaxis
- *Pleural or gastric decompression* prior to induction of anesthesia
- Volume status, coagulation profile, fluid resuscitation, and appropriate antibiotics in impending *sepsis*
- Urgent treatment of the existing uncontrolled medical comorbidities
- Differentiating chest pain caused by the perforation from a cardiac source

Lines and Monitors

Depending on the patient's comorbidities, hemodynamic parameters, and the extent of surgery planned, invasive monitoring (arterial and central venous lines) may be indicated. Even when patients are thought to be in an early phase of a septic trajectory, invasive lines and monitors aid subsequent ICU management. A central line for parenteral nutrition may be requested by the surgeon.

Regional Anesthesia

The decision to include a central neuraxial technique must be made on an individual basis considering the analgesic alternatives, the benefits of regional anesthesia, and the risk of central nervous system infection, which may occur in any bacteremic patient (5). The benefits of *thoracic epidural analgesia* or *paravertebral catheters* for thoracotomy and/or upper abdominal surgery have to be weighed against the risk of adverse patient hemodynamics and epidural abscess/hematoma. Central neuraxial blocks should not be performed in patients with untreated systemic infection or coagulopathy (5, 6). When delayed extubation is anticipated (e.g., septic or debilitated patients undergoing esophageal resection), the epidural is best postponed.

Securing the Airway

The aspiration risk is variable and must be carefully assessed. Patients with Boerhaave's syndrome or perforation from ingestion are obviously at high risk. Those with iatrogenic perforations from dilatations following a fast are at relatively lower risk. Rapid sequence induction is generally advisable as long as the airway anatomy suggests an easy intubation. Raising the head of the bed is of more value than cricoid pressure, which is not endorsed in this scenario. Inadvertent esophageal intubation may extend an esophageal tear. Maneuvers commonly employed to mitigate aspiration risk or damage (oral antacids, gastric propulsants, awake nasogastric tube evacuation of stomach contents) may be ill advised in the presence of a significant esophageal perforation. A low threshold for awake fiberoptic intubation or use of a videolaryngoscope to improve certainty of intubation is advisable if the airway anatomy is in any question.

Bronchoscopy to rule out a related injury (or tumor involvement) to the membranous trachea should be performed following intubation due to its proximity to the esophagus. This calls for a *large ETT*. If lung isolation is required and massive fluid resuscitation is anticipated, a *bronchial blocker* is recommended because it obviates the need for additional tube exchanges.

Hemodynamic Management

Patients often present with significant deficits of intravascular volume, together with various degrees of sepsis-related disruption of vascular tone and third space losses. Critical perfusion is further threatened by vasodilation, blood loss, and interference with venous return following induction (general anesthesia, positive-pressure ventilation, surgical manipulations). *Fluid resuscitation should err on the generous side* if signs of septic physiology are apparent. A history of delayed diagnosis, signs of mediastinitis, tachycardia, hypotension, oliguria, respiratory variation on arterial line tracings, depressed mental status, etc. are components of the "septic picture," which should trigger more aggressive monitoring and therapy. Maintenance of perfusion pressure and oxygen delivery is important to avoid hypoperfusion and ischemia of the flap utilized to reinforce a primary repair, as well as critical end organs. *Vasopressor and/or inotropic support* may be required in sepsis.

Postoperative Monitoring

Immediate or early extubation is reasonable in selected, hemodynamically stable patients with little or no contamination intraoperatively. More frequently, an anticipated septic postoperative course justifies postoperative intubation and aggressive fluid resuscitation. *Intensive care unit management is* usually required in major esophageal resections, sepsis, and patients with hemodynamic compromise or uncontrolled medical conditions.

Selected References

1. Lang M. H, Bruns D H, Schmitz B. Wuerl P Esophageal perforation: principles of diagnosis and surgical management Surg Today. 2006;36:332–40.

2. Jones W. G. Ginsberg R J Esophageal perforation: a continuing challenge Ann Thorac Surg. 1992;53:534–43.

3. Bufkin BL, Miller Jr JI, Mansour KA. Esophageal perforation: emphasis on management. Ann Thorac Surg. 1996;61:1447–52.

4. Brinster CJ, Singhal S, Lee L, et al. Evolving options in the management of esophageal perforation. Ann Thorac Surg. 2004;77:1475–83.

5. Wedel DJ, Horlocker TT. Regional anesthesia in the febrile or infected patient. Reg Anesth Pain Med. 2006;31:324–33.

6. Horlocker TT, Wedel DJ, Benzon H, et al. Regional anesthesia in the anticoagulated patient: defining the risks. Reg Anesth Pain Med. 2003;28:172–97.

Suggested Further Reading

Wright CD. Management of esophageal perforation. Chapter 40 in Sugarbaker DJ, et al (Editors); Adult Thoracic Surgery. McGraw-Hill, 2009, New York, p. 353-60.

Chapter 34
Lung Transplantation

Ju-Mei Ng and Vladimir Formanek

Keywords Lung transplantation • BSLT • SLT • Cardiopulmonary bypass • Bronchial anastomosis • Atrial anastomosis • HLT

Introduction

Lung transplantation is an accepted therapeutic intervention for patients with end-stage lung disease, with evidence supporting the quality of life and survival benefit for recipients. Although the modern era of lung transplantation dates back to 1983, lung transplantation remains a complex therapy with significant perioperative morbidity and mortality (1, 2). The anesthesiologist faces many challenges, including provision of stable anesthesia for patients with end-stage lung disease, management of hypoxia and hypercapnia, treatment of pulmonary hypertension and right ventricular failure, and postoperative pain management. Familiarity with the management of end-stage one-lung ventilation (OLV), cardiopulmonary bypass (CPB), inhaled nitric oxide (NO), and transesophageal echocardiography (TEE) is necessary.

P.M. Hartigan (ed.), *Practical Handbook of Thoracic Anesthesia*,
DOI 10.1007/978-0-387-88493-6_34, © Springer Science+Business Media, LLC 2012

General Considerations

Types of Lung Transplantation (Table 34-1)

Lung transplantation encompasses a group of different operations that are selected based on donor organ availability, the recipient's underlying lung disease, in some cases transplant center preferences, and evolving trends in lung transplantation.

Recent trends are for more BSLTs (fewer SLTs), especially in younger patients, even for diseases, such as pulmonary fibrosis or emphysema. Compared to SLT, long-term survival and function appear to be better after BSLT (1). However, survival curves should be interpreted with caution and multiple clinical factors appropriately influence the decision to perform a particular procedure type, including age of recipient, comorbidities, and characteristics of the donor lungs. HLTs are principally performed for congenital cardiopulmonary problems.

Indications

Lung transplant is indicated for patients with end-stage lung disease, who are failing maximal medical therapy or for whom no effective medical therapy exists (Fig 34-1). The timing of referral for transplant assessment is advisable when patients have a less than 50% 2–3-year predicted survival, New York Heart Association (NYHA) class III or IV level of function, or both. An anesthetic consultation at the time of listing is recommended. Disease-specific guidelines for transplantation continue to evolve (3).

Contraindications are listed in Table 34-2. Because donor organ availability is the limiting factor, inroads have been made in some centers by transplanting lungs from the so-called extended donors (age > 55, smoking hx, pulmonary infiltrate, purulent secretions, $PaO_2 < 300$ mmHg (at $FiO_2 = 1.0$) or utilizing living donor lobar transplants. Donation of organs after cardiac death (DCD) has further expanded the donor pool. The most common clinical scenario for DCD is the withdrawal of medical therapy and ventilator support in cases of futile therapy. After death, the donor needs to be reintubated,

Table 34-1 – Types of lung transplantation

TYPE OF LUNG TRANSPLANTATION	TECHNIQUE	COMMON INDICATIONS
Single-lung transplantation (SLT)	Left or right lung CPB required in < 10%	COPD/emyphysema Pulmonary fibrosis
Bilateral sequential lung transplantation (BSLT)	Two lungs, transplanted in sequence Often with the aid of CPB	Cystic fibrosis Bronchiectasis Pulmonary hypertension
Heart–lung transplantation (HLT)	Transplantation of the heart and lungs, en bloc, from a single donor CPB required Rarely performed	Pulmonary hypertension and congenital heart disease Eisenmenger's syndrome Primary pulmonary hypertension with right ventricular dysfunction

Table 34-1 – (continued)

TYPE OF LUNG TRANSPLANTATION	TECHNIQUE	COMMON INDICATIONS
Pediatric lung transplantation (PLT)	A double-lung transplant with the aid of ECMO	Cystic fibrosis Primary pulmonary hypertension Pulmonary hypertension secondary to congenital heart disease Bronchopulmonary dysplasia Arteriovenous malformations; hypoplastic lungs due to congenital diaphragmatic hernia
Living donor lung transplantation (LDLT)	Transplantation of two pulmonary lobes from two donors into a single recipient	Cystic fibrosis

CPB cardiopulmonary bypass, *ECMO* extracorporeal membrane oxygenator.

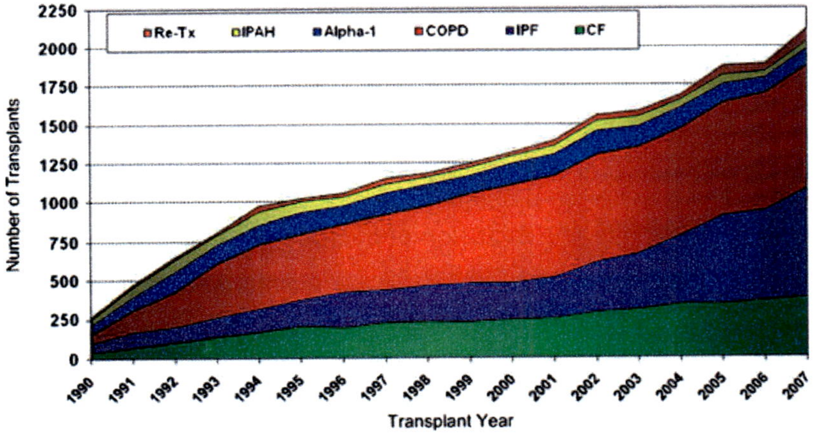

Figure 34-1 – Indications for adult lung transplantation by year (number). *CF* cystic fibrosis, *IPF* idiopathic pulmonary fibrosis, *COPD* chronic obstructive pulmonary disease, *Alpha-1* Alpha-1 antitrypsin deficiency, *IPAH* idiopathic pulmonary artery hypertension, *Re-Tx* repeat lung transplantation. From Christie JD, Edwards LB, Aurora P, et al., J Heart Lung Transplant 2009;28:1031–1049, with permission.

Table 34-2 – Contraindications to lung transplantation

Major contraindications

- Malignancy
- Untreatable advanced dysfunction of other organ systems
- Noncurable chronic extrapulmonary infection, for example HIV, hepatitis
- Untreatable psychiatric or psychologic condition with an inability to cooperate with medical therapy, including substance addiction and ongoing tobacco use

Relative contraindications

- Age; there is no set upper age limit, though older patients tend to have more comorbidities and may have less than optimal long-term survival
- Critical unstable condition
- Colonization with highly virulent microorganisms
- Mechanical ventilation or extracorporeal membrane oxygenation (ECMO) with other organ dysfunction and small chance for rehabilitation potential
- Severe chest wall deformity or pleural disease

the lungs ventilated, and harvested. Despite about an hour of warm ischemia, early results have been promising.

Donor Lung Procurement and Preservation

General donor considerations (4) include the confirmation of ABO compatibility, the exclusion of malignancy, pulmonary, or systemic infection, heavy smoking history, aspiration, or acute lung injury (contusion, ventilator-associated lung injury, neurogenic pulmonary edema, systemic inflammatory response syndrome, etc.).

Intensive management of marginal donors has been shown to improve the quality and expand the pool of donor lungs without compromising results to transplantation (5). These include:

- Strict fluid management
- Bronchoscopy to assess for bronchopulmonary infection and to provide tracheobronchial toilet
- Antibiotic therapy
- Alteration to ventilator settings (to include pressure support and increased positive end-expiratory pressure) and arterial blood gas (ABG) monitoring

Lung Preservation

The allograft is cooled, flushed with a pulmoplegic solution, and kept partially inflated with continuous positive airway pressure (CPAP). Most harvested lungs are flushed with Perfadex (Vitrolife, Gotherberg, Sweden), a low potassium dextran glucose solution. This recently introduced pulmoplegic solution has improved outcomes and significantly reduced graft dysfunction (6).

Ischemic times (the time from organ harvest to reperfusion in the recipient) of less than 6 h have been recommended, although recently it has been shown that ischemic times of greater than 8 h are possible (7, 8). Some centers add high-dose intravenous steroids or pulmonary vasodilators and either intravenous prostaglandins or prostaglandins to the pulmoplegia in an attempt to achieve better distribution, inhibition of platelet aggregation, and decreased production of neutrophil-derived free radicals. The serine protease inhibitor and antifibrinolytic, aprotinin (Trasylol, Bayer), added to the pulmoplegia have shown promising results (9). Ex vivo lung preservation is currently an area of active and promising research.

Surgical Considerations

The principal surgical concerns are to match suitable donor organs with appropriately selected recipients, and to then orchestrate efficient, viable anastomoses of the pulmonary artery, atrium, and bronchus. The most tenuous of these is the bronchial anastomosis due to the watershed blood supply of the central airways. Proximal anastomoses tend to fare better than more distal bronchial anastomoses (Fig 34-2). Remplantation of bronchial arteries is not generally considered worth the time or technical hurdles. Wrapping the anastomosis with a flap is often performed to enhance healing and buttress against the formation of a bronchovascular fistula.

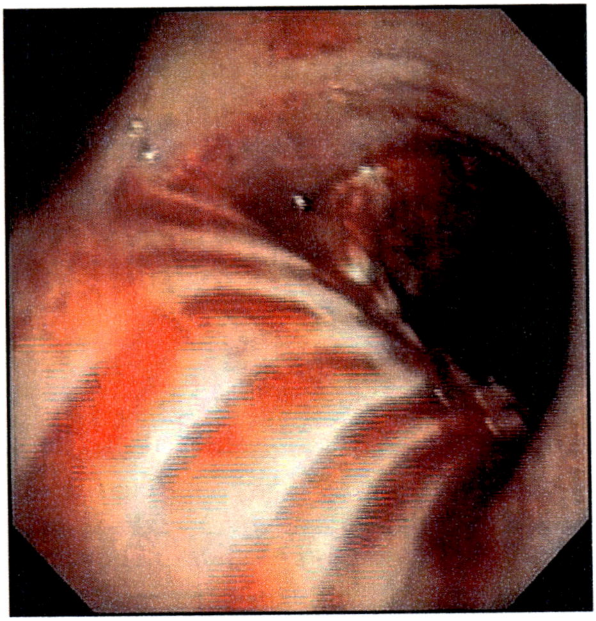

Figure 34-2 – Right mainstem end-to-end (minimally telescoped) anastomosis viewed through a bronchoscope during double-lung transplant.

The atrial anastomosis (pulmonary veins) must be performed with attention to avoid circumflex artery obstruction (by clamp) and rotational deformities leading to obstruction of pulmonary venous flow. An obstructive atrial anastomosis is clinically indistinguishable from early graft failure with pulmonary edema, and may be difficult to evaluate echocardiographically. Generally, early pulmonary edema (within first hour of perfusion) should trigger a ruling out of a technical problem with the atrial anastomosis. More delayed (>4 h following unclamping) pulmonary edema is more likely a result of cytokine-related endothelial injury.

The pulmonary artery anastomosis may be subject to kinking with chest closure if the segment is too long. Stenosis of the PA anastomosis is usually a delayed complication. Careful de-airing (either antegrade or retrograde) is essential prior to resuming circulation.

Anesthetic Considerations

Workup of the Pulmonary Transplant Recipient

The clinical evaluation and assessment of suitability for transplantation should include characterization of the underlying lung disease, evaluation for other organ system dysfunction, and the patient's suitability to tolerate long-term immunosuppressive therapy.

Essential Investigations

Chest radiographs and a *CT scan* of the *thorax* are utilized to evaluate chest cavity size so that donor and recipient lung size match is appropriate. Any unexpected mass lesions, malignancy, abscesses, pleural scarring, or adhesions can be assessed. Recipient pulmonary function tests, including *spirometry* and *V/Q scans*, are important in determining which lung to transplant if SLT is planned.

Serologic tests include ABG, electrolyte panels, and liver function test to assess renal and hepatic function, complete blood count and coagulation profile, ABO blood type and viral serology for hepatitis, cytomegalovirus (CMV), and human immunodeficiency virus (HIV).

Comprehensive cardiovascular evaluation with *EKG* and *echocardiography* is indicated to assess right and left ventricular function, exclude intracardiac shunts, unexpected valvular disease, and the calculation of PA pressures based on tricuspid regurgitation jet velocity. *Cardiac catheterization*, including coronary angiography, is indicated in patients with severe pulmonary hypertension or risk factors for coronary artery disease, especially in patients older than 50 years. If significant coronary artery disease is diagnosed, revascularization by angioplasty/stent may be considered or rarely the patient may require coronary bypass at the time of the lung transplant.

Patient Monitoring

Profound changes in pulmonary and systemic hemodynamics are common both during and after lung transplantation. Therefore, comprehensive monitoring, as for any major case, is utilized (Table 34-3).

Immediate Preoperative Preparation

Not infrequently, significant changes occur during the interim between evaluation and transplantation. Some salient points to focus on during the brief preoperative period include:

- Airway evaluation and NPO status
- Oxygen and steroid dependency
- PA pressures, cardiac (especially, right heart) dysfunction
- Other major organ system functions
- Signs or symptoms of infection
- Any other recent deterioration in clinical condition
- Pulmonary blood flow distribution (Q scan)

Table 34-3 – Specific lines and monitors

	RATIONALE AND NOTES
Pulmonary artery catheter (PAC)	Inserted routinely in most centers PA pressures reflect the load on the RV Pulmonary artery occlusion pressures (PAOP) may reflect LV filling S_vO_2 and continuous cardiac output measurement Conduit to deliver drugs to central circulation Usual caveats for PAC and pneumonectomy: ▪ Beware entrapment in staple line ▪ PAOP may spuriously lower left atrial pressures when one lung is perfused
Invasive arterial blood pressure monitoring	Serial arterial blood gasses (ABGs) Rapid-response blood pressure monitoring Large and inconsistent P_aCO_2-$P_{ET}CO_2$ gradient May be required to optimize ventilation (femoral approach may be preferred during BSLT, as radial may be damped by arm position)
Transesophageal echocardiography (TEE)	Enables continuous assessment of ventricular filling and function (RV of special interest) Assessment of pulmonary vein flow (stenosis/kinking present with increased velocity of jet flow by Doppler) (see Table 34-5)

- Recent infections and/or culture results to guide antibiotic prophylaxis

Judicious sedation may be administered for line placement, governed primarily by the functional limitations imposed by the underlying disease. Gastric acid aspiration prophylaxis, nebulized bronchodilators, and continued supplemental oxygen are recommended. Depending on the likelihood of the need for heparinization for CPB, the anesthesiologist may consider placing a thoracic epidural for postoperative pain control.

Induction of anesthesia should take place roughly 1.5 h prior to predicted arrival time of the donor lung. More time may be required if difficulty is anticipated in obtaining invasive monitoring or performing surgical dissection. It is essential to communicate with the surgeon in charge of organ harvesting, as timing may vary depending on travel times and harvest of other organs.

Conduct of Anesthesia

The choice of anesthetic technique and induction or maintenance drugs is less critical than the hemodynamic and pulmonary management. Induction and initial ventilatory settings should be tailored to the physiology (avoiding air trapping if obstructive disease). An initial bronchoscopy (via single-lumen tube) serves the purpose of assessing anomalous anatomy and clearance of secretions. The latter is particularly critical for cystic fibrosis patients and may be aided by DNAase. For lung isolation, a left double-lumen tube (DLT) is typically used for a right single-lung transplant or BSLT and a right-sided DLT for left single-lung transplants. Other preincision procedures (PAC, CVP, TEE, broad spectrum antibiotics, etc.) are performed, and the patient is positioned (Table 34-4). The timing and specific regimen of *immunosuppressive therapy* varies according to the institution. Reassessment of hemodynamic stability, gas exchange, PA pressures, and response to lung isolation following induction may alter the plan regarding the use or avoidance of CPB.

The lung allograft is very sensitive to the development of pulmonary edema. Therefore, fluid restriction, diuretic therapy, and maintaining high-volume urine output are desirable. Protective lung ventilation strategies with low tidal volumes, minimizing peak airway pressures and PEEP, are employed, as is utilizing the lowest possible FiO_2 compatible with adequate oxygenation.

Cardiopulmonary Bypass

The *use of CPB* remains inconsistent among transplant centers. Some centers attempt to do most BSLTs without CPB, and use CPB only if hemodynamic instability is encountered (or plan to use CPB

Table 34-4 – Special intraoperative considerations

SURGERY		ANESTHETIC CONSIDERATIONS
Pre-pneumonectomy	SLT: Posterolateral thoracotomy BSLT/LDLT: "Clamshell" incision Lung dissected free and exposed to hilum Cannulation of vessels (if CPB is anticipated)	Establishment of single-lung ventilation ▪ Hypoxia and hypercarbia dealt in usual ways (see Chapters 5 and 16)
	Test clamping of the PA Assess the response of the right heart to the stress of the increased afterload	Hemodynamic profile before and after test clamp Some indications for CPB (3) (controversial): ▪ SaO_2 90% on FiO_2 of 1.0 ▪ Baseline PAP greater than 40 mmHg ▪ MPAP during cross-clamp >50 mmHg ▪ Severe systemic hypotension or CI < 2 L/min/m^2

Pneumonectomy	Donor lung arrival; examined and deemed acceptable	
	Recipient pulmonary veins and artery are divided	The surgeon may need to be reminded to feel for the presence of the PA catheter prior to stapling the PA
	The bronchus is then divided, preserving as much length as possible	If a left-sided DLT is employed for a left-sided transplant, it may need to be withdrawn slightly as directed by the surgeon
	Critical juncture!	Should profound hypoxia or hypotension occur, unresponsive to vasopressors, inotropes, or optimization of ventilation to the remaining lung, it may be necessary to go onto CPB
Anastomosis	Three anastomoses (posterior-to -anterior anatomic sequence): Bronchus, PA, and pulmonary veins LA	
	Bronchial anastomosis (Fig 34-2) (telescoped if size mismatch)	
	Donor PA anastomosed to the recipient's (cross-clamp in place)	
	Cuff of donor LA containing the superior + inferior pulmonary vein entry sites anastomosed to recipient LA, isolated by a clamp	The EKG should be examined during left lung transplants because the position of the atrial "side-biter" clamp may occlude the circumflex coronary blood flow

(continued)

Table 34-4 – (continued)

SURGERY		ANESTHETIC CONSIDERATIONS
	With the recipient atrial clamp in place, the PA clamp is gradually released to fill and de-air the pulmonary circuit	Clean bronchoscope used for cleanout prior to unclamping new lung
	After thorough de-airing and confirming the absence of major leaks, LA closure is completed and the LA clamp removed	Gentle ventilation of the new lung, taking care to keep peak pressures < 25 cmH_2O Use low FiO_2 as tolerated
Reperfusion	The new lung is gently reinflated prior to releasing the PA cross-clamp in order to avoid a major shunt If post-unclamp hypotension is severe, prolonged (>minutes), or unusually refractory to vasopressor/inotrope therapy, other causes should be sought Impaired PA or pulmonary venous blood flow due to stenotic/torsed anastomoses should be excluded	Upon unclamping, variable degrees of usually transient systemic hypotension commonly occur The etiology is probably multifactorial ▪ Metabolic by-products from the ischemic lung ▪ Delayed filling of the LV as the capacity of the new lung fills up ▪ Humoral factors ▪ Reactive pulmonary vasoconstriction and pulmoplegia washout

		Typically responsive to combined use of fluids, vasopressors, and inotropes and time
		PA pressures may sometimes rise transiently during this period, but usually come down quickly after unclamping
	Ventilatory management	Peak pressures, preferably < 25 cm H_2O
		5–15-cmH_2O PEEP may minimize alveolar transudation (except in COPD patients)
		Suctioning of the new lung may be necessary
	Reperfusion injury to the new lung (see Primary Graft Dysfunction)	Inhaled NO may be started and continued in the ICU
	Electrolyte, acid–base balance	Frequent ABG's and K^+ levels should be checked
		EKG should be watched for signs of hyperkalemia.

only on select cases). Some centers always use CPB for BSLTs. The general trend is for increased use of CPB. The usual indication or predictors for the need are high PA pressures, RV dysfunction, and severely dilated pulmonary arteries in PPH (4).

Proponents of CPB cite better vascular control, better hemodynamic stability, better gas exchange, less strain to the right ventricle, easier dissection, and less stress for the first implanted lung that otherwise needs to accommodate the entire cardiac output while the second lung is implanted (10). Centers that are reluctant to use CPB routinely cite heparin and the potential for greater blood loss, need for transfusion, the systemic inflammatory response to CPB and its potential effect on the allograft, more primary graft dysfunction, and longer times to extubation (11).

A recent study showed that CPB was associated with a long period of postoperative mechanical ventilation, more pulmonary edema, more blood transfusion requirement, and increased early mortality (12).

Management of CPB

The decision to use CPB should be made in a timely fashion, with a perfusionist available. Several important points to remember are as follows.

- Anticoagulation achieved by systemic heparinization with target ACTs > 350 s.
- Cannulation sites are usually the aorta or femoral artery, RA or femoral vein for the venous cannula, although femoral artery/vein cannulation may make surgical exposure more favorable.
- Usually, warm CPB with a beating heart and venting.
- Antifibrinolytics (epsilon aminocaproic acid) are typically utilized.
- Ventilation and perfusion should be provided to the newly perfused first allograft during engraftment of the second.
- After the lungs are implanted and the patient separates from CPB, diuresis is promoted and protective ventilation strategy employed (including reduced FiO_2).

An emerging alternative to CPB is ECMO. Advantages include lower heparin levels and ACTs, and may be continued for postoperative support in the event of primary graft failure (13).

Pulmonary Hypertension and RV Dysfunction

Management principles include:

- Avoidance of hypoxia, hypercarbia, acidosis, light anesthesia, and hypothermia
- Systemic pulmonary vasodilator therapy
- Nitroglycerin, alprostadil, or sodium nitroprusside may be utilized. The major disadvantage is systemic hypotension, and in the case of nitroglycerin, increases in shunting and impaired hypoxic pulmonary vasoconstriction.
- Inotrope therapy to improve right ventricular function and cardiac output
- Inotropes, like dobutamine, milrinone, or epinephrine, are typically utilized. Milrinone may be favored for reducing PA pressure.
- Inhaled prostacyclin PGI_2 (Iloprost)

Established therapy of severe pulmonary hypertension, Iloprost, has been used with success to reduce pulmonary pressures and increase RV performance (14).

Nitric Oxide

NO (10–20 ppm), a selective pulmonary vasodilator, has been used in this setting to reduce pulmonary vascular resistance (PVR). Desirable properties of inhaled NO include:

- Reduction in pulmonary vascular tone, with improved unloading of the right ventricle
- Absence of systemic vasodilatory effects
- May effectively lower PA pressures, avoiding the need for CPB (15)
- Anti-inflammatory properties

Interferes with neutrophil adherence to endothelium, and inhibits platelet aggregation and expression of several inflammatory mediators

Currently inhaled NO is advocated for the management of a severe, established reperfusion injury (16, 17). The pre-emptive use of NO to attenuate human allograft reperfusion injury remains controversial.

Primary Graft Dysfunction

Primary graft failure is a serious complication characterized by alveolar damage, pulmonary edema, and hypoxemia due to ischemia/reperfusion injury.

The pathogenesis in the development of PGD can be grouped into the following.

1. Alloantigen dependant: A complex immune response to the allograft. Prevention and treatment stem from adequate immunosuppression with high doses of steroids, and the timely use of immunosupressive therapy, thymoglobulins, and complement inhibition.
2. Alloantigen independent: Nonimmune-mediated lung injury. This includes injury to the donor lung prior to or during harvest (mechanical trauma, aspiration, brain death, the organ harvest itself), during perfusion of the donor lung with a cold solution, or during the period of warm and then cold ischemia. Mechanical injury during surgical manipulation, reimplantation, and reperfusion may also contribute to alloantigen-independent injury.

Prevention is crucial and starts with management of the donor and donor lung using prostaglandins, steroids, and Perfadex (Vitriol, Sweden). A slow period of reperfusion, diuresis, and protective ventilation strategies has also been advocated, as has the avoidance of CPB, although the evidence basis for this is sparse. Prophylactic use of NO appeared to be an attractive option, though recent studies have not shown any benefit (18, 19).

When PGD does occur, *treatment* is supportive with mechanical ventilation, diuresis, and inhaled NO. ECMO may be a temporary lifesaving support if other measures fail.

Transesophageal Echocardiography

TEE is being used routinely at several transplant centers as a tool in the management of lung transplant patients. Assessment of cardiac anatomy and function, with focus on right-sided structures, right ventricular function, ventricular filling, interatrial septum, and

Table 34-5 – Transesophageal echocardiography in lung transplantation (20)

STRUCTURE		RATIONALE
Atrial septum	ASD or PFO	Increased risk of right-to-left shunting, especially in the event of increasing right-sided pressures, increases in PVR and RV failure This may lead to systemic hypoxemia, and right-to-left systemic embolization
Right ventricle	Function and filling	Critical at the time of PA clamping May guide therapeutic intervention or influence decision regarding the use of CPB
Cannulation sites	Ascending aorta IVC and RA	May be an aid for the process of cannulation for CPB or ECMO
Left ventricle	Function and filling	During the period of unclamping and reperfusion of the implanted lung or during separation from CPB
Anastomoses	Pulmonary artery	Evaluation of the pulmonary artery anastomosis (limited direct view)
	Pulmonary vein	Some degree of reduced venous flow may be seen in up to 29% of cases
Others		Guide the clinicians in adequate de-airing of the cardiac chambers

evaluation of pulmonary arterial and venous anastomoses, aid clinicians in decision making.

Postoperative Considerations

At the end of the procedure, the patient is reintubated with a large endotracheal tube and bronchoscopy is performed to examine the anastomoses and clean out secretions and blood. Upper airway edema may make this tube exchange treacherous. Use of a tube exchange catheter, fiber-optic bronchoscope, fiber-optic laryngoscope, and other options and backup plans should be considered. Patients typically remain intubated for 12–48 h postoperatively because of anticipated potential reperfusion injury in the new lung.

Postoperative goals are largely supportive and include:

1. Optimal management of ventilation, hemodynamics, and pain (The lowest possible FiO2 compatible with adequate oxygenation should be utilized. Peak airway pressures should be minimized (usually, limited < 25–30 cmH_2O) with 5–15 cmH_2O PEEP. Thoracic epidural analgesia, if not in situ, may be established as the patient emerges, prior to extubation.)
2. Prevention and treatment of infection
3. Optimal immunosuppression therapy

Outcome

The overall transplant half-life has improved from 4.2 to 5.7 years (Fig 34-3), and the conditional half-life among 1-year survivors has improved from 7.0 to 7.6 years. These data suggest that both short-term and, to a seemingly lesser degree, long-term survival have improved over time. Most patients with bilateral procedures had better survival within each diagnosis category. More current eras showed improved survival within each diagnosis and procedure type.

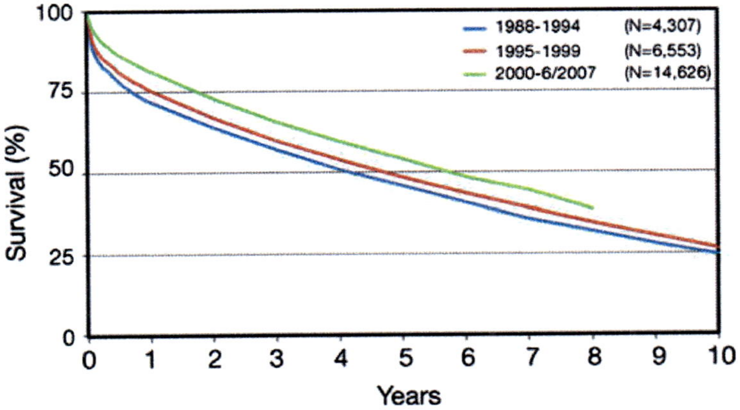

Figure 34-3 – Kaplan–Meier survival for adult lung transplants performed from January 1988 through June 2007. From Christie JD, Edwards LB, Aurora P, et al., J Heart Lung Transplant 2009;28:1031–1049, with permission.

Prolonged survival is limited by the frequent occurrence of obliterative bronchiolitis, a progressive small airways obstruction, likely the result of chronic rejection. Understanding the biology of the pulmonary allograft may enable the anesthesiologist to minimize injury to donor lungs throughout the harvest and preservation and to optimize treatment of the lung transplant recipient.

Selected References

1. Christie JD, Edwards LB, Aurora P, et al. The registry of the international society for heart and lung transplantation: twenty-sixth official adult lung and heart-lung transplantation Report-2009. J Heart Lung Transplant. 2009;28:1031–49.

2. Bracken CA, Gurkowski MA. Naples, JJ; Lung Transplantation: Historical Perspective, current concepts and anesthetic considerations. J Cardiothorac Vasc Anesth. 1997;11:220–41.

3. Orens JB, Estenne M, Arcasoy S, et al. Consensus report. International Guidelines for the Selection of Lung Transplant Candidates: 2006 Update. J Heart Lung. Transplantation. 2006;25:745–868.

4. McRae KM. Pulmonary transplantation. Cur Opin Anaesthsiol. 2000;13:53–9.

5. Gabbay E, Williams TJ, Griffiths AP, et al. Maximizing the utilization of donor organs offered for lung transplantation. Am J Respir Crit Care Med. 1999;160: 265–71.

6. Oto T, Griffiths AP, Rosenfeldt F, et al. Preservation solutions in lung transplantation: outcomes from Perfadex, Papworth, and Euro-Collins Solutions. Ann Thorac Surg. 2006;82:1842–8.

7. Ueno T, Snell GI, Williams TJ, et al. Impact of graft ischemic time on outcomes after bilateral sequential single-lung transplantation. Ann Thorac Surg. 1999;67:1577–82.

8. Novick RJ, Bennett LE, Meyer DM, et al. Influence of graft ischemic time and donor age on survival after lung transplantation. J Heart Lung Transplant. 1999;18:425–31.

9. Bittner HB, Richter M, Kuntze T, et al. Aprotinin decreases reperfusion injury and allograft dysfunction in clinical transplantation. Eur J Cardiothorac Surg. 2006;29:210–5.

10. Marczin N, Royston D. Yacoub M; Pro: Lung transplantation should be routinely performed with cardiopulmonary bypass. J Cardiothorac Vasc Anesth. 2000;13:739–45.

11. McRae K. Con: Lung transplantation should not be routinely performed with cardiopulmonary bypass. J Cardiothorac Vasc Anesth. 2000;13:746–50.

12. Dalibon N, Geffroy A, Moutafis M, et al. Use of cardiopulmonary bypass for lung transplantation: a 10-year experience. J Cardiothorac Vasc Anesth. 2006;20: 668–72.

13. Aigner C, Wisser W, Taghavi S, et al. Institutional experience with extracorporeal membrane oxygenation in lung transplantation. Eur J Cardiothorac Surg. 2007;31:468–73.

14. Rex S, Schaelte G, Metzelder S, et al. Inhaled iloprost to control pulmonary artery hypertension in patients undergoing mitral valve surgery: a prospective, randomized-controlled trial. Acta Anaesthesiol Scand. 2008;52:65–72.

15. Myles PS, Weeks AM, Buckland MR, et al. Anesthesia for bilateral sequential lung transplantation: experience of 64 cases. J Cardiothorac Vasc Anesth. 1997;44:284–99.

16. Kemming GI, Merkel MJ, Shallerer A, et al. Inhaled nitric oxide for the treatment of early allograft failure after lung transplantation. Intensive Care Med. 1998;24:1173–80.

17. Date H, Triantafillou A, Trulock EP, et al. Inhaled nitric oxide reduces human allograft dysfunction. J Thorac Cardiovasc Surg. 1996;111:913–9.

18. Botha P, Jeyakanthan M, Rao JN, et al. Inhaled nitric oxide for modulation of ischemia-reperfusion injury in lung transplantation. J Heart Lung Transplant. 2007;26:1199–205.

19. Perrin G, Rock A, Michelet P, et al. Inhaled nitric oxide does not prevent pulmonary edema after lung transplantation measured by lung water content: a randomized clinical study. Chest. 2006;129:1024–30.

20. Mypes PS. Pulmonary transplantation. In: Kaplan JA, Slinger PD, editors. Thoracic anesthesia. 3rd ed. Philadelphia, PA: Elsevier Press; 2003. p. 295–314.

Chapter 35
Miscellaneous Thoracic Surgical Procedures

Teresa M. Bean and Shannon S. McKenna

Keywords Lung cyst • Bronchogenic cysts • Pulmonary hydatid cysts • Pneumatocele • Pulmonary sequestration • Blebs • Bullae and giant bullae • Pulmonary arteriovenous malformations • Pulmonary alveolar proteinosis • Lung lavage • Idiopathic or primary hyperhidrosis • Thoracic outlet syndrome (TOS) • Radiofrequency ablation (RFA)

Introduction

The thoracic surgical procedures discussed in this chapter are bundled together because they are less commonly encountered and have limited specific anesthetic implications.

Resection of Lung Cysts and Bullae

A variety of congenital and acquired fluid and/or air-filled cystic chest lesions may require resection in adults. Resection is generally indicated for these "benign" lesions when they produce symptoms from a mass effect, infection, or rarely hemoptysis. The anesthetic considerations for this heterogenous group are sufficiently similar that they may be discussed collectively.

P.M. Hartigan (ed.), *Practical Handbook of Thoracic Anesthesia*,
DOI 10.1007/978-0-387-88493-6_35,

Lung cyst is a nonspecific term for a thin-walled, fluid and/or air-filled lesion. Lung cysts may be isolated (bronchogenic cyst) or widespread (histiocytosis X, tuberous sclerosis, leiomyomatosis, etc.). Cysts are addressed surgically for diagnosis, or to treat or prevent complications. Examples of congenital or acquired cysts occasionally encountered in adult thoracic surgery include the following:

Bronchogenic cysts (Fig 35-1) are thought to arise from primitive foregut as a developmental abnormality. The epithelial lining secretes mucous, causing the cyst to grow over time. They may be intralobar, extralobar, or mediastinal. If communicating with the tracheobronchial tree, they display air-fluid levels on CXR and are prone to recurrent infection.

Pulmonary hydatid cysts contain larvae of the dog tapeworm *Echinococcus granulosus* and are common in endemic regions (Australia, New Zealand, and Mediterranean regions) and among travelers. The cysts contain characteristically crystal clear fluid with suspended larvae, surrounded by a thin transparent membrane

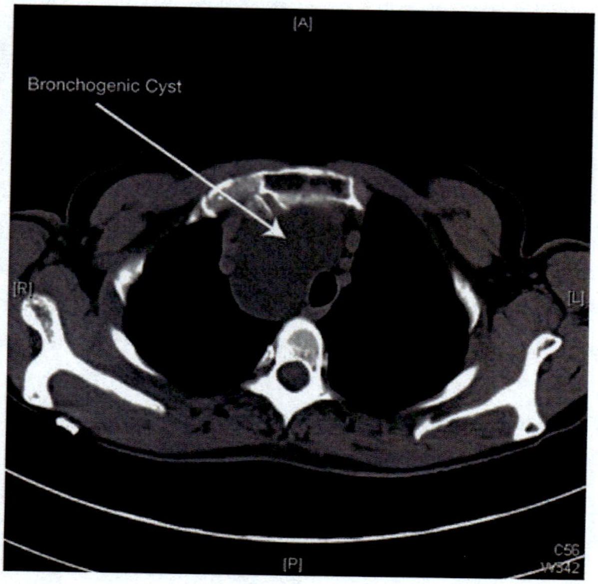

Figure 35-1 – CT scan depicting a bronchogenic cyst.

(endocyst) and an outer laminated membrane. Hydatid cysts may grow rapidly (up to 5 cm/year), exert mass effects, rupture, or cause systemic emboli. Cysts larger than 7 cm should be excised, even if asymptomatic. The surgical goal is to enucleate the hydatid cyst without rupture.

Pneumatocele is a thin-walled, mostly air-filled cyst communicating with the tracheobronchial tree, and resulting from a pulmonary infection (usually *Staphylococcus aureus*). Pneumatoceles generally resolve spontaneously over 6–8 weeks following resolution of the inciting pneumonia. Complications include enlargement and air-trapping (ball-valve effect), rupture, recurrent infection, and rarely mass effect within the chest.

Pulmonary sequestration is a congenital abnormality consisting of nonfunctioning lung parenchyma perfused by aberrant systemic circulation. Sequestrations have no functional communication with the tracheobronchial tree. They may be intra- or extralobar. The latter tends to have its own visceral pleura, making for straightforward resection. Arterial supply may be from the thoracic or abdominal aorta, or from intercostal branches. Despite their autonomy, infection can occur, presumably via pores of Kohn.

Blebs, bullae, and giant bullae are abnormal airspace collections. *Blebs* are subpleural and have a predilection for the upper lung fields. They occur as a result of rupture of neighboring alveoli. Their thin walls make them prone to rupture resulting in a spontaneous pneumothorax. Blebs may occur in the absence of diffuse underlying lung disease. A *bullae* is a larger air collection (>1 cm) within the lung parenchyma. Bullae are formed through destruction, dilatation, or confluence of air spaces distal to the terminal bronchiole. Residual parenchymal architecture may result in septations. Presenting symptoms include pneumothorax, dyspnea, and infection. They may also be associated with lung carcinoma. Bullae may occur as solitary lesions, or may be multiple, particularly in the case of underlying COPD. A bullae is termed a *giant bullae* if it occupies more than 30% of the hemithorax. Giant bullae can compress normal surrounding lung parenchyma and contribute significantly to pulmonary dysfunction.

Anesthetic Considerations for Lung Cysts and Bullae

In general, resection of small, uninfected cystic lesions which have no communication to the bronchial tree may be treated like any limited pulmonary resection (Chapter 16). Additional considerations pertain when there is infection, risk of cross contamination, significant mass effect within the chest, or communication with airways with associated risk of air trapping.

Sepsis: The clinically septic patient should be stabilized, prior to undergoing resection of the infected cyst, with antibiotics, and if feasible, percutaneous drainage. Neuraxial regional anesthetic techniques are relatively contraindicated due to risk of seeding the catheter during bacteremic episodes.

Contamination of healthy lung: When the infected cyst clearly communicates with the bronchial tree, prevention of cross-contamination is one of the principal anesthetic/surgical priorities. This may require awake placement of a double-lumen endotracheal tube (DLT) or bronchial blocker under topical anesthesia in high-risk scenarios. An alternative is to induce in rapid sequence and immediately isolate the affected lung. Patient positioning, with head of bed raised and cyst side tilted down, may offer additional protection. Double-lumen tubes offer the advantage over bronchial blockers of access to suction purulence from the effected lung without interrupting lung isolation or increasing the risk of cross-contamination.

Expansion of airspace: Air may be trapped in communicating cystic lesions by ball-valve effect or simply by the expiratory airflow resistance of the communication to the tracheobronchial tree. Positive pressure ventilation exacerbates this effect. Thus, the semistable air-filled cyst or bulla may expand or rupture with induction and mechanical ventilation. Hemodynamic compromise may occur with or without rupture (e.g., tension pneumothorax or tension pneumatocele, respectively). The greatest risk of air trapping is in large, thin-walled bullae. For such patients, many of the considerations for lung volume reduction surgery would apply (Chapter 24). Nitrous oxide should generally be avoided for lesions with closed airspaces. As above, rapid establishment of lung isolation is the best protection.

Mass effect: Large cystic lesions (particularly fluid-filled) may impose compressive effects on airways, great vessels, or the heart. Exacerbation of such mass effects within the chest can occur due to supine position, induction, and conversion to positive pressure ventilation. Large anterior mediastinal cysts are the greatest risk (see Chapter 20), but significant mass effects can occur with large eccentric fluid-filled cystic lesions as well, particularly when the patient is turned to the lateral decubitus position with the cystic lesion nondependent. The general principals of management of patients with an anterior mediastinal mass, namely, an awareness of gravitational/positional issues, cautious transition to positive pressure ventilation, and defense of airway patency and venous return, may be extrapolated to the cystic lesion which has a mass effect.

Bleeding: Congenital lesions (e.g., sequestrations) often have anomalous arterial and/or venous supply. Identifying and cleanly dividing aberrant vessels may be challenging and result in hemorrhage. Chronically infected cystic lesions are prone to bleeding from the inflammation of tissues, as well as from surgical mishap due to scarring and altered anatomy.

Resection of Pulmonary Arteriovenous Malformation

Pulmonary arteriovenous malformations (AVMs) are the abnormal communications between pulmonary arteries and pulmonary veins. Congenital lesions can be idiopathic, but most are associated with the autosomal dominant condition of hereditary hemorrhagic telangiectasia (HHT), also known as Rendu–Osler–Weber syndrome. Causes of acquired pulmonary AVMs include bronchiectasis, infection, malignancy, trauma, surgery, hepatopulmonary syndrome and schistosomiasis. Pulmonary AVMs produce a right to left shunt that does not participate in gas exchange. Very rarely, systemic pulmonary AVMs arise from abnormal communications between bronchial arteries and pulmonary veins leading to a relatively benign left to right shunt.

The consequences of untreated pulmonary AVMs can be dire. Rupture can lead to hemoptysis and hemothorax. The right to left shunt produces not only hypoxemia, but also the risk of paradoxical emboli resulting in stroke or cerebral abscess.

Anesthetic Considerations for Resection of Pulmonary AVMs

Bleeding: Blood loss can be significant depending on the surgical resection and the ability of the surgeon to identify and ligate all feeding vessels. Large bore intravenous access should be obtained and an arterial catheter may be warranted for hemodynamic monitoring and shunt comparison pre- and post-AVM excision. Other invasive monitoring like a central venous line or pulmonary arterial catheter (PAC) may be necessary depending on the patient's comorbidities. If a PAC is employed, vigilance is required to ensure it is not in the surgical field when the AVM is crossclamped.

Embolic Events: Embolic events are best avoided with air filters placed most distally on all intravenous catheters. De-airing all sources (i.e., syringes, IV fluid bags) is critical. Nitrous oxide should be avoided to prevent size increases in any air emboli. Intraoperative heparinization is often requested by the surgeon prior to cross clamping the proximal pulmonary artery and distal pulmonary vein to prevent thromboemboli.

Shunt: The degree of shunting may be complex because of multiple and/or bilateral pulmonary AVMs. AVM shunt magnitudes have been reported from a few percent to 80% of cardiac output. The surgery requires lateral decubitus positioning and lung isolation to prevent contamination of the dependent lung and provide access to the hilum. One-lung oxygenation suffers depending on the size of the AVM. An FiO_2 of 100% should be employed and nitrous oxide should be avoided. AVMs do not display HPV. Therefore hypoxemia, hypercarbia, acidosis, and increased airway pressures (including PEEP) will increase AVM shunt flow. CPAP applied to the nondependent lung may be less effective in the presence of a pulmonary AVM. Although multiple pulmonary AVMs may be present, hypoxemia should improve once the feeding arteries to the AVM are ligated.

Bronchopulmonary Lavage for Alveolar Proteinosis

Pulmonary alveolar proteinosis is a rare interstitial lung disease caused by surfactant lipoprotein accumulation in the alveoli. The buildup of surfactant lipoprotein clogs the alveolus, blocking gas exchange at the alveolar–capillary interface. The exact mechanism of the disease is still unknown; however, data suggests that abnormalities of the granulocyte-macrophage colony-stimulating factor (GM-CSF) receptor may play a role. To date, the most effective treatment is whole lung lavage (WLL).

WLL, also referred to as bronchopulmonary lavage, improves the quality of life for these dyspneic patients. For the procedure, the patient is supine under general anesthesia with a DLT. About 1 liter of warmed (37°C) saline suspended 30 cm above the patient's chest is instilled through one lumen of the DLT. With assistance of weak suction (<20 cm H_2O), the saline is drained to a container 60 cm below the patient. Repeated irrigations continue until the lavage effluent changes from a milky proteinaceous fluid to clear liquid. On average, 10–15 L of irrigation is used and at least 90% should be recovered. Usually, one lung is lavaged per session. The patient returns in about 1 week to have the opposite lung cleaned.

At our institution, some surgeons prefer to have the patient breathe spontaneously during the irrigation. The negative inspiratory pressure of spontaneous inspiration draws the irrigating fluid into the alveoli only; whereas positive pressure ventilation may increase fluid flow through the alveolar membrane causing interstitial edema.

Anesthetic Considerations of Lung Lavage

These patients have a restrictive ventilatory pattern and reduced DLCO. By the time they present for surgical intervention, they are often hypoxemic at baseline. No premedication or long-acting narcotics are necessary; these will only delay wake-up in already compromised patients.

Lung isolation: Water-tight lung isolation is required to prevent soilage of the nonlavaged lung. A left-sided DLT is most commonly employed. Inflation of the bronchial cuff while visualizing with a bronchoscope can help determine appropriate balloon inflation. Desaturation during OLV is not uncommon, depending on extent of disease. Intermittent reinflation may be necessary.

Disposition: Lung function usually takes about 24 h to the improve, so these patients often require intensive nursing in the ICU. However, depending on the degree of respiratory compromise, a thoracic step down unit may be appropriate.

Sympathectomy for Hyperhydrosis

Idiopathic or primary hyperhidrosis (abnormally excessive sweating) can occur in the face, hands, axillae, and feet. For the most part, afflicted patients are healthy, young adults desperately embarrassed by the condition. Medical treatments often fail, whereas disruption of the sympathetic chain for palmar hyperhidrosis is almost always successful, and for unknown reasons, concomitant plantar hyperhidrosis is usually also improved. Results of sympathectomy for facial and axillary hyperhidrosis are not as reliable.

In the past, sympathectomy via transection of the sympathetic ganglion was the procedure of choice. Advances in surgical technique have resulted in thoracoscopic transection of the sympathic nerve (sympathicotomy) becoming more popular.

For the procedure, the supine patient is placed under general anesthesia. A single lumen endotracheal tube may be used if the surgeon plans to insufflate the hemithorax with carbon dioxide; otherwise a left DLT can be placed so each lung can be dropped sequentially as needed. Both arms are abducted 90° and the bed is flexed into the semi-Fowler's position. A 1 cm incision is made lateral to the pectoralis major muscle on the anterior axillary line at the level of the third intercostal space. After a thoracoscope is placed in the chest, the sympathetic chain is identified and the appropriate level is transected with electrocautery or a harmonic scalpel. Once the procedure is finished, hemostasis is verified, and the lung is re-inflated under direct vision as the thoracoscope is withdrawn. No chest tubes are necessary. Small apical pneumothoraces are expected on the postoperative chest X-ray. The procedure is repeated on the opposite side.

Anesthetic Considerations for Sympathectomy for Hyperhidrosis

Communication with the surgeon is important. The surgical technique dictates whether a single lumen endotracheal tube is adequate or if a DLT is needed.

Monitoring for evidence of sympathectomy: Bilateral palmar temperature probes may be placed intraoperatively to document a rise in skin temperature. The temperature should increase 1.5–2.5°C with successful sympathectomy.

Postoperative pain control: With the small bilateral incisions and no postoperative chest tubes, PCA narcotics are generally sufficient. The sympathectomy produced by an epidural catheter makes it difficult for the surgeon to assess success of the surgery. If the procedure requires larger incisions for adequate exposure due to unexpected adhesions, aberrant anatomy, or re-operation, an epidural catheter may be placed, but should not be dosed with local anesthetic until after the surgeon documents adequate increase in palmar skin temperature as mentioned above.

Hemorrhage: The sympathetic chain lies near major vascular structures that are at risk for injury. Although significant hemorrhage is rare, adequate IV access is recommended.

First Rib Resection for Thoracic Outlet Syndrome

Compression of the subclavian artery, vein, or brachial plexus between the first rib and the scalene muscles may lead to a condition termed thoracic outlet syndrome (TOS). A cervical (supernumerary) rib arising from C7 can also lead to TOS. Symptoms may be neurogenic or vascular in origin. They are unilateral and include: paresthesias, numbness, weakness and atrophy of intrinsic hand muscles, and claudication. Nerve conduction studies and electromyography can confirm the diagnosis of neurogenic TOS. Arteriography or venography can diagnose vascular impingement.

Patients who fail conservative management may be candidates for surgical treatment. Either a supraclavicular or a transaxillary approach may be used. Significant dissection of the subclavian vessels, multiple nerves, and the scalene muscles occurs with either approach.

Anesthetic Considerations for First RIB Resection

Supraclavicular approach: General anesthesia with supine positioning and two lung ventilation is used. The incision is made in the supraclavicular fossa. Intraoperative nerve stimulation may be employed to help isolate nerves, so use of a nondepolarizing neuromuscular blocker should be specifically discussed with the surgeon. The superior aspect of the pleura may be entered. Entrained intrathoracic air may be evacuated using a drain and a Valsalva maneuver during closure. A postoperative chest X-ray should be obtained to evaluate for pneumothorax. Nitrous oxide should be avoided. Perioperative complications may include:

- *Arterial or venous injury* may occur. Rarely, sternotomy or thoracotomy may be required to gain control of a vascular injury. Adequate IV access in the contralateral extremity should be established.
- *Phenic nerve injury* or transection may result in diaphragmatic paralysis and respiratory compromise.
- *Sympathetic chain injury* may result in a Horner's syndrome.
- *Pain* and diminished sensation may occur for weeks after the procedure. Preoperatively, patients should be assessed for their level of chronic pain and current pain regimen and plans for postoperative analgesia should be tailored accordingly.

Some centers use a postoperative pain catheter embedded in the incision for immediate postoperative pain control.

Transaxillary approach: General anesthesia with lateral decubitus position and two lung ventilation is used. An axillary incision in intracostal space two is made. Arm positioning must be done in a manner to facilitate exposure. Suspension of the arm on the operative side using an orthopedic traction device with counter weights works well. Nerve stimulation is not typically used. As with the supraclavicular approach, pleural violation may occur and nitrous oxide should be avoided. Potential complications include vascular injury, sympathetic chain injury, and significant postoperative pain as detailed for the supraclavicular approach.

Radiofrequency Ablation

Radiofrequency ablation (RFA) is a percutaneous image guided intervention that can be used to treat discrete intrathoracic tumors. An electrode (probe) is placed within the tumor and electric current in the radio frequency spectrum is delivered. Resistive heating kills the surrounding cells. Large cutaneous grounding pads are used to complete the circuit and dissipate the energy.

RFA is not a first line treatment. Patients that have tumor progression despite surgery, maximal doses of radiation and chemotherapy are potential candidates. In addition, patients who are not operative candidates secondary to severe co-morbid disease may be candidates for RFA.

Anesthetic Considerations for RFA

RFA may be performed with either MAC or general anesthesia. Lung isolation is not required. Some clinicians do place double-lumen tubes for back-up, but the procedure does not require one-lung ventilation. Both patient factors and the preference of the interventional radiologist must be taken into account. Patients who are unable to lay supine and still for a prolonged period will require general anesthesia. Purported benefits to general anesthesia include optimum positioning, reliable breath holds during probe positioning, and a secured airway in the event of a cardiac or pulmonary emergency. Disadvantages include resource use, extended procedural time, potential prolonged emergence in the setting of severe obstructive lung disease, and the potential to convert a simple pneumothorax into a tension pneumothorax with positive pressure ventilation.

- *Positioning* is dictated by the exact location of the lesion and will vary according to the planned probe insertion site and anticipated trajectory. Care must be taken to pad pressure points and avoid brachial plexus injury.
- *Pneumothorax* may occur during the procedure. Reported incidences have been as high a 20–50% in small case series. The diagnosis can be made immediately by CT imaging (procedure is done in the CT scanner) and a CT-guided small bore chest tube can be placed immediately. Most pneumothoraces, however, are small and do not require drainage. Nitrous oxide should be avoided.
- *Pleuritic pain* is common postoperatively if the lesion is adjacent to or involving the pleura. Intercostal nerve blocks placed by the interventional radiologist at the time of the procedure may be of benefit for some lesions. Postprocedural pain can be treated with a combination of narcotics, acetaminophen, and nonsteroidal antiinflammatory agents.
- *Hemoptysis* in the form of blood streaked sputum is common after RFA. Massive hemoptysis is rare but has been reported.

Placement of Brachytherapy Catheters

Brachytherapy is a form of radiation treatment. The radioactive source is placed within the patient as close as possible to the lesion to be treated. It may be used intraoperatively in the surgical field as an adjunct to surgical resection. It may also be given through blind catheters placed in the tracheobronchial tree to treat endoluminal disease. This section deals specifically with the placement of catheters for endobronchial treatment.

Complications of endobronchial brachytherapy include cough, bronchitis, fistula formation (esophageal, pleural, and vascular), and hemoptysis.

Anesthetic Considerations for Brachytherapy Catheter Placement

Flexible bronchoscopy allows for visualization of the tumor and proper positioning of the brachytherapy catheter. The catheter is generally placed through the nose to allow it to be stabilized and secured postoperatively. The radiation seeds are loaded into the catheter in the radiation oncology suite after the patient has recovered from anesthesia. Optimally, the patient's naso-pharynx is well topicalized, and bronchoscopy and catheter placement proceed with only light sedation. Brief periods of deep sedation without a secured airway may also be employed if needed. It is possible to pass a brachytherapy catheter alongside an endotracheal tube but this technique is suboptimal as the catheter may be displaced at the time of extubation. Another technique sometimes used is to feed the catheter transnasally through the glottis after induction and then place an LMA. Bronchoscopy can proceed via the LMA and final positioning of the catheter can be done. There is an air leak since the catheter prevents a complete seal with the LMA and great care must be taken during LMA removal to prevent displacement of the catheter. Key concerns relevant to the anesthetic are:

- The catheter must be *precisely placed.*
- It must be *well secured* at the end of the procedure without kinking the catheter. Large coils taped to the side of the patients face work well.
- Patients must *recover rapidly* so that they can be taken to radiation oncology for treatment before the catheter moves.

Further Suggested Readings

Hartigan PM, Body SC, Sugarbaker DJ. Pulmonary resection (Chapter 11). In: Kaplan JA, Slinger PD, editors. Thoracic anesthesia. 3rd ed. Philadelphia, PA: Churchill Livingstone; 2003. p. 213–41.

Keller SM. Thoracoscopic sympathicotomy for hyperhidrosis and vasomotor disorders (Chapter 121). In: Sugarbaker DJ, Krasna MJ, Mentzer SJ, Zellos L, editors. Adult chest surgery. New York: McGraw-Hill; 2009. p. 1008–15.

Kwong KF, Krasna MJ. Dorsal sympathicotomy for hyperhidrosis (Chapter 106). In: Patterson GA, Cooper JD, Deslauriers J, Lerut AEMR, Luketich JD, Rice TW, editors. Pearson's thoracic & esophageal surgery. 3rd ed. Philadelphia, PA: Churchill Livingstone Elsevier; 2008. p. 1303–5.

McRae KM, Bussieres JS, Campos JH, Slinger PD. Anesthesia for general thoracic surgery (Chapter 4). In: Patterson GA, Cooper JD, Deslauriers J, Lerut AEMR, Luketich JD, Rice TW, editors. Pearson's thoracic & esophageal surgery. 3rd ed. Philadelphia, PA: Churchill Livingstone Elsevier; 2008. p. 39–67.

Sullivan EA, Bussieres JS, Tschernko EM. Anesthesia for specific thoracic procedures (Chapter 12). In: Kaplan JA, Slinger PD, editors. Thoracic anesthesia. 3rd ed. Philadelphia, PA: Churchill Livingstone; 2003. p. 243–68.

Zellos L. Pulmonary arteriovenous malformation (Chapter 84). In: Sugarbaker DJ, Krasna MJ, Mentzer SJ, Zellos L, editors. Adult chest surgery. New York: McGraw-Hill; 2009. p. 709–12.

Veeramachanei N, Mackinnon SE, Patterson GA. Supraclavicular approach for thoracic outlet syndrome (Chapter 122). In: Sugarbaker DJ, Krasna MJ, Mentzer SJ, Zellos L, editors. Adult chest surgery. New York: McGraw-Hill; 2009. p. 1016–23.

Urschel HC, Patel AN. Thoracic outlet syndromes (Chapter 123). In: Sugarbaker DJ, Krasna MJ, Mentzer SJ, Zellos L, editors. Adult chest surgery. New York: McGraw-Hill; 2009. p. 1024–33.

Van Sonnenberg E et al. Percutaneous thoracic tumor ablation (Chapter 77). In: Sugarbaker DJ, Krasna MJ, Mentzer SJ, Zellos L, editors. Adult chest surgery. New York: McGraw-Hill; 2009. p. 652–9.

Mutyala S, Devlin PM. Innovative radiation techniques: role of brachytherapy and intraoperative radiotherapy in treatment of lung cancer (Chapter 75). In: Sugarbaker DJ, Krasna MJ, Mentzer SJ, Zellos L, editors. Adult chest surgery. New York: McGraw-Hill; 2009. p. 639–44.

Chapter 36
Anesthesia for Pediatric Thoracic Surgery

Juan C. Ibla

Keywords Foreign body inhalation • Airway trauma • Trachesophageal fistula (TEF) • Lung parenchyma • Pulmonary cysts • Congenital diaphragmatic hernia (CDH) • Mediastinal masses • Mainstem intubation • Double-lumen tubes • Bronchial blockade

Introduction

The management of pediatric patients requiring chest surgery requires knowledge of the physiology and familiarity with the equipment and specialized techniques. This chapter reviews common clinical conditions uniquely encountered in pediatric thoracic surgery and provides practical guidance for anesthetic management. The reader is referred to other sections of this book for concepts that are not unique to pediatrics (e.g., Chapter 5 for physiology of OLV) and to standard texts for general principals of pediatric anesthesia. This chapter strictly focuses on principals unique to or principally encountered in pediatric thoracic anesthesia.

P.M. Hartigan (ed.), *Practical Handbook of Thoracic Anesthesia*,
DOI 10.1007/978-0-387-88493-6_36,

Disease Processes

Airway

Foreign Bodies

Foreign body inhalation is common and potentially a lethal emergency situation in young pediatric patients less than 1 year of age (1). The clinical presentation is not always an acute witnessed event and frequently the diagnosis can be difficult to establish. In the acute setting, the infant presents at home or emergency room with severe stridor, cyanosis, and respiratory distress, and the initial management usually involves first-response emergency personnel. In this setting, the foreign body is often in the proximal, extrathoracic airway. The reader is encouraged to review up to date principles of pediatric ACLS (http://www.aclsonline.us) for the proper management. In the subacute situation, the child presents with new onset cough and wheezing for several hours or even days suggesting an intrathoracic, more distal foreign body. CXR may reveal parenchymal collapse or signs of lobar consolidation with compensatory pulmonary overdistention and airway deviation (2). Once the diagnosis is suspected, laryngoscopy and bronchoscopy provide both confirmation of the diagnosis and definitive treatment.

Anesthetic considerations. In the acute situation when signs of respiratory distress and cyanosis are present, the goal is to maximize oxygenation until the anesthesia and surgical teams are assembled in the operating room. Maintaining a "calm" child by avoiding unnecessary painful stimulation (drawing blood or obtaining additional IV access) is essential in the initial management. Inhalational induction of general anesthesia regardless of the NPO status is the preferred practice. Allowing the patient to maintain spontaneous respiratory mechanics maximizes oxygenation and provides adequate levels of anesthesia required for laryngoscopy and bronchoscopy. In addition, spontaneous ventilation under general anesthesia minimizes aggressive coughing and valsalva maneuvers that can potentially dislodge a loose foreign body further obstructing the mayor airways or displacing it more distally. Intravenous induction and rapid-sequence intubation has also been advocated by others (3) but provides less time for laryngoscopy and requires subsequent positive-pressure ventilation. Unlike in adults, advancing an obstructive foreign body down a mainstem bronchus as a desperate rescue maneuver is less likely to succeed in pediatric patients because of the size of the airways.

Airway Trauma

Traumatic injury to the pediatric airway rarely presents as an isolated event and more frequently is associated with foreign bodies or as complication of attempts for emergent tracheal intubation. Preterm neonates are at particularly high risk of airway trauma (4). Very low birth weight patients often require endotracheal intubation and mechanical ventilation due to respiratory distress at birth and/or apnea-bradychardia. In this subset of patients, a history of multiple attempts at intubation should alert the practitioner of possible airway trauma. Descriptions of traumatic rupture of the carina, main stem bronchi, or segmental airways by airway instrumentation can be found in the literature (5). An extensive disruption of the airway is characterized by air leakage despite adequate size endotracheal tube (ETT), pneumomediastinum or pneumoperitoneum, subcutaneous emphysema, and inability to achieve adequate tidal volumes (Vt) on the ventilator. Small injuries to the trachea or airways can be asymptomatic for many days.

Anesthetic considerations. The mainstay in the ventilatory management of patients with suspected airway disruption is maintaining the lowest mean airway pressure needed for adequate ventilation until definitive and often surgical management can be accomplished. When possible, spontaneous ventilation may be beneficial, respiratory mechanics permitting (i.e., absence of pneumothorax/hemothorax). Modern ventilatory strategies include the use of pressure regulated volume control (PRVC) ventilation or high-frequency oscillatory ventilation (HFOV). In the PRVC mode, the minimum inspiratory pressure will be used to achieve a preset Vt. If the minimum inspiratory pressure (i.e., +10 cm H_2O) fails to achieve the preset Vt on the first breath, it will make small breath to breath adjustments until the preset Vt is achieved. HFOV is based on the principle that a small Vt combined with high respiratory rates results in lower mean airway pressures. Excellent practical reviews of HFOV are available (6). Other alternative ventilatory techniques are discussed further in Chapter 11.

Trachesophageal Fistula

Trachesophageal fistula (TEF) may present independently, or as part of genetic syndromes; i.e., VACTER/VACTERL associated with multiorgan malformations (vertebral/anus/cardiac/trachea/esophagus/renal and limb malformations) (7). The most common presentation involves esophageal atresia in combination with a fistulous communication of the trachea to the distal esophageal pouch (Type A). The diagnosis is usually confirmed in the delivery room due to inability to pass an orogastric tube to decompress the stomach. The neonate may present with recurrent aspiration pneumonia or respiratory failure.

Anesthetic considerations. The surgical management of TEF has evolved over the past few decades from the classic open thoracotomy to the more recent laparoscopic approach (8). The initial surgical goal is to identify and ligate the fistula; repair of esophageal atresia is often possible in the same procedure but multiple attempts at repair may be necessary. Regardless of the surgical technique used, the initial goal in managing these neonates is to maintain a low airway pressure during induction of anesthesia. A common technique involves inhaled induction and achievement of adequate anesthetic level, allowing the patient to breathe spontaneously. Next, under direct visualization with rigid bronchoschopy, the fistula is identified and occluded with a balloon-tipped embolectomy catheter; see Fig 36-2B. The embolectomy catheter is then secured in a similar fashion as an ETT. This maneuver allows the subsequent intraoperative use of positive-pressure ventilation with lower risk of insufflating the stomach via the TEF. This is mandatory if the laparoscopic technique is chosen. One-lung ventilation is usually difficult to accomplish since occlusion of the TE fistula takes precedent. Alternative ventilatory maneuvers, including high-frequency positive pressure or HFOV may be required (Chapter 11).

Lung Parenchyma

Respiratory Distress Syndrome

A multitude of etiologic factors can contribute to the development of respiratory distress syndrome (RDS) in the pediatric population. In the premature neonate, bronchopulmonary dysplasia results from a combination of lung immaturity, mechanical ventilation, and relative postnatal hyperoxia (9). This syndrome is responsible for a high acute morbidity and relatively low mortality (10) when compared to the adult population and rarely requires tissue diagnosis. In contrast, infectious etiologies of RDS or surfactant abnormality syndromes (ABC transporters) require thoracoscopic or "open-lung" biopsy (11).

Anesthetic considerations. The preoperative management of these patients involves "lung protective ventilatory strategies." These include ventilatory modalities that combine patient-triggered-pressure/volume limited ventilation, HFOV or inhaled nitric oxide (NO). In addition, reducing the FiO_2 and tolerating lower pulse oxymeter saturations (85–90%) have been demonstrated to reduce complications in this patient population (12). Lung isolation is usually requested to accomplish thoracoscopic biopsy of lung parenchyma. In some instances, HFOV must be maintained during surgery and lung isolation is difficult to accomplish under these circumstances.

Pulmonary Cysts

A number of cyst and masses of diverse embryologic origin can present at birth and are now usually diagnosed during routine prenatal ultrasonography (13). *Cystic congenital adenomatoid malformation* (CCAM) is relatively common in otherwise healthy neonates and carries the potential risk of infection and respiratory failure if not treated surgically. This lesion arises primarily from a conglomerate of dysplastic bronchial tubular structures with minimal alveolar epithelia (14). As such, this lesion carries the risk of air entrapment and pulmonary overdistention during positive-pressure ventilation. *Congenital lobar emphysema* (CLE) requires special mention in this chapter since this lesion despite being relatively uncommon can be a difficult diagnosis and often is mistaken for a pneumothorax based on radiographic appearance (15). As with CCAM, this lesion poses the risk of air entrapment during positive-pressure ventilation, with potential for hemodynamic instability and/or rupture with tension pneumothorax. *Bronchopulmonary Sequestration* is defined as an area of nonfunctioning lung parenchyma perfused by the systemic circulation (16). These lesions whether intra or extra lobar have no functional communication with the tracheobronchial tree and pose no risk of airway overdistention with positive-pressure ventilation, however, due to the potential mass effect can compress the heart, major vessels, or airways. Aberrant systemic arterial supply to sequestrations arising from the thoracic or abdominal aorta may be a significant cause of bleeding during resection.

Anesthetic considerations. As a group, cystic lesions of the lung parenchyma are managed in a similar fashion. The principal considerations are (1) the mass effect, (2) avoiding air entrapment (excluding sequestrations), (3) lung isolation (if needed), and (4) associated anomalies. The initial approach to the induction is maintaining lower airway pressures by allowing the patient to breathe spontaneously under general anesthesia until the chest is open or in severe cases a mechanism to decompress the pleural space (operating trochar, chest tube) has been established by the surgical team. Rare cases of extreme mass effects on the airway, heart, or great vessels should be treated as for anterior mediastinal masses (see below and Chapter 20). Lung isolation is usually required during thoracoscopic procedures to provide an appropriate operating field and can be accomplished in a number of ways as described later in this chapter. In addition, if the cystic lesion contains infected fluid (purulence, hydatid cysts, etc.), avoidance of cross contamination by lung isolation and patient positioning is warranted.

Esophagus

Foreign Bodies

Similarly to the airway, esophageal foreign bodies can present in all ages of pediatric patients but more frequently in the toddler group. These are characterized by acute dysphagia, drooling, and respiratory distress. More frequently they are located in the proximal 1/3 of the esophagus (73%) and are more likely to be a coin (88%) (17). These patients can present in acute distress complaining of chest pain and difficulty breathing. In the acute situation where the history is consistent with a foreign body, radiologic assessment usually confirms the diagnosis and emergent flexible or rigid esophagoscopy is indicated. In patients with minimal symptoms and a more distally located foreign body, there is controversy whether expectant management is the best treatment (18). A subset of patients suffering from eosinophilic esophagitis who have significant esophageal dismotility are at a higher risk of presenting with recurrent food impaction (19).

Anesthetic considerations. Regardless of the technique used to retrieve the foreign body, only general anesthesia is practical for pediatric patients. Patients with severe dysphagia and drooling are at high risk for tracheal aspiration during induction of anesthesia and should be considered as "full-stomach." Rapid-sequence intubation is indicated in this patient population. Foreign bodies in the esophagus rarely compromise the airway; however, fragments inadvertently left behind can pose a risk for aspiration. In the subacute situation where symptoms are not severe and there is an unclear history of a foreign body, delaying the procedure to achieve "empty stomach" conditions is a sensible choice. Surgeons must diligently search for signs of esophageal perforation or associated injury of the membranous trachea following foreign body removal from the esophagus.

Diaphragm

Congenital Diaphragmatic Hernia

Congenital diaphragmatic hernia (CDH) is a potentially lethal malformation that results from a failure of a portion of the diaphragm to form, allowing intraabdominal organs to migrate to the thoracic cavity. The left-side CDH is the most common and can result in significant pulmonary hypoplasia and pulmonary hypertension (20). Modern prenatal diagnosis can be done with the use of ultrasonography and maternal MRI can reproducibly measure fetal lung volume as indicator of postnatal survival (21). Despite improvements in the management of CDH, the mortality remains high (~10%) in most large reported series (20). The management of these neonates has undergone significant modifications as the experience with extracorporeal membrane oxygenator (ECMO) and inhaled NO has also evolved. Currently, patients with CDH are managed with lung protective ventilatory strategies and ECMO is reserved for cases of CDH with severe hypoxemia.

Anesthetic considerations. The surgical approach usually consists of "patch-repair" of the diaphragmatic defect via a lateral abdominal incision; however, recent series report excellent results with the laparoscopic technique (22). The critical consideration when taking care of these patients is to prevent pneumothorax in the contralateral side. Patients with significant pulmonary hypoplasia require high respiratory rates and low Vt to prevent over distention of the normally developed lung. The management of pulmonary hypertension may involve higher FiO_2 and inhaled NO with standard hemodynamic support. Despite successful surgical repair in the neonatal period, these patients continue to have significant pulmonary hypertension and associated comorbidities (23).

Mediastinum

Mediastinal Masses

Pediatric patients undergoing diagnostic and therapeutic procedures involving the mediastinum pose a significant anesthetic challenge. Chapter 20 discusses this topic in adults. In children, the principal concerns are the same; namely, extrinsic compression of major airways (especially at the carinal level), major vessels (pulmonary artery, superior vena cava), and the heart or right ventricular outflow tract. Anesthesia may exacerbate such mass effects to a life-threatening degree as discussed in Chapter 20. Some important differences in the pediatric population include the following:

Pediatric mediastinal tumor types are different (neuroblastomas, lymphomas, etc.) and tend to be rapidly growing and more responsive to radiatiotherapy (24).

- Obtaining a reliable history of subtle positional symptoms is more difficult in children.

- Pediatric chest walls are more compliant than adults.
- Pediatric airways are smaller at baseline, and less weight is required to extrinsically compress them.
- Pediatric patients are less tolerant of biopsy or imaging procedures under sedation, and more likely to require general anesthesia for such.
- Pediatric patients are less likely to tolerate awake fiberoptic bronchoscopy.
- Rescue maneuvers for the collapsed trachea situation (endobronchial intubation, rigid bronchoscopy, etc.) may be technically more difficult with pediatric airways than adults.
- The majority of case reports of anesthesia-related disasters in patients with anterior mediastinal masses have been in children.

Anesthetic considerations: While the mechanisms and anesthetic management principles are the same for children and adults, the practice patterns tend to differ. The default approach in adults when perceived risk is high (namely awake, sitting fiberoptic bronchoscopy, and stenting open the airway with an ETT) is not as feasible with young children. This together with the fact that pediatric anesthesiologists tend to be more comfortable and facile with awake, spontaneous breathing inhalational inductions, makes this the more frequent approach in children.

Efforts to stratify the risk of airway/vascular compression in pediatric patients with mediastinal masses undergoing general anesthesia have described the perioperative evaluation of baseline pulmonary function tests and airway dimensions. In children, the presence of symptoms does not correlate with the degree of airway compression and does not predict airway collapse under anesthesia except when severe orthopnea is present at baseline (25). CT quantification of tracheal-cross section has been used as a general guide to determine whether patients will tolerate general anesthesia. Children with preoperative tracheal narrowing of more than 50% are at high risk of developing complete airway collapse with induction and maintenance of general anesthesia. In such patients, most procedures should be performed with local anesthesia and sedation when possible. Patients with less than 50% cross-sectional area tracheal narrowing tolerate inhaled anesthesia and endotracheal intubation if free of symptoms (dyspnea and orthopnea) (26). Patients with severe respiratory distress at baseline often need radiotherapy before they can be safely anesthetized. The threshold for preoperative echocardiographic studies to evaluate cardiac and vascular compression should probably be lower for small children than adults.

Lung Isolation in Pediatric Patients

General Considerations

The principal differences from adult lung isolation are the limitations imposed by the sizes of airways and equipment. The lung isolation plan depends on assessments of the patient's airway dimensions (based on age, size, airway history, pulmonary function tests, and radiologic data), as well as the side of surgery and specific patient airway anatomic features.

It should be evident that the technical feasibility of lung isolation does not guarantee tolerance of one-lung ventilation. Conditions such as single ventricle physiology, cyanotic heart disease, and pulmonary hypertension do not tolerate the relative hypoxia and hypercapnea of OLV. Table 36-1 provides other examples of pediatric medical conditions which may preclude safe OLV in children.

The remainder of this chapter provides technical guidance for lung isolation in children.

Assessment of Airway Dimensions

The estimated airway dimensions are derived from the following information:

- Historical data (Table 36-2) may suggest subglotic stenosis or other relevant abnormalities.
    - Prematurity
    - History of tracheostomy

Table 36-1 – Medical history

Heart disease	▪ Cyanosis from mixing lesions or decreased pulmonary blood flow may not tolerate single lung ventilation ▪ Single ventricle physiology may not tolerate high $ETCO_2$ ▪ Systemic or supra systemic right ventricular pressure ▪ Decreased ventricular function as found in cardiomyopathies
Vascular disease	▪ Right aortic arch with anomalous left subclavian artery can create vascular rings and airway compression ▪ Double aortic arch ▪ Vascular sling (right pulmonary artery from left PA or vice versa)
Genetic syndromes	▪ Trisomy 21 patients have a small subglottic diameter ▪ Pierre–Robin syndrome
Severe lung disease	▪ Cystic fibrosis ▪ Pulmonary vein stenosis ▪ Pulmonary artery hypertension

    - Neonatal history of stridor
    - Previous airway surgery
- Radiologic data (CXR, CT Scans, 3-D Reconstructions, MRI)
    - Direct measurements may slightly underestimate actual airway diameters.
    - Stenosis or other abnormalities should be sought along entire trachea and both mainstem bronchi.
- Population normal values by age (Tables 36-3 and 36-4)
- Prior anesthetic records and tube sizes utilized.
- Peak expiratory flow rate (correlates with airway dimensions)

Table 36-2 – Airway history

Prematurity	▪ History of prolonged intubation and mechanical ventilation predispose to subglottic stenosis ▪ High incidence of past instrumentation to the airway, balloon dilation, etc. ▪ History of previous tracheostomy
Subglottic stenosis	▪ Can present in term neonates without associated anomalies ▪ Can present without major symptoms affecting the airway dimension
Stridor	▪ Can resolve spontaneously as the patient grows ▪ Maybe a symptom of trachea or bronchomalacia resulting in a partially occluded airway
Severe gastroesophageal reflux	▪ Increases the risk of aspiration during thoracic procedures ▪ Can be a result of vocal cord paresis/paralysis, cleft vocal cord, etc.

Table 36-3 –Predicted airway size in normal children

AGE	I.D. (MM)
Premature	2.5–3.0
Term (40 ± 2) week gestation	3.0–3.5
1 Year	4.0
2 Years	4.0–4.5
3 Years	4.5
4–5 Years	4.5–5.0
6 Years	5.0–5.5
8–10 Years	5.5–6.0
10–17 Years	6.0–7.0

Consider the following formula: Age/4 + 4 = I.D. in mm

Table 36-4 – I.D. and O.D. comparison in pediatric endotracheal tubes

I.D. (MM)	O.D. (MM)
3.0	4.3
3.5	4.9
4.0	5.6
4.5	6.2
5.0	6.9
5.5	7.5
6.0	8.2

For simplicity, airway dimensions may be subdivided into the following useful categories and techniques:

AIRWAY SIZE (MM)	TECHNIQUE MOST COMMONLY USED
3.5–4.5	Mainstem intubation
4.5–6.0	Bronchial blocker or mainstem intubation
>6.0	Double-lumen tube

Fiberoptic Bronchoscopy

Whatever technique is used, size permitting, fiberoptic bronchoscopic (FOB) guidance and confirmation is preferred. Table 36-5 provides sizes of common pediatric fiberoptic bronchoscopes and relates them to single-lumen and double-lumen tubes. For airways too small to accept a DLT, bronchial blockers may be placed either through or alongside single-lumen tubes (SLT), with the FOB passed through the SLT. Alternatively, the FOB may guide endobronchial intubation with a SLT.

Table 36-5 – Size comparison of pediatric fiberoptic bronchoscopes

BRONCHOSCOPE O.D. (MM)	ETT I.D. (MM)	DLT FR
LFP (2.2 mm)	3.0 and greater	26 and 28 Fr
DP (3.1 mm)	3.5 and greater	32 Fr and greater
GP (4.1 mm)	4.5 and greater	37 Fr and greater

Table 36-6 – Double-lumen tube size guide in pediatric patients

AGE (YEARS)	SINGLE-LUMEN ETT SIZE	DTL SIZE
8–12	6.0	26
10–12	6.5	26–28
12–14	6.5–7.0	32
14–16	7.0	35
16–18	7.0	35–37

Double-Lumen Tubes

Aside from size issues, the technical aspects of DLT placement in children are not different from adults (Chapter 9). Generally, DLTs are feasible for patients with airways >6.0 mm. The smallest DLT commonly available is 26 Fr. Table 36-6 correlates DLT size with age and SLT size. *In children, airway size correlates with age better than body weight or height*. Difficulties in placing DLT may occur when the distance between the bronchial and tracheal lumens do not match the anatomy. In addition, the pediatric airway is more elastic than in adults, and rotational forces applied to the proximal end may not transmit to the distal end; rather the entire airway may rotate with the ETT.

Mainstem Intubation

This is a relatively simple technique, most useful for patients with airways between 3.5 and 6.0 mm. Use of modern cuffed ETTs (Mallinckrodt I.D. 3.0–7.0 mm) allows for the use of smaller O.D. and better seal. Right endobronchial intubation is easier than left, due to the angle of the left mainstem. FOB guidance is recommended when possible.

- The appropriate sized ETT (Tables 36-3 and 36-4) is initially placed to mid-tracheal depth by direct laryngoscopy. (*Note*: the ETT I.D. multiplied by three times provides the approximate depth (cm) for mid-tracheal intubation)
- ETT size appropriateness is confirmed by performing leak test (auscultation of air leak with positive pressure) and by passing fiberoptic scope.
- FOB is advanced into the target mainstem bronchus.
- ETT is advanced over bronchus to depth guided by FOB.
- For left mainstem intubations, turning head to the right as the ETT is advanced improves the angle and success rate.
- For right mainstem intubations with a short right mainstem (or tracheal bronchus), the ETT should be advanced into the bronchus intermedius. Often patients will tolerate OLV with just the middle and lower lobes ventilated.

Bronchial Blockade

This technique provides a safe alternative for any size airway independent of the side to be isolated. We discuss the Arndt Pediatric Endobronchial Blocker System (Cook Medical) as well as an alternative technique using a Fogarty arterial embolectomy catheter (Edwards Lifesciences).

Arndt Pediatric Endobronchial Blocker

Technical principles for safely positioning an Arndt bronchial blocker are not different in children than adults (see Chapter 9) excepting the minor variations discussed below. This blocker is manufactured in 5.0 Fr/50 cm and 7.0 Fr/65 cm. When using the 5.0 Fr/50 cm system, the smallest ETT size (I.D.) recommended is 4.5 mm and should result in a peak airway pressure no more than 20 cm H_2O. When using the 7.0 Fr/65 cm system the smallest ETT size (I.D) recommended is 6.0 mm and should result in a peak airway pressure no more than 25 cm H_2O. *Higher peak inspiratory pressures or absence of normal $EtCO_2$ tracing alert to the possibility of an incorrect positioning of the blocker.* Inability to ventilate implies tracheal occlusion by proximal migration of the blocker and should prompt deflation of the balloon.

Bronchial blockade in airways between 3.5 and 4.5 mm. (Placement outside the ETT):

When faced with the need of lung isolation in young child (neonate to 2–3 years old) whose airway may not accommodate an ETT of at least 4.5 mm, we use the 5.0 Fr/50 cm system with the following steps:

Right main stem blockade (Arndt system)

1. Select the adequate ETT size guided by Tables 36-3 and 36-4.
2. Select the adequate bronchoscope according to the endotracheal size, Table 36-5.
3. *Perform laryngoscopy and advance gently the Arndt Blocker through the vocal cords until resistance is met.* This is usually found from 3 to 5 cm deeper than the mid-tracheal level. In our experience, this maneuver results in right main intubation in over 95% of the cases.
4. While keeping a direct view of the vocal cords, advance the appropriate size ETT to the mid-tracheal level. Consider using 1/2 size smaller ETT than predicted for the age.
5. Ensure adequate ventilation of both lungs.
6. Perform flexible bronchoscopy to verify that the bronchial blocker is placed in the right main bronchus and withdraw the blocker until a rim of the blue cuff is seen. Insuflate 0.5 cc to a maximum of 2 cc (Fig 36-1A, B) into the cuff and

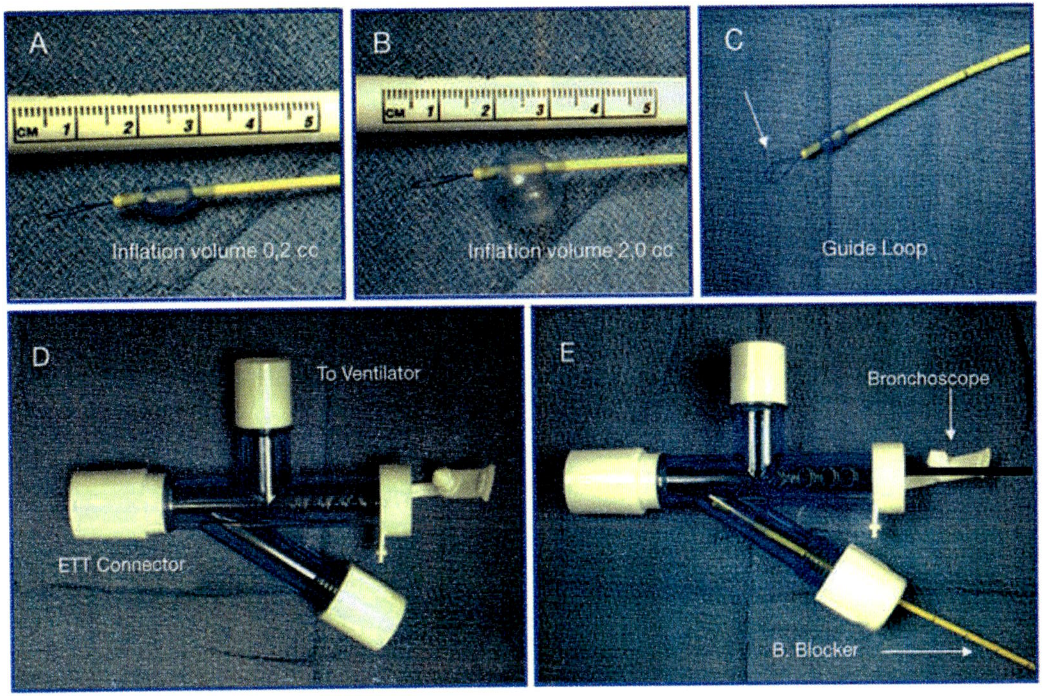

Figure 36-1 – Arndt pediatric endobronchial blocker set. (**A**) Minimal inflation volume of 0.2 cc of air enables its use in small pediatric airways (term newborn). (**B**) An inflation volume of 2 cc provides ideal bronchial occlusion conditions in older children (up to 12 years of age). (**C**) The guide loop is useful when directing the endobronchial blocker to the left main stem bronchus. (**D**) The airway multiport airway adaptor allows simultaneous placement of the endobronchial blocker and adequate ventilation even during spontaneous breathing. (**E**) Assembly of the endobronchial blocker outside the ETT guarantees its proper placement. Generous lubrication is essential for its success.

observe complete occlusion of the bronchus. Note and record the distance of the blocker necessary to obtain the desired position.

Left main stem blockade (Arndt system)

- As above for steps 1–5, except that the blocker is only advanced to the estimated mid-tracheal level.
- Perform flexible bronchoscopy to visualize the blocker and carina (Fig 36-1C). With head turned to the right, try to advance the blocker into the left mainstem bronchus.
- If this fails, drive the bronchoscope through the blue guide loop and into the left main bronchus.
- Advance the Arndt Blocker until the blue guide loop is visible beyond the scope, within the left mainstem bronchus (turning head to the right may help).
- Withdraw the scope to view the carina and fine tune the depth of the blocker.
- Inflate 0.5 cc to a maximum of 2 cc into the cuff and observe complete occlusion of the bronchus (Fig 36-1A, B).

Bronchial blockade in airways between 4.5 and 6.0 mm. (Placement inside the ETT):

When faced with the need of lung isolation in child (3–12 years old) whose airway can accommodate an ETT of at least 4.5 mm but no more that 6.0 mm, we use the 5.0 Fr/50 cm Arndt system with the following steps:

- Select the appropriate ETT size (Tables 36-3 and 36-4) and bronchoscope (Table 36-5).
- Intubate to mid-tracheal level and confirm ventilation.
- Attach the Arndt Multiport Airway Adapter (Fig 36-1D) onto the ETT.
- Lubricate the bronchoscope and bronchial blocker.

- Advance the endobronchial blocker through the blocker port and control the air leakage by screwing down the cap on the blocker port (Fig 36-1D).
- Place the bronchoscope through the diaphragm of the bronchoscope port of the adapter (Fig 36-1E) until the guide loop comes into view.
- Use the bronchoscope to guide or direct the blocker into the target mainstem bronchus as described above or in Chapter 9. Tightly screw closed the blocker orifice to eliminate air leak and fix the blocker's position to the adapter.

Bronchial Blockade in Airways Larger Than 6.0 mm

For this size airway, we use the 7.0 Fr/65 cm system. Otherwise, the steps are identical to the above or as described for adults in Chapter 9.

Bronchial blockade using the Fogarty arterial embolectomy catheter:

Fogarty arterial embolectomy catheters are an alternative to the Arndt system which is particularly useful for very small airways. Size ranges between 2.0 and 7.0 Fr are typically used for pediatric lung isolation. This technique can be used for placement outside or inside the ETT. Some particular disadvantages can be circumvented but include: (a) no guide loop or central lumen, (b) no multiport adapter is provided (but an equivalent can be easily assembled (Fig 36-2A)), (c) *the balloon is designed for intravascular procedures and tears easily if not handled with caution*, and (d) left main bronchial blockade can be difficult to accomplish in airway less than 4.5 mm. The 2 Fr/60 cm catheter uses a maximum of 0.1 ml of air/saline inflation volume, 3 Fr/80 cm, 0.2 ml and the 4 Fr/80, 0.75 ml (Fig 36-2B).

Embolectomy catheters with a malleable central wire stylette allow one to create a 45° bend at the tip to facilitate steering it under bronchoscopic guidance. Alternatively, the embolectomy catheter may be passed through the ETT and out through the Murphy Eye to create a 30° bend at the tip (Fig 36-3). By advancing

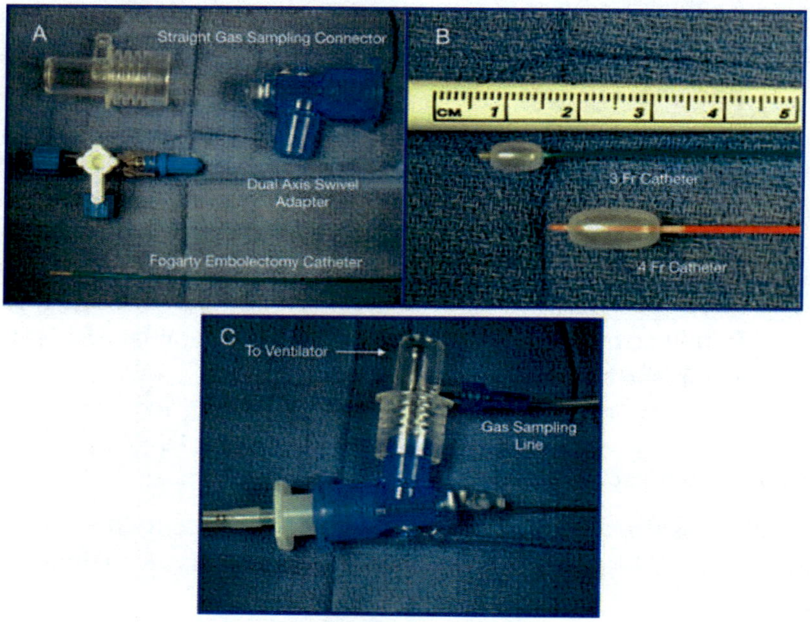

Figure 36-2 – Bronchial blockade using the Fogarty arterial embolectomy catheter. (**A**) Additional components in this technique need to be gathered before hand and are easily obtained in the standard operating room. (**B**) The 3 Fr Fogarty catheter is ideal for bronchial blockade in small infants (newborn). The 4 Fr Fogarty catheter can be used in children from 2 to 4 years old. (**C**) Assembly of the bronchial blockade system is easy and allows adequate placement and simultaneous ventilation.

the ETT/catheter assembly close to the carina, and rotating the proximal end of the ETT/catheter/swivel adapter, the catheter tip can be directed into either mainstem bronchus under bronchoscopic guidance.

Double-lumen ETT (for airways of 6.0 mm or more)

The proper technique and basic principles of placement of a double-lumen tube (DLT) are reviewed in detail in Chapter 9 of this book and are the same used for pediatric patients. When deciding on a DLT, airway size consideration is of prime importance. Pediatric DLT are manufactured from 26 to 42 Fr and a guide of the approximated airway size comparison is shown in Table 36-6.

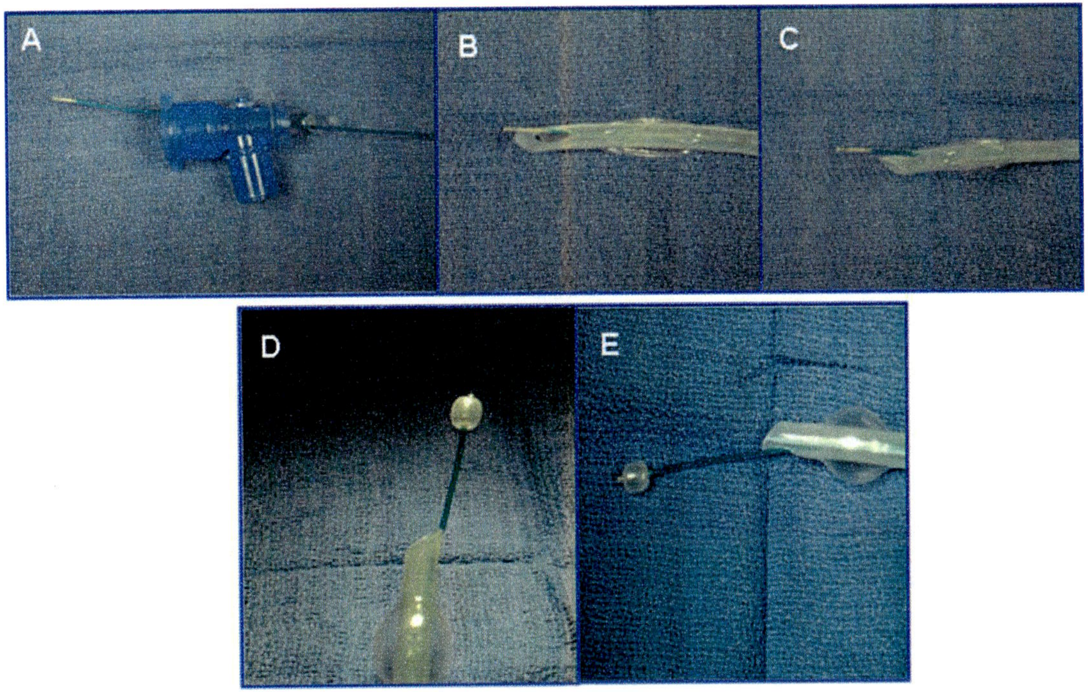

Figure 36-3 – Steps necessary for adequate placement of the Fogarty embolectomy catheter. (**A**) Initially, the Fogarty catheter is placed through the diaphragm of the dual-axis dual adaptor. (**B**) Next, the Fogarty catheter is advanced through the lumen of the ETT and until it reaches the Murphy eye. (**C**) The ETT/Fogarty assembled catheter is advanced through the vocal cords into the mid-tracheal level. (**D**) Right-ward rotation of the ETT directs the Fogarty catheter toward the right main stem bronchus. (**E**) Left-ward rotation (180°) aligns the Fogarty catheter with the left main bronchus.

It is important to remember that airway size correlates with age and not body weight or height.

Selected References

1. Chen LH, Zhang X, Li SQ, Liu YQ, Zhang TY, Wu JZ. The risk factors for hypoxemia in children younger than 5 years old undergoing rigid bronchoscopy for foreign body removal. Anesth Analg. 2009;109(4):1079–84.

2. Mu LC, Sun DQ, He P. Radiological diagnosis of aspirated foreign bodies in children: review of 343 cases. J Laryngol Otol. 1990;104(10):778–82.

3. Soodan A, Pawar D, Subramanium R. Anesthesia for removal of inhaled foreign bodies in children. Paediatr Anaesth. 2004;14(11):947–52.

4. Holzki J, Laschat M, Stratmann C. Stridor in the neonate and infant. Implications for the paediatric anaesthetist. Prospective description of 155 patients with congenital and acquired stridor in early infancy. Paediatr Anaesth. 1998;8(3):221–7.

5. Chiou HL, Diaz R, Orlino Jr E, Poulain FR. Acute airway obstruction by a sheared endotracheal intubation stylet sheath in a premature infant. J Perinatol. 2007;27(11):727–9.

6. Stawicki SP, Goyal M, Sarani B. High-frequency oscillatory ventilation (HFOV) and airway pressure release ventilation (APRV): a practical guide. J Intensive Care Med. 2009;24(4):215–29.

7. Al-Malki TA, Ibrahim AH. Esophageal atresia with tracheoesophageal fistula and early postoperative mortality. West Afr J Med. 2005;24(4):311–5.

8. Holcomb III GW, Rothenberg SS, Bax KM, et al. Thoracoscopic repair of esophageal atresia and tracheoesophageal fistula: a multi-institutional analysis. Ann Surg. 2005;242(3):422–8. discussion 428–30.

9. Demirel N, Bas AY, Zenciroglu A. Bronchopulmonary dysplasia in very low birth weight infants. Indian J Pediatr. 2009;76(7):695–8.

10. Randolph AG. Management of acute lung injury and acute respiratory distress syndrome in children. Crit Care Med. 2009;37(8):2448–54.

11. Willson DF, Chess PR, Notter RH. Surfactant for pediatric acute lung injury. Pediatr Clin North Am. 2008;55(3):545–75. ix.

12. Stevens TP, Harrington EW, Blennow M, Soll RF. Early surfactant administration with brief ventilation vs. selective surfactant and continued mechanical ventilation for preterm infants with or at risk for respiratory distress syndrome. Cochrane Database Syst Rev. 2007;4:CD003063.

13. Zeidan S, Hery G, Lacroix F, et al. Intralobar sequestration associated with cystic adenomatoid malformation: diagnostic and thoracoscopic pitfalls. Surg Endosc. 2009;23(8):1750–3.

14. Guo H, Cajaiba MM, Borys D, et al. Expression of epidermal growth factor receptor, but not K-RAS mutations, is present in congenital cystic airway malformation/congenital pulmonary airway malformation. Hum Pathol. 2007;38(12):1772–8.

15. Ulku R, Onat S, Ozcelik C. Congenital lobar emphysema: differential diagnosis and therapeutic approach. Pediatr Int. 2008;50(5):658–61.

16. Zeidan S, Gorincour G, Potier A, et al. Congenital lung malformation: evaluation of prenatal and postnatal radiological findings. Respirology. 2009;14(7): 1005–11.

17. Turkyilmaz A, Aydin Y, Yilmaz O, Aslan S, Eroglu A, Karaoglanoglu N. Esophageal foreign bodies: analysis of 188 cases. Ulus Travma Acil Cerrahi Derg. 2009; 15(3):222–7.

18. Waltzman ML, Baskin M, Wypij D, Mooney D, Jones D, Fleisher G. A randomized clinical trial of the management of esophageal coins in children. Pediatrics. 2005;116(3):614–9.

19. Luis AL, Rinon C, Encinas JL, et al. Non stenotic food impaction due to eosinophilic esophagitis: a potential surgical emergency. Eur J Pediatr Surg. 2006;16(6):399–402.

20. Abdullah F, Zhang Y, Sciortino C, et al. Congenital diaphragmatic hernia: outcome review of 2,173 surgical repairs in US infants. Pediatr Surg Int. 2009;25(12):1059–64.

21. Kilian AK, Busing KA, Schuetz EM, Schaible T, Neff KW. Fetal MR lung volumetry in congenital diaphragmatic hernia (CDH): prediction of clinical outcome and the need for extracorporeal membrane oxygenation (ECMO). Klin Padiatr. 2009;221(5):295–301.

22. Gourlay DM, Cassidy LD, Sato TT, Lal DR, Arca MJ. Beyond feasibility: a comparison of newborns undergoing thoracoscopic and open repair of congenital diaphragmatic hernias. J Pediatr Surg. 2009;44(9):1702–7.

23. Muratore CS, Kharasch V, Lund DP, et al. Pulmonary morbidity in 100 survivors of congenital diaphragmatic hernia monitored in a multidisciplinary clinic. J Pediatr Surg. 2001;36(1):133–40.

24. Dubashi B, Cyriac S, Tenali SG. Clinicopathological analysis and outcome of primary mediastinal malignancies – a report of 91 cases from a single institute. Ann Thorac Med. 2009;4(3):140–2.

25. Shamberger RC, Holzman RS, Griscom NT, Tarbell NJ, Weinstein HJ, Wohl ME. Prospective evaluation by computed tomography and pulmonary function tests of children with mediastinal masses. Surgery. 1995;118(3):468–71.

26. Shamberger RC, Holzman RS, Griscom NT, Tarbell NJ, Weinstein HJ. CT quantitation of tracheal cross-sectional area as a guide to the surgical and anesthetic management of children with anterior mediastinal masses. J Pediatr Surg. 1991;26(2):138–42.

V

Essential of Pain Management Following Thoracic Surgery

Chapter 37
Acute Postoperative Pain Control Following Thoracic Surgery

Peter Gerner and Philip M. Hartigan

Keywords Thoracotomy • Thoracotomy pain • Thoracic epidural analgesia • Intercostal nerve injury • Pleural injury • VATS incisions • TEA • Thoracic paravertebral block • Percutaneous TPB • Intercostal nerve blocks • Cryoanalgesia • Interpleural Catheter Technique • Transcutaneous electrical nerve stimulation

Introduction

Thoracotomy is among the most painful of all surgical incisions. Necessary motions of respiration exacerbate that pain. It is no surprise that the most frequent perioperative complications following thoracic surgery are pulmonary in nature, or that good control of thoracotomy pain improves pulmonary outcome. The fact that IV narcotics also inhibit respiratory function has driven the development of alternative solutions to pain control following thoracic surgery. Thoracic epidural analgesia (TEA), the most prominent modality in current practice, may have additional outcome benefits. Essential knowledge of TEA, as well as alternative modalities is summarized here, while the technical aspects are covered in Chapter 13.

P.M. Hartigan (ed.), *Practical Handbook of Thoracic Anesthesia*,
DOI 10.1007/978-0-387-88493-6_37, © Springer Science+Business Media, LLC 2012

Mechanisms of Pain Following Thoracic Surgery

Thoracotomy Pain

Acute pain after thoracotomy is due to multiple causes: soft tissue trauma, osseous trauma (rib retraction, resection, or fracture), dislocation of costovertebral joints, intercostal nerve injury, and pleural injury or irritation by thoracostomy tubes. Depending on the surgery, other sources of pain may contribute, including lung parenchymal staple lines, diaphragm injury, transection of the tracheobronchial tree, or injury to other mediastinal structures (pericardium, esophagus, etc.). Afferent pain pathways involve somatic sensory dermatomes (C3-T10), and travel with intercostal, vagus, and phrenic nerves. A robust inflammatory response accompanies thoracic surgery. Local mediators of inflammation (prostaglandins, bradykinin, histamine, nerve growth factor, cytokines, etc.) lead to peripheral sensitization, and amplified pain (primary hyperalgesia) at the affected site (1). Intense and prolonged noxious stimuli or tissue injury also cause central sensitization, hyperactivity of spinal cord dorsal horn neurons and other CNS neurons, through activation of *N*-methyl-D-aspartate (NMDA) receptors leading to chronic post-thorocotomy pain (see Chapter 38). Central sensitization is especially important for the pain in the unaffected tissue surrounding the injury site (secondary hyperalgesia) (2).

Compared to thoracotomy, VATS incisions result in less chest wall soft tissue injury and a reduced inflammatory response. Acute pain after VATS is generally less severe than thoracotomy, but angulation of the instruments may crush intercostal nerves and severely bruise the periosteum of ribs.

Shoulder Pain

Up to 75% of thoracotomy patients report constant severe ache in the ipsilateral shoulder following thoracic surgery (3). The mechanism of this pain is controversial, and likely multifactorial. Shoulder pain is not typically relieved by TEA. Often, with a working epidural, shoulder pain is the dominant complaint of thoracic surgery patients in the early recovery period.

Postulated mechanisms include transection of a major bronchus, ligamentous strain from malposition (during lateral decubitus position) or surgical mobilization of the scapula, pleural irritation due to the thoracostomy tube, or referred pain from irritation of the pericardium or mediastinal and diaphragmatic pleural surfaces. It appears that the most important origin of shoulder pain is referred pain via the phrenic nerve. Periphrenic infiltration with local anesthetic eliminates shoulder pain in some, but not all patients (4). This could be due to anatomical variations in the emergence of the sensory fibers from the phrenic nerve, or to alternative sources of shoulder pain in some patients. While phrenic nerve infiltration helps shed light on the mechanism, it is clinically impractical because of the rapid absorption and limited duration of local anesthetic in the phrenic bed.

It is likely that a proportion of patients with shoulder pain have a significant contribution from position-related mechanical stress of the shoulder (coracoid impingement syndrome and coraco-clavicular ligament strain). Evidence favoring this comes from the partial relief of shoulder pain in some patients by interscalene brachial plexus block. Adjuncts with anti-inflammatory effects (NSAIDS) are particularly effective in helping relieve shoulder pain.

Overview of Strategies for Post-Thoracotomy Pain

In general, a multimodal approach, combining regional anesthesia techniques and systemic therapy is preferable, in order to improve efficacy and decrease side effects.

Thoracic Epidural Analgesia

TEA is the most widely utilized mode of treatment for acute pain following thoracic surgery, and currently regarded as the "gold standard" against which other modalities are compared. Technical aspects of TEA are discussed in Chapter 13. Indications, efficacy, physiology, and pharmacology are summarized here.

Indications: TEA is generally employed for thoracotomies, and selected VATS approaches (those with anticipated significant utility ports such as VATS lobectomies). TEA may also be advantageous with lesser incisions when a narcotic sparing technique is desired (e.g., severe pulmonary disease, obstructive sleep apnea, etc.).

Efficacy of TEA: No other single modality provides superior control of acute incisional pain following thoracotomy. Consensus on this is sufficiently widespread that randomized comparisons between TEA and other modalities following thoracotomy are now difficult to acquire approval for. Distinctions have been made between static (pain at rest) and dynamic pain (e.g., during deep breathing and coughing). Even when sufficient parenteral narcotics are administered to achieve comparable static pain relief, TEA provides superior dynamic analgesia following thoracotomy (5).

Other positives of TEA are that it has a long track record, and high safety index. Success rates depend on operator experience, but approach 96% in centers with significant volume. Importantly, the physiologic effects of TEA may improve pulmonary and cardiovascular outcome as well as the incidence of chronic post-thoracotomy pain (see below). Disadvantages include the need for institutional infrastructure to manage and adjust dosages, monitor for complications (infections, etc.), and remove catheters at the appropriate time and coagulation status. The list of complications is well known (Table 37-1), but the incidence is low. Contraindications (Table 37-2) are no different from any neuraxial regional technique. The definition of acceptable coagulation status should be a matter of judgment, individualized to the patient, and guided by published recommendations (see American Society of Regional Anesthesia website guidelines at www.asra.com) (Table 37-3). Interestingly, the incidence of epidural hematoma is lower following the thoracic compared to lumbar epidural approach (6).

Respiratory Effects of TEA

Respiratory muscle function: Thoracic epidural blockade in healthy volunteers results in decreased lung volumes (VC, TLC, FRC, and FEV_1) due to modestly decreased intercostal muscle motor strength. Diaphragm function is preserved, and may be enhanced

Table 37-1 – Complications of thoracic epidurals

- Inadequate analgesia/failed block
- Hypotension
- Infection (superficial vs. epidural abscess)
- Accidental dural puncture/spinal block
- Postdural puncture headache
- Epidural hematoma
- Spinal cord or root injury
- Urinary retention
- Local anesthetic toxicity
- Horner's syndrome
- Backache/transient radicular irritation (TRI)
- Epidural narcotic-related effects:
  - Pruritis
  - Nausea/vomiting
  - Respiratory depression
  - Drowsiness, delirium

Table 37-2 – Contraindications to thoracic epidurals

- Patient refusal
- Coagulopathy (see Table 37-3)
- Infection or tumor at insertion site or needle pathway
- Bacteremia/sepsis
- Cardiovascular instability or intolerance of sympathetic blockade (relative)
  - Critical aortic stenosis
  - Severe hypertrophic subaortic stenosis (IHSS)
  - Severe hypovolemia

Table 37-3 – Recommended duration to hold anticoagulants prior to epidural catheter placement

ANTICOAGULANT		DURATION
Nonsteriodal-related	NSAIDS, ASA, COX-2 Inhibitors	0
	Aggrenox (ASA + dipyridamole)	0
Unfractionated heparin	Prophylactic BID SQ dose (total daily dose <10,000 U)	0
	Therapeutic IV	4 h
Low-molecular weight heparin	High dose	24 h
	Low dose	12 h
Warfarin		4–5 days (or normal INR)
Selective ADP inhibitors	Clopidogrel (Plavix®)	7 days
	Ticlopidine (Ticlid®)	14 days
Glycoprotein IIb/IIIa inhibitors	Tirofiban (Aggrastat®)	4–8 h
	Eptifibatide (Integrilin®)	4–8 h
	Abciximab (ReoPro®)	24–48 h
New anticoagulants	[a]Desirudin (Revasc®)	12 h
	[a]Lepirudin (Refludan®)	6 h
	[a]Bivalirudin (Angiomax®)	2 h
	[a]Argatroban (Acova®)	4 h
	[a]Fondaparinux (Arixtra®)	4 days
	[b]Rivaroxaban (Xarelto®)	18 h

Adapted from American Society of Regional Anesthesia and Pain Medicine Evidence-Based Guidelines (Third Edition). Note, combining agents likely results in increased risk. See complete guidelines for important details and caveats (See Horlocker TT, Wedel DJ, Rowlingson JC, et al. Reg Anesth Pain Med 2010;35:64–101 or www.asra.com).

Variance from these recommendations:

[a]These estimates are based solely on individual drug pharmacokinetic data (i.e., 4× elimination half-life). Patients with delayed drug elimination (e.g., renal impairment) may require longer intervals.

[b]Adapted from the Scandinavian Society of Anaesthesiology and Intensive Care Medicine guidelines.

by the altered chest wall conformation and resting length. Following thoracic surgery, the respiratory benefits of TEA (improved dynamic analgesia, decreased splinting, etc.), outweigh the negatives such that function is enhanced compared to that with systemic opioid analgesia (7). Even in patients with severe COPD, concerns regarding TEA-induced impairment of respiratory muscle strength are unwarranted when using conventional, dilute solutions.

Bronchial tone: TEA variably blocks sympathetic supply to the lungs. In theory, unopposed parasympathetic tone would predispose to bronchoconstriction. Thoracic surgical patients are at particular risk for bronchospasm. In practice, even patients with severe asthma tolerate TEA well without evidence of increased airways resistance or reactivity. It has been speculated that deafferentation, and the systemic effect of absorbed local anesthetics may blunt airway reactivity, counteracting the autonomic effect.

Gas exchange: TEA shifts the CO_2 response curve mildly to the right in awake volunteers. There is no direct effect on HPV and V/Q matching is preserved. Following thoracic surgery, TEA improves gas exchange (compared to systemic opioids) by reducing splinting and atelectasis, through improved diaphragm function and dynamic analgesia which is essential for effective deep breathing, coughing, and participation in respiratory physiotherapy.

Cardiovascular Effects of TEA

Pump function: Thoracic epidural local anesthetics cause preganglionic sympathetic blockade. The extent of sympatholysis may be variable, and only loosely related to the sensory level. TEA sympathetic blockade extending to the "cardiac accelerators" (T1–T4) likely exerts a negative inotropic effect, (8) in addition to effects on loading conditions.

Vascular tone: TEA sympatholysis results in vasodilation and increased venous and arterial capacitance. The hemodynamic effect depends not only on the extent and density of the block but also on the pre-existing tone. Severe dilation of a previously constricted splanchnic bed will impair venous return and preload more significantly than if the splanchnic bed had been dilated and full. Thus, the effect on preload may be difficult to predict.

Heart rate and rhythm: TEA generally causes a mild reduction in heart rate, or blunting of the HR response to surgical stimulation. Atrio-ventricular (AV) nodal conduction time and AV node refractoriness are prolonged. Some studies found a decrease in perioperative supraventricular tachyarrhythmias with TEA, (9) while others did not.

Hemodynamic effect: The net effect of the above is generally a mild to moderate depression of blood pressure with TEA (10). The magnitude depends on the level and density of sympatholysis, the preexisting tone and volume status, and other factors. The predominant mechanism may either be through reduction of venous return, or negative inotropy. It is often not apparent which mechanism is dominant. Thus, a poor response to maneuvers which augment venous return (vasopressors, fluids) should prompt a trial of mixed alpha-beta adrenergic agonist to augment contractility as well.

Other Effects

Gastrointestinal: TEA has been associated with more rapid return of bowel function, presumably related to reduction of splanchnic sympathetic tone.

Stress response to surgery: TEA is associated with reduced catecholamine levels and other stress hormones following surgery. It may also favorably affect the balance between pro- and anti-inflammatory mediators, as well as the immunologic response to the stress of surgery.

Choice of Epidural Agents

No single best recipe has been established. There is general consensus on the following statements:

- The initial (test) dose should contain a short acting local anesthetic with epinephrine to rule out an intravascular or subarachnoid catheter (e.g., 3 ml of 2% lidocaine with epinephrine 1:200,000).

- Longer acting amide local (anesthetics, bupivacaine, ropivacaine) anesthetics are more commonly used for maintenance infusions.
  - Bupivacaine is a racemic mixture, while ropivacaine is marketed as the *S*-enantiomer of its racemate.
  - Ropivacaine is less potent than bupivacaine, and has lower cardiotoxicity and possibly greater differentiation between motor/sensory block.
  - The differences between equipotent doses of bupivacaine and ropivacaine are modest, and rarely of clinical significance.
- Overall, the dosage, not the concentration, of local anesthetic determines the extent of block, density, and quality of analgesia (11).
- Synergy occurs between epidural local anesthetics and narcotics. (Local anesthetics may facilitate entry of narcotics in to the CSF) (12).
- The choice of epidural narcotics is primarily based on lipophilicity which determines rate of systemic uptake and neuraxial dwell time. Other factors include duration of action, and institutional preferences.
  - Lipophilic: fentanyl and sufentanyl
  - Hydrophilic: morphine
  - Intermediate: hydromorphone
- Most centers prefer lipophilic or intermediate epidural narcotics out of concern that hydrophilic agents (morphine) may be more apt to spread cephalad and cause delayed respiratory depression.
- Side effects common to all epidural narcotics include nausea, pruritis, urinary retention, drowsiness, and respiratory depression (by neuraxial ascention or systemic absorption).
- Other agents (clonidine, neostigmine, etc.) have potential use as replacements for, or adjuncts to epidural local anesthetics and narcotics.

Compared to continuous infusion, patient-controlled epidural analgesia (PCEA) results in improved patient satisfaction, lower total drug utilization, and lower incidence of rescue interventions for inadequate pain control in some studies.

Based on the above, choice of epidural agents and combinations may be customized to the patient, the operation, and institutional preferences. For example, despite the advantages of synergism, some centers may utilize narcotic-free epidural local anesthetics when they anticipate the need for combined TEA/IV PCA (e.g., for shoulder pain or for the narcotic addicted patient), thus obviating confusion and excessive narcotic effect.

Asleep vs. Awake Technique

The safety of thoracic epidural placement in anesthetized patients is a matter of debate. In the USA, asleep thoracic epidural placement is not the routine, except in specific circumstances where the risk of awake placement is increased. Pediatric or mentally challenged patients who might become panicked or combative during placement are examples of such situations. In contrast, a survey of practice in the UK revealed that thoracic epidural cannulation is usually (60%) performed after induction of anesthesia (13). The risk of thoracic spinal cord or root damage is very low, but nonzero, and potentially of serious consequence. Cryomicrotome sections of human epidural anatomy revealed that the ligamentum flavum was more frequently discontinuous at the thoracic level compared to the lumbar level (14). Case reports of complications prompted the statement by Horlocker in the American Society of Anesthesiologists Newsletter that "techniques above the termination of the spinal cord…should be avoided [in anesthetized patients]" (15). In the situation where a minimally invasive approach unexpectedly turns into a thoracotomy, intercostal blocks can be used as a bridge to comfortably awaken and extubate patients for placement of an awake thoracic epidural in the PACU.

Thoracic Epidurals and Outcome

Outcome studies are challenging to conduct and interpret. Randomized controlled trials are legion, but heterogenous, underpowered, and contaminated by unreported variables. Meta-analyses achieve substantial power, but are only as valid as their component studies. How epidurals are managed, and the agents used in them, are more important than the presence or absence of a catheter, yet such differences are rarely accounted for. Despite these caveats, the following conclusions are reasonably well founded in evidence.

Pulmonary Outcomes

Compared to systemic opioid analgesia, epidural analgesia is associated with a lower incidence of perioperative pulmonary complications in general, and specifically of pneumonia, and atelectasis (16–18). The most important complication, pneumonia, has recently been meta-analyzed specifically with reference to thoracic and abdominal surgery. In that study, Popping confirmed that TEA was associated with lower rates of perioperative pneumonia, but found that the relative protective effect has lessened over the past 35 years because of reduced baseline pneumonia levels in the comparison group (due to improvements in perioperative care and alternative analgesic regimens) (18). The presumptive mechanism of protection is the superior dynamic analgesia allowing for deeper volitional breathing, stronger cough, and better participation in respiratory physiotherapy. Diaphragm shortening is improved with TEA, though the precise mechanism of this is a matter of debate (19). In a number of human studies, tidal volume, vital capacity, and oxygen saturation are improved with TEA following thoracic surgery.

Cardiovascular Outcomes

Specific evidence that TEA reduces perioperative myocardial infarction (MI) after thoracic surgery is lacking. However, meta-analyses culling data from multiple types of surgery indicate that postoperative MI rates are reduced when TEA is employed and extended at least 24 h postoperatively (20). There is also consistent evidence from randomized controlled trials that epidurals reduce perioperative MI following major abdominal surgery. The cardioprotective effect of TEA is presumed related to sympatholysis, favorably altering myocardial oxygen supply–demand, and redistributing coronary blood flow in favor of subendocardium. In experimentally induced ischemia in animals, epidural blockade has been associated with less ST depression, smaller infarct size, improved endocardial blood flow, reduced postinfarction myocardial stunning, and fewer malignant ventricular arrhythmias (21). In humans with coronary artery disease, TEA reduces anginal pain and improves treadmill exercise tolerance, as well as echocardiographic results during stress testing. It is essential to understand that mismanagement of TEA such that coronary perfusion pressure is reduced, may counteract any cardioprotective effects of TEA.

TEA has been associated with reduced postoperative supraventricular arrhythmias, (9) but does not appear to reduce atrial fibrillation following thoracic surgery.

Gastrointestinal Outcomes

Epidural analgesia is associated with reduced duration of postoperative ileus. Mechanisms include reduced narcotic consumption, splanchnic sympathetic blockade, suppression of surgical stress response, and altered inflammatory response to surgery. Whether there is benefit to anastomotic healing in esophagectomy patients is unclear.

Mortality

There is currently insufficient evidence to confirm or deny that TEA improves mortality following thoracic surgery. The low mortality rates, the pervasiveness of TEA, and the inherent difficulties of clinical outcome studies make this unsurprising. A potential mortality benefit is suggested by the cardiorespiratory outcome advantages above.

Thoracic Paravertebral Block

Thoracic paravertebral block (TPB) provides unilateral analgesia of the chest either by catheter or multiple injections (see Chapter 13).

TPB is comparable to TEA in quality of analgesia (pain scores) and respiratory benefits. Although first introduced in 1905, it is unfamiliar to many practitioners, and has a failure rate of 10%. Advantages of TPB are that hemodynamic effects are minimal (unilateral sympathetic block), and the risks of spinal compression from hematoma are less. TPB has been advantageous to thoracic surgeons where epidural services are unavailable, because the catheter can be surgically positioned (approximately) through a flap in the parietal pleura prior to chest closure. Percutaneous TPB is useful for thoracoscopic procedures where early chest tube removal and discharge are anticipated, or where TEA is contraindicated or technically unfeasible.

Local anesthetic introduced into the paravertebral space anesthetizes the dorsal and ventral spinal rami, and the proximate sympathetic chain. Contrast studies indicate that fluid ascends and descends within the paravertebral space without spreading medially to the epidural space. In practice, bilateral analgesia and sympathectomy can occur. Whether this is from technical error or medial diffusion in certain cases is unclear. Among the technical challenges of TPB is the fact that loss of resistance is more subtle than with TEA, it is difficult to thread the catheter, and it is easy to transgress the endothoracic fascia with the needle, which hinders diffusion of drug into the paravertebral space (Fig 37-1).

Intercostal Nerve Blockade

Intercostal nerve blocks are technically simple (Chapter 13), and when successful, provide good, but seldom complete chest wall analgesia. The simplest technique is a single injection of local anesthetic into multiple intercostal spaces before closure of a thoracotomy (usually 2–3 interspaces above, below, and at the level of incision). Duration is limited to 4–10 h, even with long acting local anesthetics, necessitating repeat blockade (often in the middle of the night). A longer lasting method involves continuous infusion of local anesthetic through an indwelling catheter placed in a subpleural/extrapleural pocket, from which local anesthetic diffuses to the nerves.

The proximity of intercostal vessels to nerves raises the risk of accidental intravascular injection and also accelerates absorption

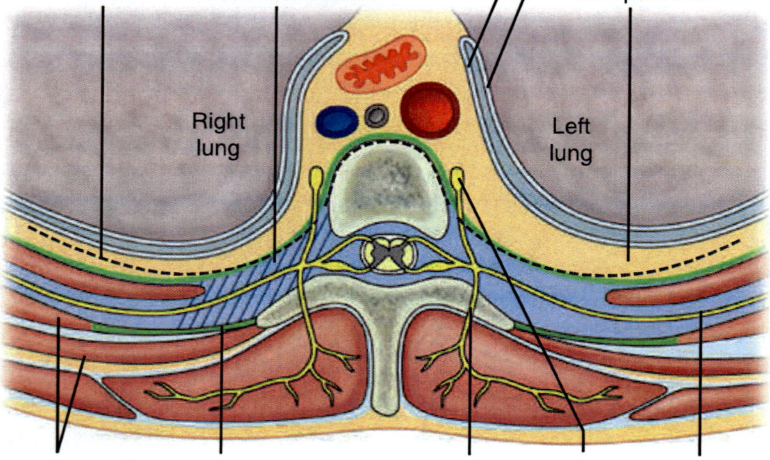

Figure 37-1 – Thoracic paravertebral compartment. Midthoracic coronal view demonstrating the thoracic paravertebral compartment and its relations to adjacent structures.

which limits duration and predisposes to toxicity. Intercostal blocks which are not placed sufficiently posterior will fail to block the posterior branch of the lateral cutaneous nerve (Fig 37-2). The posterior cutaneous nerve which supplies innervation to the posterior portion of posterolateral thoracotomies, is not blocked by intercostal nerve blocks. Intercostal blocks are a poor substitute for TEA, and do not compare favorably in outcome studies following thoracotomy. However, they are useful as an adjunct to PCA for lesser incisions, or as a bridge to allow comfortable emergence and extubation before placing a thoracic epidural postoperatively. A common scenario is the patient whose minimally invasive approach unexpectedly converted to an open thoracotomy. When a percutaneous approach is used, pneumothorax is a potential complication, though the needle is small and there is often a chest tube in that hemithorax.

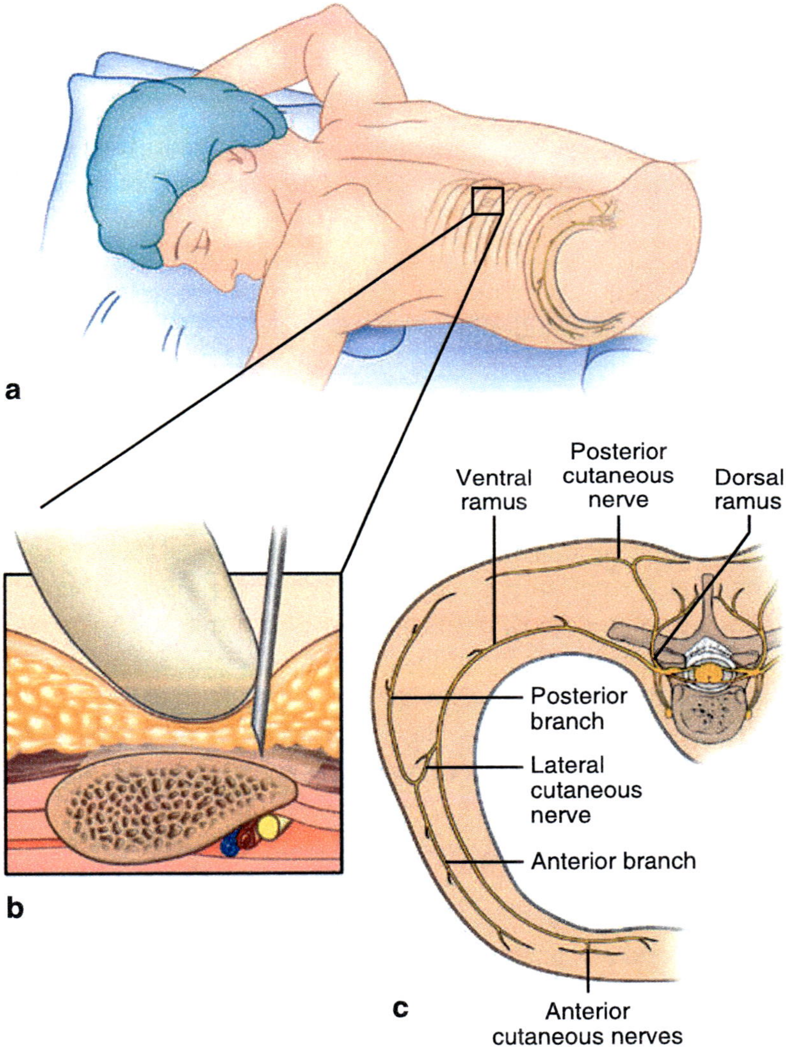

Figure 37-2 – Intercostal nerve anatomy. Note in C that the lateral cutaneous nerve (with anterior and posterior branches) departs from the ventral ramus at a relatively posterior point. It is recommended that intercostal blocks be placed posterior to the posterior axillary line in order to include the lateral cutaneous branches. The posterior cutaneous nerve is not blocked by intercostal nerve blocks.

Cryoanalgesia

Cryoanalgesia is achieved by application of a cold probe (usually –60°C) directly to the intercostal nerves prior to chest closure. As with intercostal blocks, the cryo probe is applied posteriorly, to approximately five interspaces around the level of incision. General application times are 30 s, with a 5-s pause, followed by a second set for 30 s. This leads to axon degeneration, but endoneurium and perineurium are preserved allowing axon regrowth in the ensuing 1–3 months. Although nerve transmission is interrupted for much of this period, the high incidence of dysesthesia and neuropathic pain have limited acceptance of this technique.

Interpleural Catheter Technique

Catheters may be placed into the space between the visceral and parietal pleurae either by percutaneous approach, or open technique (by surgeons prior to chest closure). A third technique is to inject local anesthetic through indwelling chest tubes, and then clamp the tube for a period of time. Local anesthetic delivered through interpleural catheters may provide a measure of analgesia. The density and distribution of analgesia are affected by gravity and chest drains. When patients are semiupright, pooling in the costophrenic angle occurs. When positioned in trendelenberg, a Horner's syndrome may result. Local anesthetic is frequently poorly distributed and partially lost to suction via chest tubes. Comparative studies consistently find interpleural analgesia to be inferior to TEA.

Transcutaneous Electrical Nerve Stimulation

Transcutaneous electrical nerve stimulation (TENS) is a noninvasive analgesic technique in which pads placed over the affected dermatomes deliver high frequency (>50 Hz), low intensity (below muscle contraction threshold) electrical impulses. More widely used in chronic pain scenarios, the efficacy of TENS for acute post-thoracotomy pain is not well established. The mechanism is thought to involve activation of CNS opioid receptors, reduced spinal glutamate release, and increased spinal GABA release ("gate theory"). As a sole modality, the intensity of analgesia from TENS units is inadequate for thoracotomy pain, but it may have a role as an adjunct.

Systemic Therapy

Parenteral Narcotics

As a sole modality, IV narcotics are generally not ideal for thoracotomy incisions because the doses required for satisfactory analgesia induce drowsiness, respiratory depression, and other side effects. Pulmonary complications are greater following thoracic surgery with parenteral narcotic analgesia compared to TEA (16, 18). As mentioned above, dynamic analgesia with narcotics is inferior to that with TEA. As an adjunct, or as the sole modality in lesser incisions, IV patient-controlled narcotics have a role.

Other Adjuncts are listed below:

COX-2 inhibitors

NSAID

Acetaminophen

Dexmedetomidine

Ketamine

Transdermal local anesthetic or narcotic patches

Use of COX-2 inhibitors has been limited due to possible cardiovascular side effects. NSAIDS can be a valuable addition if not contraindicated by renal insufficiency or bleeding. Rectal acetaminophen is effective as an adjunct for shoulder pain in the immediate postoperative period. Dexmedetomidine is widely used as part of a TIVA regimen, or for postoperative sedation for intubated patients. There is little literature on its utility as an adjunct for post-thoracotomy pain. Ketamine's NMDA receptor blocking activity makes it a potent analgesic and effective adjunct. At low infusion doses, side effects, including flashbacks and hallucinations are minimal. Respiratory drive is well preserved with low dose ketamine infusions.

Selected References

1. Cheng JK, Ji RR. Intracellular signaling in primary sensory neurons and persistent pain. Neurochem Res. 2008;33(10):1970–8.

2. Ji RR, Kohno T, Moore KA, Woolf CJ. Central sensitization and LTP: do pain and memory share similar mechanisms? Trends Neurosci. 2003;26(12):696–705.

3. Burgess FW, Anderson DM, Colonna D, Sborov MJ, Cavanaugh DG. Ipsilateral shoulder pain following thoracic surgery. Anesthesiology. 1993;78(2):365–8.

4. Danelli G, Berti M, Casati A, et al. Ipsilateral shoulder pain after thoracotomy surgery: a prospective, randomized, double-blind, placebo-controlled evaluation of the efficacy of infiltrating the phrenic nerve with 0.2%wt/vol ropivacaine. Eur J Anaesthesiol. 2007;24(7):596–601.

5. Boisseau N, Rabary O, Padovani B, et al. Improvement of "dynamic analgesia" does not decrease atelectasis after thoracotomy. Br J Anaesth. 2001;87(4):564–9.

6. Popping DM, Zahn PK, Van Aken HK, Dasch B, Boche R, Pogatzki-Zahn EM. Effectiveness and safety of postoperative pain management: a survey of 18 925 consecutive patients between 1998 and 2006 (2nd revision): a database analysis of prospectively raised data. Br J Anaesth. 2008;101(6):832–40.

7. Groeben H. Epidural anesthesia and pulmonary function. J Anesth. 2006;20(4):290–9.

8. Goertz AW, Seeling W, Heinrich H, Lindner KH, Schirmer U. Influence of high thoracic epidural anesthesia on left ventricular contractility assessed using the end-systolic pressure-length relationship. Acta Anaesthesiol Scand. 1993;37(1):38–44.

9. Oka T, Ozawa Y, Ohkubo Y. Thoracic epidural bupivacaine attenuates supraventricular tachyarrhythmias after pulmonary resection. Anesth Analg. 2001;93(2):253–9.

10. Jideus L, Joachimsson PO, Stridsberg M, et al. Thoracic epidural anesthesia does not influence the occurrence of postoperative sustained atrial fibrillation. Ann Thorac Surg. 2001;72(1):65–71.

11. Dernedde M, Stadler M, Taviaux N, Boogaerts JG. Postoperative patient-controlled thoracic epidural analgesia: importance of dose compared to volume or concentration. Anaesth Intensive Care. 2008;36(6):814–21.

12. De CG, Congedo E, Mascia A, Adducci E, Lai C, Aceto P. Epidural infusion of levobupivacaine and sufentanil following thoracotomy. Anaesthesia. 2007;62(10):994–9.

13. Romer HC, Russell GN. A survey of the practice of thoracic epidural analgesia in the United Kingdom. Anaesthesia. 1998;53(10):1016–22.

14. Hogan QH. Epidural anatomy examined by cryomicrotome section. Influence of age, vertebral level, and disease. Reg Anesth. 1996;21(5):395–406.

15. Horlocker TT. ASA Newsletter. ASA Newsletter Jan 4 2001.

16. Ballantyne JC, Carr DB, deFerranti S, et al. The comparative effects of postoperative analgesic therapies on pulmonary outcome: cumulative meta-analyses of randomized, controlled trials. Anesth Analg. 1998;86(3):598–612.

17. Liu SS, Wu CL. Effect of postoperative analgesia on major postoperative complications: a systematic update of the evidence. Anesth Analg. 2007;104(3): 689–702.

18. Popping DM, Elia N, Marret E, Remy C, Tramer MR. Protective effects of epidural analgesia on pulmonary complications after abdominal and thoracic surgery: a meta-analysis. Arch Surg. 2008;143(10):990–9.

19. Polaner DM, Kimball WR, Fratacci MD, Wain JC, Zapol WM. Thoracic epidural anesthesia increases diaphragmatic shortening after thoracotomy in the awake lamb. Anesthesiology. 1993;79(4):808–16.

20. Beattie WS, Badner NH, Choi P. Epidural analgesia reduces postoperative myocardial infarction: a meta-analysis. Anesth Analg. 2001;93(4):853–8.

21. Ng JM, Hartigan PM. Pain management strategies for patients undergoing extrapleural pneumonectomy. Thorac Surg Clin. 2004;14(4):585–92.

Further Suggested Reading

Clementi A, Carli F. The physiological effects of thoracic epidural anesthesia and analgesia on the cardiovascular, respiratory, and gastrointestinal systems. Minerva Anestesiol. 2008;74:549–63.

DeCosmo G, Aceto P, Gualtieri E, Congedo E. Analgesia in thoracic surgery: review. Minerva Anestesiol. 2009;75:393–400.

Joshi G, Bonnet F, Shah R, et al. A systematic review of randomized trials evaluating regional techniques for postthoracotomy analgesia. Anesth Analg. 2008; 107:1026–40.

Horlocker TT, Wedel DJ, Rowlingson JC, et al. Regional anesthesia in the patient receiving antithrombotic or thrombolytic therapy. American society of regional anesthesia and pain medicine evidence-based guidelines (3rd edition). Reg Anesth Pain Med. 2010;35:64–101.

Breivik H, Bang U, Jalonen J, et al. Nordic guidelines for neuraxial blocks in disturbed haemostasis from the Scandinavian Society of Anaesthesiology and Intensive Care Medicine. Acta Anaesthesiol Scand. 2010;54:16–41.

Chapter 38
Chronic Postthoracotomy Pain Syndrome

Peter Gerner

Keywords Postthoracotomy neuralgia • Postthoracotomy pain syndrome • Chronic postthoracotomy pain • Central sensitization • Intercostal nerve damage • Cryoanalgesia/cryoablation • Preemptive analgesia

Introduction

Postthoracotomy pain syndrome (PTPS), also known as chronic postthoracotomy pain or postthoracotomy neuralgia, is defined by the International Association for the Study of Pain (IASP) as "pain that recurs or persists along a thoracotomy incision at least 2 months following the surgical procedure." In general, it is burning and stabbing pain (spontaneous pain) with dysesthesia and thus shares many features of neuropathic pain. The sensation of evoked pain, in response to a normally nonpainful stimulus (*allodynia*), such as tactile allodynia, or an exaggerated response to a slightly painful stimulus (*hyperalgesia*), such as mechanical and thermal hyperalgesia, especially when accompanied by numbness, is considered diagnostic for nerve injury. These symptoms occur frequently along the innervation area of the intercostal nerves and are the most frequent feature of postthoracotomy pain. PTPS is increasingly acknowledged by anesthesiologists and surgeons as significant and potentially modifiable (1).

P.M. Hartigan (ed.), *Practical Handbook of Thoracic Anesthesia*,
DOI 10.1007/978-0-387-88493-6_38, © Springer Science+Business Media, LLC 2012

Incidence and Severity

Chronic postthoracotomy pain was commonly noted by surgeons during the Second World War in men who had had a thoracotomy for chest trauma; it was called chronic intercostal pain. Progress has been hampered by the fact that the majority of patients did not seek help for their pain, but mentioned it only when specifically asked. A common misconception was that postthoracotomy pain was uncommon and transient. The incidence of long-term postthoracotomy pain has been reported to be 80% at 3 months, 75% at 6 months, and 61% at 1 year after surgery. The incidence of severe pain is 3–5%, and pain that interferes with normal life is reportedly about 50% of patients (2). In one study, over 70% of the patients with PTPS received three or more of the treatment regimens that have been reported to be of value. More than 50% needed to be referred to three different types of specialists. Nevertheless, no patient claimed to have become free of symptoms as a result of treatment, and a significant proportion implied that therapy was either more disabling than PTPS or made it worse (3). For many patients, even the gentlest stimulation provokes intense pain, impairing participation in routine daily activities.

Although there is a wide variation in the reported incidence (probably attributable to differences in the definition of pain), postthoracotomy pain is the most common complication of thoracotomy, and its impact on patients is significant.

Mechanisms

There are several potential mechanisms for PTPS. No consensus exists regarding causality. Understanding of that mechanism is currently evolving and almost entirely derived from animal data. Central sensitization is widely considered integral to the development of PTPS. It has been shown that circulating proinflammatory cytokines lead to COX-2 induction, (e.g., interleukin-1β-mediated induction of

COX-2) and NMDA receptor sensitization (4) in the CNS, thereby contributing to pain hypersensitivity. Activation of microglial cells in the spinal cord also contributes to central sensitization and neuropathic pain by producing proinflammatory cytokines (5).

Therefore, in order to achieve optimal outcomes based on the concept of preventive analgesia, a complete "humoral blockade" by means of regional anesthesia and systemic pain therapy would be necessary to prevent central sensitization, a task that is difficult to achieve clinically.

Intercostal Nerve Damage

Surgery routinely crushes intercostal nerves between instruments and ribs. It is also common for the nerve to be totally severed or included in a suture when closing the chest. Among the many possibilities for nerve injury are mechanical damage during rib resection and compression with a retractor. Furthermore, incidental rib fractures may damage the intercostal nerve immediately or entrap an intercostal nerve during healing, leading to neuropathic pain symptoms.

Neurophysiological assessment of the intercostal nerve during thoracotomy has demonstrated total conduction block, implying nerve injury during rib retraction (6). In another study, the authors performed recordings on 24 patients 1 month after thoracotomy and found that patients with a higher degree of intraoperative intercostal nerve impairment had greater postthoracotomy pain (7).

Injury to Structures Other than Intercostal Nerves

The costochondral and costovertebral junctions may be disarticulated due to extensive rib retraction. Ipsilateral shoulder disability is common as a result of division of serratus anterior muscles and latissimus dorsi. Injuries to the muscles responsible for moving the shoulder as well as insufficiently treated pain lead to inadequate rehabilitation and may produce frozen shoulder.

Tumor Recurrence

Many studies have shown that increasing postthoracotomy pain is associated with tumor recurrence. The relationship (cause vs. effect) and mechanism is unclear. Increasing PTP may be an early sign of tumor recurrence.

Type of Incision

Many surgical techniques have been correlated with the amount of postoperative pain. Even muscle-sparing incisions appear to have no major advantage over posterolateral incisions (8). The rate of long-term persistent pain (3–18 months) has been found to be the same after both thoracotomy and thoracoscopic procedures (9). However, other authors concluded that the use of video-assisted thoracic surgery for pulmonary resection may decrease the incidence of chronic pain and disability when compared with thoracotomy (10). Overall, type of surgical technique does not appear to be a powerful predictor of PTPS.

Psychological Factors

Studies suggest that personality traits are strong modulatory factors in the overall postthoracotomy pain experience. Preoperative anxiety appears to play a major role.

Treatment

The PTPS remains a daunting treatment challenge. Modalities which have been employed, with varying success include:

- Intercostal nerve blockade.
- Cryoanalgesia/cryoablation.
- Epidural steroids.
- Neuropathic pain medications (antidepressents, anticonvulsive agents, NSAIDS).

- Opioids.
- Lidocaine transdermal patch.
- Radiofrequency ablation.
- Spinal cord stimulator.

Prevention/Preemptive Analgesia

The concept of sensitization has led to an increased effort to control acute pain by a more or less total afferent blockade, with the goal of reducing the development of postthoracotomy pain.

Preemptive analgesia is intended to prevent the establishment of central sensitization caused by incisional and inflammatory injuries. Evidence from basic research has indicated that analgesic drugs are more effective if administered before, rather than after, a noxious stimulus (11). The benefit of preemptive analgesia has been supported by some clinical studies using local anesthetics, opioids, and nonsteroidal antiinflammatory drugs (12, 13). However, the clinical usefulness of preemptive analgesia has remained controversial, (14) probably due in part to the wide variation in study conditions such as surgery, drugs, doses, routes of administration, and treatment duration as well as pain assessment methods used in different studies (15, 16).

Previous studies comparing the effects of preoperative and postoperative epidural block in abdominal surgery have failed to demonstrate any benefit of preemptive analgesia. This lack of benefit was partly attributed to the less discrete, visceral nature of pain after abdominal surgery. Thoracotomy produces high-intensity noxious stimuli sufficient to cause central sensitization, (17) and the area of postthoracotomy pain is more discrete and largely restricted to the site of surgery. Hence, it was hoped that preemptive epidural analgesia might be more effective in thoracic surgery than in abdominal surgery.

Though results from clinical studies so far have not shown a major impact of preemptive epidural analgesia on postoperative pain after thoracic surgery, (18) the concept remains compelling, especially in preventing the development of chronic postthoracotomy pain (19).

It has also been suggested that while preemptive analgesia is beneficial in some surgical procedures, it is ineffective in others. One explanation offered is that the respective surgical area is innervated by multiple segmental and cranial nerves (20).

The degree of acute pain after thoracic surgery may predict long-term postthoracotomy pain, and hence aggressive management of early postoperative pain should reduce the likelihood of long-term postthoracotomy pain (17). A good analgesic regimen not only reduces pulmonary complications in the immediate perioperative period, but also helps in early mobilization (21). As mentioned in this chapter, the most common technique for pain relief is a thoracic epidural, with the catheter in the mid-thoracic region with a continuous infusion of local anesthetic and narcotics.

Some recent studies (19, 22, 23) have shown beneficial effects (both immediate and late) when preemptive analgesia (nerve blockade either by epidural or intercostal nerve block) was begun before the surgical incision. However, other researchers have found marginal or no benefits even when a multimodal approach was used (18, 24).

In summary, PTPS is a common and significant complication of thoracic surgery. Its etiology is complex and incompletely understood. Central sensitization from neural and humoral influences is integral to its development. Interruption of central sensitization through preemptive analgesia is challenging because it would require dense, and possibly prolonged (days) suppression of both neural and humoral responses to thoracotomy. It is nonetheless an area of active and promising research (25).

Selected References

1. Gottschalk A, Cohen SP, Yang S, Ochroch EA. Preventing and treating pain after thoracic surgery. Anesthesiology. 2006;104(3):594–600.

2. Perttunen K, Tasmuth T, Kalso E. Chronic pain after thoracic surgery: a follow-up study. Acta Anaesthesiol Scand. 1999;43(5):563–7.

3. Conacher ID. Therapists and therapies for post-thoracotomy neuralgia. Pain. 1992;48(3):409–12.

4. Kawasaki Y, Zhang L, Cheng JK, Ji RR. Cytokine mechanisms of central sensitization: distinct and overlapping role of interleukin-1beta, interleukin-6, and tumor necrosis factor-alpha in regulating synaptic and neuronal activity in the superficial spinal cord. J Neurosci. 2008;28(20):5189–94.

5. Suter MR, Wen YR, Decosterd I, Ji RR. Do glial cells control pain? Neuron Glia Biol. 2007;3(3):255–68.

6. Rogers ML, Henderson L, Mahajan RP, Duffy JP. Preliminary findings in the neurophysiological assessment of intercostal nerve injury during thoracotomy. Eur J Cardiothorac Surg. 2002;21(2):298–301.

7. Benedetti F, Vighetti S, Ricco C, et al. Neurophysiologic assessment of nerve impairment in posterolateral and muscle-sparing thoracotomy. J Thorac Cardiovasc Surg. 1998;115(4):841–7.

8. Ochroch EA, Gottschalk A, Augoustides JG, Aukburg SJ, Kaiser LR, Shrager JB. Pain and physical function are similar following axillary, muscle-sparing vs posterolateral thoracotomy. Chest. 2005;128(4):2664–70.

9. Maguire MF, Ravenscroft A, Beggs D, Duffy JP. A questionnaire study investigating the prevalence of the neuropathic component of chronic pain after thoracic surgery. Eur J Cardiothorac Surg. 2006;29(5):800–5.

10. Landreneau RJ, Mack MJ, Hazelrigg SR, et al. Prevalence of chronic pain after pulmonary resection by thoracotomy or video-assisted thoracic surgery. J Thorac Cardiovasc Surg. 1994;107(4):1079–85.

11. Yashpal K, Katz J, Coderre TJ. Effects of preemptive or postinjury intrathecal local anesthesia on persistent nociceptive responses in rats. Confounding influences of peripheral inflammation and the general anesthetic regimen. Anesthesiology. 1996;84(5):1119–28.

12. Fridrich P, Colvin HP, Zizza A, et al. Phase 1A safety assessment of intravenous amitriptyline. J Pain. 2007;8(7):549–55.

13. Dahl JB, Kehlet H. The value of pre-emptive analgesia in the treatment of postoperative pain. Br J Anaesth. 1993;70(4):434–9.

14. Kissin I. Preemptive analgesia. Why its effect is not always obvious. Anesthesiology. 1996;84(5):1015–9.

15. Senturk M. Acute and chronic pain after thoracotomies. Curr Opin Anaesthesiol. 2005;18(1):1–4.

16. Bong CL, Samuel M, Ng JM, Ip-Yam C. Effects of preemptive epidural analgesia on post-thoracotomy pain. J Cardiothorac Vasc Anesth. 2005;19(6):786–93.

17. Katz J, Jackson M, Kavanagh BP, Sandler AN. Acute pain after thoracic surgery predicts long-term post-thoracotomy pain. Clin J Pain. 1996;12(1):50–5.

18. Kavanagh BP, Katz J, Sandler AN, et al. Multimodal analgesia before thoracic surgery does not reduce postoperative pain. Br J Anaesth. 1994;73(2):184–9.

19. Obata H, Saito S, Fujita N, Fuse Y, Ishizaki K, Goto F. Epidural block with mepivacaine before surgery reduces long-term post-thoracotomy pain. Can J Anaesth. 1999;46(12):1127–32.

20. Aida S, Baba H, Yamakura T, Taga K, Fukuda S, Shimoji K. The effectiveness of preemptive analgesia varies according to the type of surgery: a randomized, double-blind study. Anesth Analg. 1999;89(3):711–6.

21. Schultz AM, Werba A, Ulbing S, Gollmann G, Lehofer F. Peri-operative thoracic epidural analgesia for thoracotomy. Eur J Anaesthesiol. 1997;14(6):600–3.

22. Katz J, Kavanagh BP, Sandler AN, et al. Preemptive analgesia. Clinical evidence of neuroplasticity contributing to postoperative pain. Anesthesiology. 1992;77(3):439–46.

23. Senturk M, Ozcan PE, Talu GK, et al. The effects of three different analgesia techniques on long-term postthoracotomy pain. Anesth Analg. 2002;94(1):11–5. Table.

24. Doyle E, Bowler GM. Pre-emptive effect of multimodal analgesia in thoracic surgery. Br J Anaesth. 1998;80(2):147–51.

25. Kissin I. Preemptive analgesia. Anesthesiology. 2000;93(4):1138–43.

Index

P.M. Hartigan (ed.), *Practical Handbook of Thoracic Anesthesia*,
DOI 10.1007/978-0-387-88493-6, © Springer Science+Business Media, LLC 2012

C

P

T